'Dr Sharma has been a vital part of my own 'healthy ageing', and I know that his book will be invaluable to a lot of people.

Hayley Mills, actress

I have for 25 years benefited immeasurably from Dr Sharma's insight into and understanding of health and well-being. I look forward to making the *Living Longer, Living Younger* wisdom part of my life and to undiminished vitality with Dr Sharma's guidance.

Alice Krige, actress

Dr Rajendra Sharma's book *Live Longer, Live Younger* is a clear and concise guide to optimizing health as we age. I am pleased to see an anti-ageing/healthy ageing book promoting health from within, allowing self-regeneration using emerging techniques born out of exciting science. At a time when gene assessment looks capable of giving us advanced notice of our areas of risk, Dr Sharma provides us with the information and tools to prevent and heal premature ageing and disaeases – and the sooner we start, the easier it is.

Fouad I. Ghaly, MD, leading expert in regenerative medicine therapies, Diplomat of the American Board of Anti-Aging Medicine

Dedication

Emily – Live Long!
Liam, Maddie and Bryony – Live Young!

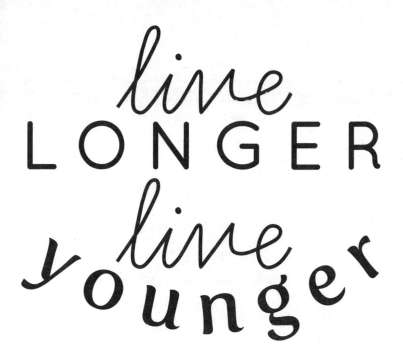

live LONGER live younger

DESIGN YOUR PERSONAL PLAN FOR A LONG AND HEALTHY LIFE

DR RAJENDRA SHARMA

MB BCh BAO LRCP&S (Ire) MFHom

WATKINS PUBLISHING

LONDON

This edition first published in the UK and USA 2014 by
Watkins Publishing Limited
PO Box 883
Oxford, OX1 9PL
UK

A member of Osprey Group

For enquiries in the USA and Canada:
Osprey Publishing
PO Box 3985
New York, NY 10185-3985
Tel: (001) 212 753 4402
Email: info@ospreypublishing.com

XX, 332 : ILL   1 3 5 7 9 10 8 6 4 2

Typeset by Jerry Goldie Graphic Design

Illustrations by the Gallery Bude

Printed and bound in the UK by CPI Group (UK) Ltd, Croydon, CR0 4YY

A CIP record for this book is available from the British Library

ISBN: 978-1-78028-510-8

Watkins Publishing is supporting the Woodland Trust, the UK's leading
woodland conservation charity, by funding tree-planting initiatives and
woodland maintenance.

www.watkinspublishing.co.uk

Contents

Acknowledgements

Emily, thank you. No you, no book. My inspiration and drive are all down to you. Liam, Maddie and Bryony – you have been my reasons for doing the work. Thank you to Alex Oakes, who kept reminding me 'I can' and Hans Snook for all his support over the years. Love and huge respect to the following for their constant support and reassurance: Chandra Ashfield, Adrian, Marina, Suzanne and Wendy at the Accounting Bureau for managing my practice, Andy Wren at NutriGold, Mark Givert and Robyn at Get-fitt, Yehudi Gordon and Megan Fensom Turner, Faith Cole and her team Dhara and Mahi at Independent Nursing Services, Geeta Sidhu-Robb at NOSH Detox and Justin Price at Regenerus Labs. For helping me clear my head, thanks to Mike B and my Arsenal buddies and Richard Berenson. Thank you, Susan Mears, for finding my publishers, Watkins Publishing Limited, and thank you to their team for editing, formatting and helping the project along.

And, most importantly, thank you to my ultimate teachers – my patients.

Foreword

Ageing starts at birth, and the sooner we can focus on health, the less likely we are to struggle with age-related issues and a shorter life span. As co-founder and chairman of the world's largest preventative medical society in Anti-Ageing and Regenerative Medicine, I have focused and promoted healthy ageing for the best part of my career. While I am working at the cutting edge in areas of anti-aging science, including brain resuscitation, organ transplant and blood preservation technologies, I value and recognize the need to make healthy ageing advice available to the public, practitioners and doctors.

Dr Rajendra Sharma's book particularly succeeds in this area. *Live Longer, Live Younger* is a clear and concise guide, whether you are dedicated to healthy living or not. Dr Sharma points out that many age-related problems can be attributed to vitamin and mineral deficiencies (heart and arterial disease reduced by antioxidants, osteoporosis by minerals as examples), and that avoiding environmental toxins can make a profound difference. Chapters on nutrition and diet as well as lifestyle provide simple steps that will help you make fundamental changes.

I am particularly pleased to see a broad anti-ageing/healthy ageing book promoting exercise. I have a special interest in this area, having received an International Olympic Committee Tribute Diploma and being an inductee into the Martial Arts Hall of Fame as well as the Guinness Book of World Records for sports endeavours. Dr Sharma quite rightly cites exercise as perhaps the most important factor in healthy ageing.

I was introduced to Dr Sharma in 2008 when he was invited onto the Review Board for London's annual Anti-Ageing Conference, and we have crossed paths occasionally since. His lecture that year focused on the use of food and food-based supplements in healthy ageing, and highlighted the minimum requirements we all need but may not obtain without careful scrutiny of our intake. *Live Longer, Live Younger* has expanded on this theme to provide the basics as well as the advanced options in supplementing our intake in these environmentally polluted and deficient times.

As one of my roles as co-founder of The American Anti-Aging Academy of Medicine, I visit over 20 counties a year and lecture on the very areas Dr Sharma's book focuses on. By highlighting the risks of a lack of exercise, toxicity, poor lifestyle and deficiencies, this book shows us how we can recognize and understand our areas of weakness. As he puts it, 'How old is our oldest part?'

Live Longer, Live Younger subdivides into the main areas of age-related health, including heart and arteries, nervous system, detoxification and hormones. The book focuses our attention on areas of risk and encourages discussion with doctors and practitioners to perform available investigations and consider advanced therapeutic options.

At a time when gene assessment looks capable of giving us advanced notice of our areas of risk, Dr Sharma provides us with the information and tools to prevent and heal premature ageing and diseases – and the sooner we start, the easier it is.

Dr Robert M Goldman MD, PhD, DO, FAASP

Dr Robert M Goldman MD, PhD, DO, FAASP has spearheaded the development of numerous international medical organizations and corporations. Dr Goldman has served as a Senior Fellow at the Lincoln Filene Center, Tufts University, and as an Affiliate at the Philosophy of Education Research Center, Graduate School of Education, Harvard University. He is Clinical Consultant, Department of Obstetrics and Gynaecology, Korea Medical University; and Professor, Department of Internal Medicine at the University of Central America Health Sciences, Department of Internal Medicine. Dr Goldman holds the positions of Visiting Professor, Udayana University School of Medicine, Indonesia; Visiting Professor, Huazhong University of Science & Technology Tong Ji Medical School, China; Visiting Professor, The Wuhan Institute of Science & Technology, China; Visiting Professor at Hainan Medical College, China; and Visiting Professor, School of Anti-Aging, Aesthetics and Regenerative Medicine, UCSI University, Malaysia. Dr Goldman is a Fellow of the American Academy of Sports Physicians and a Board Diplomat in Sports Medicine and Board Certified in Anti-Aging Medicine. Dr Goldman is a Fellow of the American Academy of Sports Physicians and a Board Diplomat in Sports Medicine and Board Certified in Anti-Aging Medicine.

Introduction

We are as old as our oldest part

I t's a fact: one part of us is wearing out faster than the rest. We have to know which organ or system this is if we want to remain as well as possible for as long as possible. Armed with this knowledge there is much we can do to slow down the ageing process and even reverse any damage that has already taken place.

We need to explore how to maintain optimum health and longevity to enhance personal performance at work and in play, including sports activities, relaxation, socializing, relationships and any other area you can think of – and we need to do so at the earliest opportunity to avoid the effects of ageing.

The anti-ageing business is thriving. It is, however, predominantly concerned with outward appearance. There are many 'miracle creams' available that claim to lift and firm sagging skin, decrease the appearance of wrinkles, banish cellulite or restore a youthful glow. The efficacy of many such creams may or may not be clinically proven; and as there are already so many toxins absorbed from everyday skin products, why worry about introducing even more to your system? For those of you considering more radical or even surgical treatments, remember that products introduced into the body in cosmetic procedures such as breast and lip augmentation can have dire effects. Going under the knife always carries risks, and you should be aware of potential problems such as scarring and tissue damage.

There is an abundance of books and magazine articles on how to prevent the signs of ageing, and I am in awe of how health journalists are able to update us so effusively, week in and week out, on all the developments. After all, cosmetics and cosmetic surgery aside, surely it all boils down to:

- Eat well – stay thin.
- Exercise – stay fit.
- Avoid bad habits – stay away from toxins.
- Be happy – stay positive.

Oh, and let's hope your genes are good and … that's it, isn't it?

Well, yes, frankly it is. However, the trouble is this: the majority of my friends and family (myself included) like an alcoholic drink or two and live in a world that is rather polluted and filled with convenience food. I don't know anyone who is not affected by the stress of everyday life. A few of my crowd still smoke – bless them! We don't, as a group, exercise quite as much as we should, and, frankly, weight-wise there is more of each of us individually than there should be.

But I don't want my tribe to head off into the Himalayas to eat brown rice and meditate for eight hours a day. I take pleasure in seeing them on an afternoon or evening at the football or the theatre … and going for a pre-match/show drink with them. I want to enjoy a glass (or more) of wine with my wife over an occasional overindulgent meal and sometimes have a fast-food treat with my children.

Furthermore, I would like to do so for as long as possible in as good a state of health as possible.

To do that, I need to know some facts about how I am dealing with this lifestyle:

- How toxic am I and how efficiently can I remove toxins from my body?
- How undernourished or deficient is my lifestyle is making me?
- Which part of me is failing?
- What can I do to compensate for my 'evils'?

I do not wish to deny myself my indulgences, so by recognizing my personal limits and utilizing functional medical investigations to define my boundaries and capabilities, I can establish a *life plan* to allow me to live in this ecologically unsound world with my unsound, unhealthy attitude.

Want to join me? If so, you need to know which are your oldest parts, what acceptable lifestyle changes you as an individual need to make and what you need to supplement in your system to allow you to go on for as long and in as healthy a state as possible.

This book is dedicated to simplifying the process of:

- understanding your body;

- establishing a lifestyle that fits into your busy schedule; and
- giving basic information on a supplemental programme to cover the deficiencies created by a non-perfect lifestyle in a polluted world.

The integrated approach to health

My professional life's work has been as a fully qualified doctor with a chosen interest in the field of complementary and alternative medicine (CAM). My peer group are integrated or integrative physicians (IPs) who always consider environmental effects on health conditions, with recourse to our training in conventional, traditional and CAM options of healthcare.

I, for one, have acted as an advisor to those wishing to stay well as much as I have helped restore health in those that are ill. My father, a physician before me, styled himself as a specialist in chronic disease and used homoe-opathy and Ayurvedic knowledge to support his conventional training. My upbringing has given me a similar approach to healthcare.

Ecological medicine is not yet a recognized speciality. Yet, unless more doctors and health-governing authorities start to focus on this new medical arena, current healthcare systems – in the countries that are sufficiently developed to have a healthcare system – will soon run out of money to

---

WORLD POPULATION AND HEALTH EXPENDITURE

World population (past):
1960 – 3.0272 billion
2010 – 6.8405 billion
Estimated world population (future):
2025 – 8 billion
2042 – 9 billion
2083 – 10 billion
Health expenditure
According to the Organization for Economic Co-operation and Development (OECD), the UK Government's spend in 2009 on social health structure was 9.8 percent of gross domestic product (GDP). In the USA, Congressional Budget Office figures (2011) show that annual healthcare expenditure is projected to exceed $4 trillion by 2015 and that the national healthcare budget will be responsible for 19.6 percent of the US GDP by 2019.

finance the increasing number of people our planet has to support. Ecological medicine is described as a form of healthcare that considers the interactions between individuals and the environment, and the consequences to health. It focuses on three areas:

- INPUTS: the impact of nutritional and environmental factors on the individual
- PROCESSING: the way we handle inputs and how that determines our health
- OUTPUTS: the impact of each of us, individually and collectively, by our actions on the environment upon which, ultimately, we all depend[1]

Prevention is better than cure

Groups of scientists and doctors worldwide have researched and developed a wealth of knowledge and experience in therapeutic and, more importantly, preventative healthcare that can optimize human performance, reduce the speed and rate of the development of disease and offer a range of treatments with and without the use of drugs. To date, this has been shrouded in what is perceived as a predominantly commercial and 'faddy' branch of medicine known as Anti-Ageing Medicine.

The leading lights of anti-ageing medicine, in particular those involved via the USA through the American Academy of Anti-Aging Medicine, provide research and training worldwide in the most advanced diagnostic, preventative, therapeutic and curative healthcare programmes available. Integrated physicians can be found in most parts of the world through this organization.

Such physicians believe that the answer to defying age lies in what is termed functional medicine. This focuses on the normal functioning of the body, the cellular metabolism, the healthy activity of tissues and organs, and the use of natural approaches as much as possible to harness the body's evolutionary and phenomenal ability to repair and maintain optimum function.

The conventional medical paradigm today is to treat illness once it has set in. Screening is geared toward early detection rather than on prediction or prevention. Of the thousands of drugs available, the vast majority are there to alleviate pain and discomfort and to provide support to failing organs, not to cure or restore the normal, unaided capability of a failed system. It may sound cynical, but companies do not make money if they don't sell drugs. The healthy and well have no commercial value, so little money is provided to research into the prevention of disease.

This orthodox attitude to medicine (that is, treatment through drugs and intervention, but not prevention) has led us all down a path where we expect to become ill and infirm as we age, but hope that, if we are lucky, we will be given a drug or provided with a technique or procedure that will keep us going. Here, in the high-tech developed world, we watch our elderly population deal with unproductive years in care homes or in isolation or both. The concept that it takes a village to bring up a child extends in many parts of the world to 'we need a village to help us age'. We are losing that village, that attitude, and with it our capability to enjoy our later years in good health. Now, more than ever, we need to focus on *healthy ageing and optimizing performance* as we live longer and are expected to work longer, too.

The modern medical world has made great strides with regard to the treatment of diseases associated with ageing (geriatrics), yet we have no real focus or set-up – and, possibly, no current plans – to expand healthy ageing (gerontology) to frontline medicine. Apart from a few leading experts in theoretical research at our top universities, who can we turn to? There are no doctors in our health services or in mainstream medicine specializing in healthy ageing.

The majority of us do not have access to a doctor to whom we can turn and ask, 'How can I stay well, please?'

Yet, these days, *healthy ageing* is a far more relevant term than anti-ageing, and it is possible to achieve this much more easily than many people think through simple changes to life patterns and the use of supplements and certain procedures. It is my aim in this book to show you how.

Why do we age?

I hope that understanding the theoretical reasons behind ageing may help you focus on the necessary changes you need to make and encourage you to focus on your health. Providing reasons for why particular actions are important frequently makes the job seem a lot easier.

If we know why we have to do something, and there is purpose behind it, we feel far more motivated to fulfil the task.

Many people, including some doctors, believe that longevity and remaining healthy into old age is predominantly down to individual genes – but this is not the case. It is now known that the way we live and what we put into our bodies have a direct influence on our genes and alter their behaviour, as much as our habits influence the ageing of the organs and cells in our bodies. As you will see throughout this book, good nutrition, avoidance of toxins and the use of supplements, exercise, good lifestyle habits, relaxation, meditation and breathing techniques are all vitally important.

A *laissez-faire* attitude, assuming your longevity and health are all down to heredity, is abrogating responsibility and wrong.

The more we understand about why we age, the more we can do to prevent the dysfunction that comes along with advancing years. Scientists are taking an interest in healthy ageing with the intention of engineering drugs that can slow down the degenerative processes that lead to age-related disease.

Nobody has yet developed a unified theory that explains ageing. Why do cells and metabolic processes function efficiently until we are fully grown, maintain that function for two or three decades and then start to decline? The human body is remarkably efficient, having evolved to make us, arguably, the most successful species on the planet. However, unlike a car, which can have worn-out parts replaced and so potentially run forever, something happens with the self-repairing process in the body that prevents it carrying on.

It may be a surprise to find that, despite our advances in science, we have *theories of ageing* but not a clearly understood collection of facts. By 2007, there were over 300 theories of ageing![2] A theory is defined as 'a set of statements or principles devised to explain a group of facts or phenomena'. A theory is an assumption based on current information, but, at the end of the day, it is speculative and a conjecture.

Intracellular and extracellular theories of ageing

Whatever causes ageing to occur must happen inside cells or in the space outside known as 'extracellular space' (the body tissues). My classification allows a certain unification of all the main theories of ageing so that, from a practical point of view, we are able to understand why we need to follow the advice in the rest of this book.

Intracellular Ageing Processes
1. The Free Radical Theory of Ageing
All the metabolic processes that go on inside every cell create free radicals. These damage the DNA found in the nucleus of a cell (the command centre) and the DNA in the mitochondria, which provide the cell with energy. Free radicals also damage the cell walls and the many different structures important to cell function. One researcher coined the phrase 'garbage catastrophe theory' referring to the junk or gunk that collects in cells and prevents normal function.[3]

A GLOSSARY OF ANTI-AGEING TERMS

Senescence – senescent cells are those that have lost the ability to reproduce themselves. They are dysfunctional or useless, secrete abnormal proteins that are harmful to themselves and surrounding cells, and break down tissue structure around them.

DNA (deoxyribonucleic acid) – carries genetic information in the body's cells.

Gene – a string of DNA that passes information to proteins, which activate cell function.

Chromosomes – bundles of genes.

Telomere – a sequence of DNA at the end of a chromosome. Telomeres do not transmit instructions to the cell as other parts of the chromosome do, but they prevent the chromosome from becoming entangled or joining up with other chromosomes. Each time our cells divide, which they do by replicating chromosomes, part of the telomere is broken off. When the telomere gets to a particular short length, usually after about 50 replications (the Hayflick limit, named after the scientist who discovered it), the chromosome can no longer divide and the cell stops replicating itself – a good thing if the replication has changed the cell to a cancerous or useless one.

Mutation – each time a chromosome or a DNA strand replicates itself, small changes occur. The majority of these changes throughout our life do not affect the functioning of the cell, but occasionally they can be harmful. A cancerous change, for example, would be one that allows the cell to replicate at too fast a rate. Telomeres are there to protect us from that happening.

Telomerase – an enzyme that restores the length of telomeres, effectively stopping the shortening and therefore risking overproduction of potentially mutated cells.

Free radicals – many (if not most) biochemical pathways include the production of molecules that are missing an electron (a negatively charged particle whizzing around the nucleus of atoms). Such molecules are known as free radicals and can be damaging because they will try to pull away an electron from another molecule, thereby disrupting important function or structure.

Oxidative damage – the term given to the damage caused by free radicals.

Rather than this being a disease process, the age-related failure of cell function is related to the waste products of normal functioning and the inevitable production of free radicals leading to eventual dysfunction. In other words, cells age because they make 'garbage' from their normal function that is going to destroy them eventually.

2. The Telomere Theory of Ageing

Telomeres prevent chromosomes from fusing together, bending or unravelling incorrectly and also stop chromosomes and DNA binding to each other. If abnormal patterns occur in DNA or chromosomes, instructions to the cell go wrong and these mutations may render the cell useless or dangerous.

Cells should multiply only a certain number of times (the Hayflick limit) and then die off. The telomere theory of ageing simply defines the process as one that is set in our genes and, provided nothing interferes, only healthy cells will exist. As we age, the cellular pattern of cleaving off telomeres becomes compromised, thereby allowing cells to multiply with ever-increasing mutations.

Telomerase is an enzyme that rebuilds telomeres, and healthy cells make a certain amount. There is a gene – *hTERT* – that turns telomerase activity on or off. Damage to this gene by pollutants sticking to it (adducting) stops normal telomere repair.

3. Immune System Theory of Ageing

Senescent cells need to be removed by the immune system, which should recognize that these are altered cells that are not functional. Unfortunately,

RESEARCH INTO CELL REPAIR

At first glance it would appear that if we could encourage telomerase activity, cells would continue to replicate, and provided they were not damaged, these would remain healthy and longer living. There is considerable ongoing research into drugs that activate telomerase activity. However, we must be wary as cancer cells also have active *hTERT* genes, suggesting that such treatment may risk encouraging, if not forming, cancer.

Research shows that a plant extract called TA 65, from the astragalus plant, appears to activate telomerase and may be proven to benefit our cells by encouraging normal function of replication in tissues. Let's wait and see.

as we age, our immune system develops faults (described fully in Chapter 8), leaving useless and potentially dangerous senescent cells in place. These cells continue to produce proteins in an attempt to become functional again, but the proteins tend to be damaged and trigger an inflammatory response. Inflammation encourages white blood cells into the area to kill off the senescent cells, but the process of inflammation is damaging to surrounding cells and a domino effect takes place, weakening the organs involved.

4. The Mitochondrial Free Radical Theory of Ageing[4]
This theory appears in a book of the same name. The mitochondria in cells contain DNA that may be slightly different from the nuclear DNA. This becomes damaged through free-radical activity as described above. Unfortunately, damaged mitochondria, through a complex biochemical pathway, make more free radicals as they attempt to correct themselves. When the damage is too great, the cell breaks down, releasing free radicals in the process to damage the neighbouring cells and tissues. Low-density lipoproteins, which most of us have heard of in association with their carriage of LDL cholesterol, mop up these free radicals. As more low-density lipoproteins are produced, damage to arteries occurs, leading to a reduction in oxygenation and nutrition to most parts of the body.

5. DNA Damage Theory of Ageing
The attachments of toxic compounds are known as DNA adducts. Heavy metals and many of our pollutant chemicals are now known to attach to DNA and can be tested for. In 1973, Leslie Orgel, a British chemist, described this as the 'Error Catastrophe Theory'. When DNA is damaged, errors occur in the transmitting of information to the cell, leaving it unable to function properly.

Extracellular Ageing Processes
1. The Glycosylation Theory of Ageing
Sugars in the form of glucose are a cell's main source of energy. Mitochondria combines glucose with oxygen to free up electrons that activate metabolic pathways. This process creates byproducts known as advanced glycation end products (AGEs). These are generally dealt with by the house-cleaning elimination process and, provided not too much sugar is introduced into the tissues, AGEs are not troublesome. Unfortunately, we tend to ingest too much sugar and AGEs start to attach to the proteins in the body's tissues.

They act a bit like glue, forming so-called crosslinks between proteins. This meshwork stiffens tissues, damages cells and blocks the flow of oxygen and nutrients through the arteries. Furthermore, carbon dioxide and waste products are not as easily removed by the lymphatic system.

Reducing the amount of sugar available may therefore be the key. It is known that calorie restriction enhances the length of life in mice, and observation in humans suggests that calorific restriction is a mainstay of longevity. If you look around at our nonagenarians and centurions, they are rarely overweight, and most of the active elderly people we know tend to eat less as they have aged.

Research is being conducted to see if drugs can block or break down crosslinking, and it is worth keeping a lookout for results from one such study on Alagebrium. Another manufactured drug, Aminoguanidine, which has been touted as a potential anti-ageing drug since 1986, may also work in the same way.[5]

L-carnosine, a naturally occurring amino acid in the body, also appears to interfere with crosslinking.

2. Reproductive Cell Cycle Theory of Ageing

Instead of considering ageing as being an occurrence of changes at a bio-chemical level of the cells or extracellular space, this theory considers that if all chemical reactions in a cell were stopped, other than those that maintain the structure, then the cell would not age. So, whatever controls the chemical reactions is responsible for ageing. Hormones are governed to a great degree by what is known as the hypothalamic-pituitary-gonadal (HPG) axis, the first two being part of the brain. The HPG axis, in conjunction with the brain's control of sugar and insulin levels, are theorized to control cellular function and therefore ageing.

Women taking hormone replacement therapy, those who reach menopause later in life and men replacing testosterone all show longevity and a reduction in the speed at which age-related diseases are reached. These facts support the theory. Calorie restriction suppresses the HPG axis and might be one of the reasons why low food intake is associated with longevity.

3. Non-Biological Theories of Ageing

Researchers in biology are rather critical of psychologists who put forward theories of ageing based on mind rather than matter. Theories such as Disengagement Activity, Selectivity and Continuity are all terms speculating that specific activities, or disengaging from them as we age, or maintaining other habits and personality traits lead to less disease and therefore healthier ageing and longevity. The effects of psychology on nerve function and particularly on the immunity are unquestioned, and I therefore do not think we can dismiss the mind-body effect on ageing. I am sure that, as science gets closer to understanding mind and consciousness, we will find practical methods of slowing the ageing process through mind control.

Summary

No one theory has all the answers, and because of the disparity between just the few theories I have commented upon, the chances are that they are all interrelated. However, from a physical perspective, free radicals seem to be responsible at a core level of disrupting our mitochondria, our DNA and our cell function. For this reason, avoiding the toxins that trigger free-radical activity and ensuring high quantities of nutrients, particularly antioxidants, that neutralize free radicals, seem to present the bottom line when it comes to healthy ageing.

How to use this book

Enough about the theory … it's time to put anti-ageing into practice!

My aim in this book is to help you to identify which part or parts of your body you particularly need to focus on, make you aware of the many diagnostic tests that are available to clarify why these are your problem areas and show you how to slow down and even reverse the ageing process while continuing to enjoy life, too! My recommendations range from simple lifestyle changes, including diet, exercise and avoiding toxins and pollutants, to advice on supplements, therapies and medical interventions.

I strongly advise you to read Chapters 1–5 in order as these contain information about the building blocks for optimum health. Chapter 1 explains the various diagnostic tests and lifestyle changes that everyone should consider; Chapter 2 contains essential nutritional advice, some of it very new; Chapter 3 outlines the importance of exercise, arguably the most important area for healthy ageing, and if you are not already an exercise devotee, you may change your mind after reading this chapter!); Chapter 4 describes how to reduce your exposure to everyday toxins and to repair damage; Chapter 5 contains information about the minerals we all need. After that, please feel free to read the chapters on body systems in any order according to your individual concerns. Each chapter describes age-related problems and how to prevent or treat them and, building on the basic advice given in Chapter 1, provides further information on boosting or repairing whichever body system you wish to focus on. Because everyone has different needs and priorities, within each chapter you will find different levels of tests (first- and second-line investigations) and advice on which supplements to take (Dr Sharma's Maintenance, Advanced and Repair Programmes).

Chapter 1

Know your body

N ow that I have stated my position, I will start by addressing healthy ageing from three angles:

1. *Dr Sharma's Diagnostic Programmes* – how best to assess your current health and predict the arrival of problems through functional testing
2. *Dr Sharma's Healthy Ageing Lifestyle Guide* – basic life tips that we can all abide by
3. *Dr Sharma's Supplemental Advice* – nutritional advice and information about the supplements we should be taking

1. Dr Sharma's Diagnostic Programmes

The diagnostic programmes described here incorporate a broad range of functional and structural tests, some at a cellular level using a highly refined blend of common conventional medical screening and pioneering methods of health prediction. My *Regenerus Programme*, as well as establishing a flash view of your health now and providing early diagnosis of illness, aims to predict your weakest areas of health, identifying causes for concerns and establishing the need for change or further investigation.

With the help of your preferred CAM healthcare provider or doctor or through simple exploration on the Internet, you can obtain and organize these tests wherever you live.

Conventional screening is geared only toward early detection of a problem. My programmes aim to predict the potential for ill-health as well, and this is the mainstay of healthy ageing. The principle of the *Regenerus* programme is to examine your current health proactively and your functional state comprehensively to see what your personal major health issues are or are likely to be. Recommendations can then be made to optimize your health and performance in a clear, concise and determined effort to head off potential health problems *before they set in*. By following essential advice and support tailored to your individual results, you will optimize your mental acuity, become physically fit and restore sexual drive, and remain disease-free for as long as possible.

My suggested programmes investigate the unique function of your body and mind. A few tests can establish how your psychology, habits, diet and lifestyle are directly influencing your genetic makeup (your personal genome).

Your very own specific life plan means you can keep, or moderate, at least some of your 'bad habits' by reducing their effects!

The programmes provide a wealth of information about you, including:
• existing and potential nutritional deficiencies;
• toxins and detoxification capability;
• effects of stress;
• metabolic dysfunctions;
• digestive and absorption problems.

These investigations are described in detail in chapters of this book that cover specific organs and systems. Remember, you are as old as your oldest part, so recognition of which part of your body this is allows you to place your focus where you need to in order to achieve healthy ageing.

Once you know about your body, you can choose to focus on:
• structure and bone density (Chapter 5);
• arteries and heart (Chapter 6);
• brain and neurological system (Chapter 7);
• hormones (Chapter 8);
• immune system (Chapter 9).

Your own personal 'prescription' is developed through this programme – as unique to you as your own internal blueprint. Ideally, you will be able to discuss one of the following options with your primary healthcare provider or preferably an integrated physician. It is to be hoped that you will be able to access the tests locally; if you fail to obtain such support, go through the Resources section toward the end of the book of local health organizations, or the equivalents in your part of the world, and visit a practitioner.

The following are three screening programmes designed to review your body in different ways:

- *The Optimum Performance Screen*
- *The Healthy Ageing Risk Analysis Profile*
- *Regenerus – The Life Extension Programme* (a combination of both the above with an extensive health screen to establish current well-being)

The Optimum Performance Screen

This programme of tests and investigations analyzes your individual ability to perform. The results lead to the design of a programme to help you achieve your optimum physical and psychological levels. The quality of all your work, rest and play is improved enormously when your body and mind are working at their maximum capacity. Putting this into effect as soon as possible makes a profound difference to how you age. The programme establishes your nutrition and metabolic functional status, investigates bowel function, toxicity levels, hormone levels (which govern so much of our function, including mood and sleep patterns) and evaluates your current physical strength, fitness, posture and balance.

The programme includes the following components:

1. A comprehensive medical history and examination by an anti-ageing or integrated doctor who will know how to access the tests needed.
2. A fitness and structure analysis by specialized personal trainers, fitness physiotherapists – Corrective Holistic Exercise Kinesiologists (CHEK) are well-respected – or you can find an osteopath or chiropractor trained in such areas.
3. Heart rate variability – this is a specific stress test that monitors your heart beat to assess how you deal with chronic stress (both physical and psychological).
4. Full nutritional evaluation through blood and urine samples, looking at nutrients in the body at an intracellular level.
5. Metabolic evaluation of toxins and heavy metals.
6. Blood/urine analysis to establish your body's ability to detoxify.
7. Stress neurohormone evaluation.
8. Energy production capability (mitochondrial function).
9. Digestive and absorptive capabilities and the measurement of beneficial and pathogenic bowel bacteria (comprehensive stool analysis).
10. A comprehensive hormonal profile.

The Healthy Ageing Risk Analysis Profile

This programme investigates the areas of risk that influence your personal ageing process and helps define which is/are your 'oldest part(s)'. An understanding of where your risks lie allows you to focus on maintaining optimum health in those areas – it is no good having the heart and arteries of someone 10 years younger than you if your immune system is 20 years older.

By reviewing how your genes interact with your environment (genomics), it is possible to dedicate a programme to optimize the health of your heart and arteries, brain and nervous system, provide hormonal balance, strengthen your immune system, encourage your ability to detoxify and maintain your structure, bones and joints.

This programme includes:

1. A comprehensive medical history and examination by an anti-ageing or integrated doctor who will know how to access the tests needed.
2. Blood tests for cardiovascular risk.
3. Arteriograph (if available). This is a non-invasive and simple test employing a blood-pressure cuff and computerized system to measure the flexibility of your arteries.
4. Bone-density analysis of a compound called deoxypyridinoline (DPD) through a urinary test and bone-scanning with ultrasound or low-level X-ray.
5. Fitness and structure analysis as in the Optimum Performance Screen.
6. A comprehensive hormonal profile.
7. Brain function assessment through hemoenecephalography, quantative electro-encephalograpy (QEEG) or other locally available 'brain mapping' techniques.
8. Genomic anti-ageing analysis – a blood or cheek cell test looking at your personal gene makeup from the point of view of how it interacts with the environment (that is, not looking at genetic disease). Testing all genes is potentially prohibitively expensive. Many laboratories will have an anti-ageing profile that looks at a selection of genomes to give an overview of genetic tendencies toward problems in the following areas:
   - heart and arteries;
   - neurological system;
   - bone density;
   - hormonal control;
   - immune system.

Further tests can then be focused on any identified risk areas.

Regenerus – The Life Extension Programme

This is the most extensive of the programmes and is a combination of:
* the Optimum Performance Screen

    +
* the Healthy Ageing Risk Analysis Profile

    +
* a full conventional medical screen

    +
* an extensive predictive medical screen

This screening programme highlights any current areas of ill-health you may have and provides you with a uniquely designed health programme that includes:
* lifestyle advice;
* diet and general nutrition;
* a bespoke exercise programme;
* specific nutritional and supplemental advice.

In addition to the components listed under the Optimum Performance Screen and the Healthy Ageing Risk Analysis Profile, the *Regenerus* screen includes the following:

1. A sensitive blood test to detect cancer cells – the blood test is capable of detecting one cancerous cell in 25ml of blood – and cancer gene markers (see Chapter 10).
2. Insulin levels and adiponectin for sugar control.
3. Insulin-like growth factor 1 (IGF1) – as a measurement of human growth hormone.
4. sIgA – immune status marker.
5. Full conventional blood and urine analysis to detect diseases such as diabetes, liver and kidney dysfunction, anaemia, and so on.
6. Stool analysis to detect bowel inflammation, evidence of food allergy and bowel cancer.
7. A urinalysis to detect increased intestinal permeability (the leaky gut test).

As you read through the simple explanations I give in each chapter, the relevance and benefits of this extensive range of tests becomes clear and leads to a full understanding of why we can all enjoy our less-than-per-fect lifestyle by following simple rules (described next), and by taking the nutrients and specific protective functional medicine – much of it natural – described at the end of this chapter and throughout the book.

2. Dr Sharma's Healthy Ageing Lifestyle Guide

There are so many things that we all do, blissfully unaware of their harmful effects on our health. These inevitably move us more swiftly toward age-related conditions. If we add in the 'naughty' things that we *know* are detrimental to our health, we end up with a cumulative effect that increases the risks of us facing age-related dysfunction earlier than necessary.

This book is not about the *perfect* lifestyle: it is about helping you achieve *optimum health* for as long as possible within your *normal life patterns*. If we are made aware of simple changes that we can make, we can continue to inhabit our polluted environment, live on imperfect diets and enjoy, in moderation, our bad habits.

If you are of the ilk to regularly and persistently meditate, eat predominantly non-processed and organic foods, exercise and ensure optimum levels of sleep, you have a level of dedication that only a few of us can achieve.

I would like to take you through a 24-hour period, offering simple and practical advice on a range of changes that you can easily integrate in your everyday life. You will see, as you read through this book, that small, seemingly innocuous things may have a negative influence on ageing healthily. In addition, resting, exercising, eating correctly, and so on, all have to fit in realistically with normal life.

Your time in bed

If you wake up aching or stiff, with no known or obvious condition such as arthritis or a strained muscle, you are probably sleeping on the wrong mattress. Highly technical mattresses are now available although some people do better simply sleeping on the floor. As you go through life, you will probably spend time with friends, at hotels, in guest houses, but always on different mattresses. When you come across one that you feel is right, try to recognize its qualities such as firmness and size and buy the same or similar for your regular bed. A quarter to a third of your life may be spent in bed, so it is well worth getting that environment right.

Sleep in a room that is as dark and quiet as is feasible. Light and noise pollution stop you from dropping into the necessary deeper levels of sleep, thus preventing biochemical and hormonal changes that are vital to regeneration and detoxification through the night.

Do not go to bed for any reason other than to sleep or to have sex. Avoid reading, listening to the radio or watching TV in bed as your brain will start to associate bedtime with activity, and normal sleep patterns will be disrupted. Sex is allowed as it is effectively a form of exercise that is beneficial to the sleep process.

Many of us sleep with a partner. Snoring (and other noises!), excessive movements, different times of going to sleep and waking up are all disruptive. If your partner markedly disturbs your sleep, consider separate beds or even bedrooms. The comfort of sleeping with a loved one is valuable, of course, but do not underestimate the benefit of moving into the spare room or even onto the sitting room couch, if comfortable, once or twice a week to allow undisturbed sleep.

Consider asking your GP for a prescription for melatonin after you have read about this sleep hormone in Chapter 8.

Make sure that your bed is not placed within 3 metres (10 feet) of the electrical input or mains boxes in the house. Think what is below your floor as you may be sleeping above the fuse box. High levels of electromagnetic radiation emanate from here that, if close to your head for 6–10 hours per night, is likely to be causing damage. Keep electrical gadgets such as alarm clocks, electric radios and mobile phones at least 1 metre (3–4 feet) away. Bear in mind that most of us live within an electromagnetic ring, courtesy of the plug sockets in the skirting of our rooms. We do not need to have further electromagnetic influence on our nervous system.

Upon waking

Drink a glass of water, preferably with a squeeze of lemon. This has a cleansing effect on the body.

Consider a healthy, stimulating herbal tea such as green tea. Avoid highly caffeinated drinks (accepting that green tea has a certain amount of caffeine) until you are about to eat something as this artificial jolt speeds up the metabolism, thereby depleting some of the biochemical preparation for the day more quickly than is desirable. The body's natural stress-coping hormone, cortisol, reaches a peak prior to awakening and drops to its lowest level in late afternoon/early evening. A hit of caffeine may alter this hormonal rhythm, leaving you less capable of coping at the end of the day.

Stretching

If you watch any animal or baby waking up, you will see that their natural instinct is to stretch. Stretching removes metabolic products that build up during the night – particularly advanced glycation end-products (AGEs; *see* pp xvii–xviii) and protein bonds (crosslinks) that are a fundamental part of the ageing processes. A simple 3–5-minute programme of stretching, yoga or tai chi can minimize the effects of AGEs by increasing blood flow and waste drainage through the lymphatic system (see diagrams opposite).

Breathing

Breathing exercises are an integral part of most yoga and tai chi techniques. A few minutes spent aerating the body and moving life energy (from an Eastern perspective) is invaluable to health.

Exercise

The best time of day for exercise depends on each individual, so up to a point I suggest you follow your instinct. Some people do well to burn up the adrenalin they have derived through the day by exercising in the evening, whereas others are better off using up energy reserves that have amassed during the night. However, if at all possible, do not get up too early and sacrifice sleep for exercise. Your choice of exercise can range from 12 minutes-per-week programmes through to longer aerobic and strengthening sessions in the gym or playing your favourite sport. A mix of aerobic, stretching, balancing and strengthening is undoubtedly best (see Chapter 3). Finally, make sure that you shower or bathe as soon as you can after exercise. A lot of water-soluble toxins come out with the sweat, but your body will reabsorb them if they are left to sit on your skin.

Ablutions

Cleansing your body of toxins and pathogens occurs in many and varied ways, including going to the toilet and washing your body. The bladder will look after itself, as will your bowel, unless you suffer from health problems. However, constipation is, unfortunately, too common a problem – particularly for those of us eating an overrefined Western diet. As you will discover in Chapter 10, the bowel does not only carry the toxins and unwanted nutrients that we do not absorb from food but also a majority of the waste products that are eliminated through the liver. Holding on to these toxins throughout the day is not a good thing. We often create habits simply by persisting with current behaviour, so even if your usual regime does not have

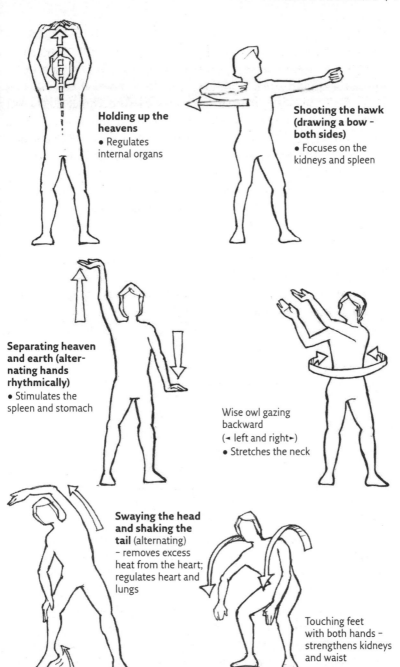

Holding up the heavens
• Regulates internal organs

Shooting the hawk (drawing a bow – both sides)
• Focuses on the kidneys and spleen

Separating heaven and earth (alternating hands rhythmically)
• Stimulates the spleen and stomach

Wise owl gazing backward
(◄ left and right►)
• Stretches the neck

Swaying the head and shaking the tail (alternating) – removes excess heat from the heart; regulates heart and lungs

Touching feet with both hands – strengthens kidneys and waist

Figure 1: **Qi Gong Ba Duan Jin, exercises**

you sitting on the toilet, start trying to empty your bowels in the morning, before breakfast.

Taking a bath or shower to remove toxins that your body eliminates through sweat during the night is as important as doing so after exercise. Dry your skin briskly with a roughish towel as skin brushing further helps remove surface toxins.

Clean your teeth regularly. Some age-related health conditions, particularly arterial and heart health, have a direct link with poor oral hygiene, infections and inflammation in the gums (gingivitis or periodontal disease).

You could even try nasal washing with salt water. This yogic technique, known as *jala lota*, carries very little risk if performed properly, and the health benefits to be derived from it are supported by many studies and traditional values from the East.

I would strongly advise against applying deodorants, especially antiperspirants, directly on the skin. The chemicals they contain are artificial and are absorbed into the bloodstream. Natural plant extracts are unlikely to cause problems unless they are in the form of gels or ointments that may plug the pores. Armpit sweating is an important part of detoxification. Many deodorants carry metals either as part of the product manufacture or leeched from the metal container. Spraying yourself daily with a toxin that is capable of being absorbed through the skin will take its toll as metals are associated with so many age-related conditions.

Breakfast

Do not miss this meal. If you do not feel hungry, it means that you have detrimentally retrained your evolutionary, natural instinct to break the nighttime fast, and you need to reprogramme your appetite centres. Breaking the fast has many beneficial consequences. If you do not eat until midday and had your supper early the previous evening, you may be going 14–16 hours without eating. After about six hours, your body's metabolism alters to a default setting of 'starvation'. This means that the next meal you eat is going to be considered as a break from famine and you will store as much as is possible as fat. The idea that cutting back on calories by missing breakfast will help you lose weight is a falsehood – any decrease in calories is more than overcompensated for by a downturn shift in metabolism that leads to weight gain. Skipping a meal, particularly breakfast, will push you toward obesity and the health issues associated with that. One study actually suggests that increased carbohydrate intake at breakfast time might even help weight loss.[1]

Chapter 2 will guide you to better foods and menus, but the simple rules are:
- Avoid refined foods such as sweetened cereals.
- Go easy on cow's products, preferably using soy, almond, rice, goat's or sheep's milk instead.
- Eat some food with any caffeinated drinks.
- Consider having a freshly made fruit or vegetable juice or smoothie as an integral part of every breakfast (there are a couple of delicious recipes in Chapter 2).

Getting to work

Many of us have to commute and soon after getting up in the morning. Many of us support those who leave the home, and many of us now work from home. Whatever your movements are, you can follow some basic rules to turn the start of the day into a positive health environment.

If travelling, avoid mechanized transport for the first or last 10 minutes of the journey. Get off the train, bus or tram one or two stops before your place of work. Aim at 10–15 minutes of brisk walking (100 steps/minute) as part of your 30–40 minutes/day of exercise. Keep your 'work shoes' at work and make the journey to and from your workplace in trainers so that this regime is easy on your feet.

Through the morning

If you are a sedentary worker, ensure that you sit on your chair at a height where your elbows are above your keyboard or writing level, but not so high that you have to slouch forward to rest your arms on the desk. Try to walk about every 15–20 minutes. During this break, stretch your back and limbs, do neck rolls, flap your hands and wriggle your toes in this break. Recognize those muscle groups that tighten up when you sit for long periods and focus on them. Find out about ergonomics in a book or on the Internet. This is the study of equipment and devices that fit the human body, its movements and its cognitive abilities. Here are a few important tips:
- Try to keep your computer at least 1 metre (3 feet) away from you even if the screen is closer.
- Obtain an electro-magnetic-absorbing front screen if you spend more than 2–3 hours a day in front of the computer.
- Ensure good aeration to avoid volatile oxidative compounds produced by house-cleaning solvents and the heat within the computer. If you are in an environment with many computers, point out the implications for your health (for example, free-radical damage to your

arteries and nervous system) to your employers or suggest the use of filters or ionizers in your section of the office.

When doing physically active jobs such as housekeeping, building and decorating, landscaping, plumbing, and so on, ensure that you use both sides of your body equally. Hold the shovel or push the vacuum cleaner with different hands. It will feel strange at first, but it is important to balance your muscular development as it will improve your sense of balance and your overall strength. Do not forget to stretch regularly.

Keep hydrated, especially in warm, stuffy environments or if your work builds up a sweat. You need to be aiming to drink at least 0.5 litre (1¼ pints) of water during the morning, the afternoon and, again, during the evening.

Glass obstructs many of the healthy wavelengths of light, but natural light through a window will still influence brain activity for the better. If you cannot be close to natural light, try to have natural spectrum light bulbs wherever possible.

Try to absorb some sunlight during your breaks. Roll up your sleeves, undo the top buttons on your shirt and expose as much skin to the vitamin D-forming ultraviolet light as is sensible as discussed in the section on skin (see Chapter 10).

Keep caffeine intake from colas, tea or coffee to a maximum of 2–3 cups of medium strength daily. Use the quick-fix caffeine kick as you would alcohol or drugs – sparingly – with recognition of the consequences to your health.

Sweet drinks (often caffeinated) such as colas and 'sodas', are associated with an increased risk of some cancers.[2]

Morning snack

Avoid anything containing highly refined sugars such as biscuits, although some enjoyment is never a bad thing! Remember, sugar turns to fat, damages arteries, increases diabetes risk and ages tissues and cells. Try keeping a variety of nuts to hand, including pine nuts mixed with pumpkin and sesame seeds. A handful of this combination when you feel hungry, and a delay of five minutes before enjoying any sweet food, will lead to a reduction in the amount of the 'bad stuff' you ingest as hunger hormones will be satiated by the 'healthy stuff' hitting the bloodstream. Although there is some controversy about the dangers of salt intake, avoid foods with a high salt content.[3] It is also sensible to avoid saturated fats.

Lunchtime and the afternoon

Avoid skipping lunch for the same reasons as not missing breakfast. Try to have a midday meal consisting of protein and vegetables instead of carbohydrate. Carbohydrate is absorbed quickly into the bloodstream and raises your blood-sugar levels, which, in turn, causes an outpouring of insulin. High insulin drags down your sugar levels, and this slump will occur within 1–2 hours of eating carbohydrates or sweet food. Ideally, have a siesta – as is enjoyed by many parts of the world. (In evolutionary terms, think about what animals and babies do after a meal: they sleep.) A power nap of a few minutes after a meal can be helpful in balancing the hormone levels.

Afternoon snack

Reach for those nuts and seeds and try to eat some fruit at around 4 pm – bananas are especially good as the sugar content gives a quick energy boost, while the starch content releases energy more slowly and so will stave off hunger pangs until the end of the workday. Grab another handful of nuts and seeds half an hour before you are due to leave your workplace or as you prepare for the evening after a day at home. This will reduce any craving for a quick fix of alcohol, unhealthy, processed salted nuts and crisps, or snacking on the kids' early tea or supper.

Ending the day

Now that your stomach is somewhat lined by healthy complex carbohydrates and proteins, the bad effects of that sociable after-work drink or that glass of wine as you prepare to face the hordes returning from school and the office is much reduced!

Repeat the morning travel advice and put on your trainers – aim for a 15-minute brisk walk to wherever you pick up your transport or allow yourself 15 minutes at the end of your journey. If you are an 'evening exerciser', get on your bike!

Your evening at home

Try as much as possible to leave work in the workplace. When you get home, focus on your family and social life and try to discuss only positive aspects of work in the evening. By all means, bring up concerns in the morning or possibly set time aside during the day to make a phone call if you wish to off-load to family or friends. We must remember that we work to live, not live to work, and longevity has been shown to be related to the time we spend relaxing.

Supper and afterward

Your healthy evening meal, governed by the nutritional advice in Chapter 2, should be followed by relaxation time. Even if you are tempted by the crime-thriller series, try to end your TV watching with a comedy. Socializing, reading, playing games and interacting are vitally important for calming the mind and encouraging healthy ageing. Research clearly shows that a day made up of both productive activity and times of rest and relaxation can optimize health.

Going to bed

Ablution time again! Clean those teeth – get the bristles between your teeth to protect the gums and floss regularly.

Wash your face and body. If you have been in a polluted environment and have sweated while doing your one (or preferably two) 15-minute invigorating walks, five minutes under the shower at the end of your day, followed by a brisk rub-down, will enhance detoxification, which, over a lifetime, will maintain health and add healthy years.

Try not to go to bed feeling cross – it is a simple but important rule as your brain will not respond well to the adrenalin associated with anger.

And that's it, really! As you read around the subject of healthy ageing, you will come across lots of other tips and you may already have many of your own.

3. Dr Sharma's Supplemental Advice

As you read this book, you will see that I have provided specific recommendations for supplementation for the different organs and systems because our food no longer carries all the vitamins and minerals, EFAs and amino acids we need to maintain optimum heath. We need to take supplements to achieve healthy ageing and enhance longevity.

Wherever possible, I recommend that patients take organic or citrate forms of nutrients or natural food-state (NFS) products. These are easily absorbed both by the gut and by cells, they are recognized by the cell receptors as food, they do not block receptors as pharmaceutical nutrients are theorized to do and have shown better effects in some studies. (*See* useful websites for more information.)

In the conventional, orthodox medical profession there is some controversy over the use of supplements. A recent study shows a moderate decrease in rates of cancer in those taking supplements; however, other studies disagree.[4] I believe that pharmaceutical-grade supplements, making up 98 per cent or so of those available to the public, are potentially dangerous. Moreover, analysis of published medical papers suggests that some nutrients are dangerous in some circumstances.[5] The press certainly enjoyed scare-mongering by providing headlines on 28 February 2008, such as:

'Supplements raise death rate by 5 per cent' (*The Times*, UK)

'Des vitamines dangéreuses pour la santé?' (*Le Soir*, France)

'Another knock on antioxidants' (*Los Angeles Times*, USA)

However, in reality, what the headlines should have suggested is:
'A selective study of certain research papers has found that you have an increased risk of dying if you take:
- pharmaceutical-grade supplements rather than plant extracts;
- supplements at non-individualized dosages;
- supplements with no regard of whether or not you are deficient;
- particular supplements that are unlikely to benefit you;
- supplements that are taken at the wrong dosage when you are already struggling with a serious illness.'
… *Not quite the same thing, is it?!*

Dr Sharma's Maintenance Programme

The following list of supplements is the minimum I think we all need to be taking every day. In this book, I give dosages of supplements where I think appropriate. These are aimed at adults, male and female, but should be discussed with your primary healthcare practitioner, especially if you are already taking a supplement. At some points, I do not give a dosage for these supplements as you should discuss a specific dose with your practitioner.

I direct you to various websites if I do not think there is a range of supplement options, and you need to be specific in your acquisition. I also make the following statement: *At first glance, the following extensive list seems daunting, but remember: many of these nutrients can be found in the same tablet or capsule as multivitamin/mineral complexes.*

Health professionals can advise you and they too will have their favourites; however, you can tell them about my preferences for organic citrates and NFS.

MINERALS
- *Calcium and magnesium* – at a ratio of 1:2
- *Selenium* – best taken nightly

- *Zinc/copper* – ratio 15:1 before bedtime
- *Iron* – particularly if your diet avoids, or is not high on, red meat (discuss iron supplementation with a professional if you are over 50 years old)

VITAMINS
- *B-complex* – one that specifically includes vitamin B6 and folic acid
- Vitamins C, D, E and K

ESSENTIAL FATTY ACIDS
- *Omega-6 and omega-3* – mix at a ratio of 4:1

AMINO ACIDS
- *Amino acid combination* – whey extract or a vegetable-based whole amino acid complex

OTHER NUTRIENTS
- *Probiotics* – a combination product containing a mix of beneficial bacteria and the food they eat (known as prebiotics)
- *Coenzyme Q10*
- *Melatonin* – no more than 2–3 mg nightly unless prescribed by a practitioner
- *Resveratrol*
- *Alpha lipoic acid*
- *Phytoestrogens* (for women) – such as genistein and/or daidzein
- *A joint-support formula* – one containing a combination of some or all of the following: glucosamine sulphate, methylsulfonylmethane (MSM), silica, calcium and manganese

THERAPEUTIC INTERVENTIONS
Far infrared sauna therapy – discussed in Chapter 4

Dr Sharma's Advanced Programme
The supplements listed are necessary only for people who have established risk factors or those who simply want an advanced programme of nutrients to decrease the likelihood of age-related conditions occurring.

You may well be a walking natural pharmacy, but the evidence supports my learned hypothesis that taking this full range of supplements will improve the quality of your life and increase longevity.

In an ideal world, you should discuss taking these supplements with a health professional to ensure correct dosage and use. In the case of hormone replacement, this needs to be prescribed – do not try to self-prescribe even through what may appear to be reputable Internet sources.

MINERALS
- *Iodine* – promoted by some authorities but not by others – low dose 2–3 times a week is an option (see discussion in Chapter 5)

VITAMINS
- *Mixed carotenoids* – particularly lutein, zeaxanthin and astaxanthin (for those with eye or visual issues)
- *Vitamin B12 injection* – minimally every three months, after discussion with an integrated practitioner, if persistently tired and fatigued

ESSENTIAL FATTY ACIDS (EFAs)
- Phosphatidylcholine

AMINO ACIDS
- *L-carnosine* – provides arterial and cardiovascular protection
- *Glutathione* – should be taken sublingually or as an oral spray to enhance antioxidant activity and detoxification

OTHER NUTRIENTS
- *Hyaluronic acid (HA)* – for the health of hair follicles, skin and joints
- *Collagen (hydrolized form)* – for hair follicle activity and maintenance of skin and joints
- *Gingko biloba* – for memory and arterial protection
- *Huperzine* – for mental acuity, but not to be taken before bedtime

MEDICAL PRESCRIPTIONS
- *Aminoguanadine* – should be considered by borderline diabetics in particular or those with peripheral vascular disease
- *Thyroid replacement* – after testing and discussion on its use if in the lower regions of normal reference range
- *Female hormones* – oestrogen and progesterone, preferably in bioidentical form

- *Testosterone* – for men, particularly if tests show lower-than-normal range levels (women lacking libido can also discuss the use of testosterone with an expert)
- *Chelation therapy* – to remove heavy metals to which we are all exposed daily (see Chapter 4)
- *Blue green algae or zeolite* – oral daily intake
- *IV therapy* – consider discussion with a specialist about occasional courses
- *Human growth hormone (HGH)* – secretagogues or discuss HGH injections with an expert or experienced practitioner (see Chapter 8)

THERAPEUTIC INTERVENTIONS

- *Pulsed electro-magnetic frequency* – discussed in Chapter 4
- *Various small self-help 'stress-busting' gizmos* – useful for relaxation or enhancing meditation

STEM CELL THERAPY

This chapter would not be complete without a discussion of the role of stem cells in longevity. Stem cells are found in most multicellular animals and are identified by their ability to grow into any number of different cell types. Humans (and all mammals) have embryonic and adult stem cells. As the names suggest, the former are involved in our development from embryo, while the latter are involved in repairing and replenishing mature tissues.

Adult stem cells are few in number, but are found in many different tissues. A stem cell can become a particular type of cell or tissue according to local chemical and hormonal influences from the surrounding cells. A stem cell placed in the brain will become nervous tissue, while another placed in the heart will become a myocardial cell, and so on.

Controversy surrounds embryonic stem cell research, and there is considerable religious and political obstruction regarding its use. Research with adult stem cells is not such an emotive issue – destroying a potential life is not quite the same as extracting stem cells from bone marrow, the root of the lower-jaw third molar tooth and adipose (fat) tissue. However, despite greater freedom to operate in this area, pharmaceutical companies are not too keen on finding methods of repair that may hamper the sale of drugs.

Stem cell research continues, and centres around the world aim to offer more widely available treatments for a range of conditions, many of which are age related. Research suggests that there may be benefits from stem cell therapy in:

STEM CELLS

There are two main types of stem cells. One known as totipotent grows into embryonic cells that can build a complete body with many different organs; the other type – pluripotent stem cells – can differentiate into most forms of cell. There are also subdivisions of pluripotent cells such as multipotent, unipotent and oligopotent, but that is getting too technical!

- Alzheimer's disease;
- Parkinson's disease;
- motor neurone disease;
- multiple sclerosis;
- post-stroke recovery;
- traumatic brain injury;
- wound healing;
- arthritis (osteoarthritis and rheumatoid arthritis);
- heart tissue damage (including post heart attack);
- muscle diseases;
- Crohn's disease;
- cancers;
- vision issues and blindness;
- deafness.

Watch this space – stem cell therapy may well become a mainstay in the treatment of most conditions and many age-related diseases.

Chapter 2

Diet and nutrition

There is a proliferation of nutrition-based research highlighting diseases linked to nutritional status: for example, a single search on the web for 'diets and longevity' provided 140,000 research papers. Not so very long ago, in 1988, the Surgeon General Dr Evert Koop concluded that 15 out of 21 deaths in the USA were related to diet. There is clearly no 'one size fits all' diet. For example, Eskimos living in cold polar regions require high-energy food such as blubber and would not fare well on a macrobiotic diet as followed by someone from the Far East.

Experimenting in a controlled manner with the variety of foods available in the developed world should enable us to establish what suits us as individuals. Even within the same family, some people will be better off as vegetarians, while others will benefit from being predominantly carnivorous.

The principle rule in your nutritional plan for healthy ageing and longevity is finding the right balance of carbohydrates, proteins and fats. The *optimum* proportion of each depends very much upon individual requirements. As a rough guide, ideally you should make up your diet along the following lines:
* vegetables and fruits – 50 per cent
* proteins – 35 per cent
* grains – 15 per cent

This clearly contradicts much of the advice given over the last three or four decades – a period that has seen exponential rises in the developing world of diabetes, arterial disease, strokes, heart attacks and cancers (Harvard School of Public Health).[1]

Put simply, half of our diet should be fruit and vegetables, and we should eat twice as much protein as grain. There, that saves you reading any more books on nutrition – the rest is just detail!

How important is nutrition for healthy ageing?

I think the World Health Organisation (WHO) sums it up best:

> *Every structure and function in the body is dependent upon a*
> *vitamin or mineral. These nutrients, along with proteins and fats,*
> *are derived from our diet. Nutritional deficiencies are one of the most*
> *researched and best established causes of diseases world wide. It is*
> *estimated one third of the world population is deficient.*[2]

Most of us are unaware that nutritional deficiency is prevalent in the overfed and developed countries.

You have probably heard about scurvy, caused by a lack of vitamin C, and blindness arising from vitamin A deficiency; other conditions caused by an inadequate intake of vitamins, such as beriberi (lack of vitamin B1) and pellagra (lack of vitamin B3) are common in developing countries. Vitamin D deficiency is associated with diabetes, cancer, asthma, poor immunity and the bone-deforming disease rickets. Furthermore, vitamin D is necessary for calcium absorption. Vitamin D levels are largely dependent on receiving enough sunlight directly onto the skin, and so it is important to spend time outside (in the UK, more than 70 per cent of the population are vitamin D deficient in mid-winter). It is a surprising fact that, from a nutrient point of view, 10 per cent of the population in the UK have dietary intakes similar to that of populations in some developing countries[3] and the UK is now seeing a resurgence in rickets,[4] and scurvy in children.[5]

Selenium deficiency leads to cancer and arterial disease; yet the daily selenium intake in the USA and UK is below baseline recommendations.[6]

Magnesium is thought to be deficient in 57 per cent of the UK's population; such deficiency has been associated with high blood pressure, chronic fatigue, insulin resistance and heart failure (USDA, 2009).[7]

You can argue that many, if not most, age-related health issues are caused by nutritional deficiency, particularly a lack of minerals. If we simply acknowledge this scientifically proven link and adjust our diets or take supplementation if necessary, we can prevent or improve many common conditions such as:

- Arthritis – associated with deficiency in selenium, zinc, copper and sulphur;
- Arterial disease (heart attacks and strokes) – associated with deficiency in selenium, magnesium, vitamin C;
- Cancer – associated with deficiency in selenium, magnesium and many antioxidants;

CHRONIC FATIGUE SYNDROME

Chronic fatigue syndrome (CFS) may affect as much as 3 per cent of the population in the US[8], and 250,000 people in the UK, including 1 per cent of children. According to the Centers for Disease Control and Prevention, 80 per cent of cases of CFS have undiagnosed causes.[9]

- Chronic fatigue syndrome (CFS) – associated with deficiency in magnesium, essential fatty acids, coenzyme Q10 and vitamin B complex (Werbach, 2000);[10]
- High blood pressure – associated with deficiency in vitamin B3, vitamin C, magnesium and selenium;
- Osteoporosis – associated with deficiency in calcium, magnesium, manganese, boron and silicon.

The Eastern approach to healthy eating

The Eastern philosophies consider all food to have a variety of 'energies'. Foods may have masculine or feminine energy or a mixture of both. Foods contain different elements and states found in our universe – space, air, fire, earth, wood, metal and water. Food is sweet, bitter, sour, salty or spicy and may be hot, warm or cold.

Diet is not only about calorific input and output and nutritional balance. It must include an understanding of the 'vital force' (energy known as *prana* in Sanskrit or *qi* in Chinese culture) imparted from foods. There needs to be a spiritual and psychological connection with nutrition. The most reliable way for a person to feel a food's energy involves instinct when choosing and preparing food.

Yin and yang foods

Eastern philosophies consider that conditions of ill-health are created by excess of or deficiency in *yin* or *yang* leads leading to ill health. Put simply, *yin* is the fluid of the body, which acts as our fuel reserve and lubricant within the system, whereas *yang* is the heat or fire. *Yin* is the fuel and *yang* is the spark that ignites it.

Depending upon your specific symptoms, you might wish to increase or decrease the type of energetic food you eat. Instinct is usually a good guide to individual requirements at any given time in relation to the balance of *yin* and *yang*. Often the body (when healthy) will automatically balance and absorb what it needs.

Yin foods tend to be sweet and cool. They create dampness (which is why they include foods such as mucus-producing milk products) and contain a variety of nutrients. Examples of *yin* foods are:

- most fruits (especially apple, pineapple, citrus fruits, pears and watermelon);
- eggs, oysters, rabbit, duck and pork;
- tofu, yam, tomatoes, asparagus, kidney beans and peas;
- milk, yoghurt and cheese;
- honey (a particularly good source of *yin*).

Yang foods are principally warming. They are foods that benefit from being cooked and have strong flavours. *Yang* foods include:

- most herbs and spices (especially ginger, garlic, clove and nutmeg);
- lamb, lobster and shrimp;
- nuts (especially chestnut and walnut);
- offal (such as kidney).

Foods to avoid

The following foods are considered to be lacking in *qi*, and as many of them have contraindications for health from a Western medicine point of view, they are best avoided:

- Fried foods
- Foods containing refined sugars, such as chocolates and sweets
- Jams, marmalades and preserves with added white sugar; foods made from refined flour, including white bread
- Non-organic meat and all pig products as pigs are mostly fed on our leftovers
- Caffeine-containing drinks (coffee, strong tea, chocolate and many carbonated drinks)
- Squashes and most pre-prepared juices (most contain extra sugar regardless of the labelling because manufacturers are allowed to replace an estimated amount of sugar that may be lost in the manufacturing process)
- Smoked foods where the fumes come from chemically treated charcoal
- Alcoholic beverages
- Products with added salt
- High-fat foods such as pizzas, processed burgers and French fries

TIPS FOR BALANCING ENERGY

Keep in touch with your instincts. Eat what you feel like eating, but ignore unhealthy cravings. If you long for a piece of chocolate, your body is suggesting a need for sweetness and energy – so have some fruit instead. If the craving is for pasta, make sure it is wholegrain.

Balance temperatures – on a hot, sunny day enjoy a salad; in the depths of winter, prepare soup. The rule of thumb is that raw and steamed foods are cooling, while stewed, baked and stir-fried foods are warming, and deep-fried, roasted, grilled and barbecued foods are heating.

Balance raw and cooked foods, depending upon the temperature in the environment. Even a very warm day requires some heating foods, but a predominantly raw diet is best. *'Predominant' is the operative word here.*

Try to balance your flavour combinations throughout the day or even at each meal: for example, you could balance the saltiness of fish with the sourness of some lemon sprinkled over.

Eat foods with vital force. Organic food, grown locally, imparts energy from the part of the world in which you live. Organic food is also probably better for you.

Traditional Chinese medicine states that 'the stomach has no teeth'. Chew food well and conserve energy by lessening the work of the digestive system.

- Mass-produced eggs and poultry
- Any food with additives or preservatives
- Any tinned foods and any coloured or flavoured foods

Psycho-spiritual attitudes to eating

Try to be happy around food. Biochemical reactions abound when you eat and prepare to eat – saliva and stomach-acid production increases, digestive enzymes are churned out, and the gut starts to contract. Stress hormones decrease all these activities, inhibiting digestion and absorption, so set aside time in the day to eat without any disturbances.

If allowed to eat according to instinct, without time constraints or issues of food availability, the human body will set its own pattern. Whenever possible, select your food according to its smell and appearance; note that your choices will be affected by how you feel at that particular time.

Ensure that your kitchen and eating area are hygienic and comfortable and that they have a happy atmosphere. Very often the family gathers only around food, so make sure that this happens in bright and airy surroundings. Eating is not just about obtaining calories. It is about ingesting energy and undertaking social interaction. 'Table culture' is something that many parts of the world excel at, but which others substantially lack. The fast-food and TV-dinner concept is removing the important time for 'herd communication'. Children improve their language, social and communication skills around a table, and bonding also occurs at mealtimes. It is worth remembering that the human body derives pleasure from both input and output. Spend time with your food. Make time for contemplation or worship while you prepare and eat food – you are what you eat, and how you relate to what goes into you is a major part of that.

How much should you eat?

You should aim to feed your body an appropriate amount for its requirements. If you are in a sedentary job, eat less. Restricting what you eat has been proven to create changes in cells associated with increasing longevity.[11]

Be aware of when you have eaten enough at any meal. Leave the table slightly hungry if possible. One simple trick is always to leave a small portion of food on the plate – perhaps enough to add to the next meal so as not to be wasteful. Do not eat anything on your plate that you do not feel like eating.

Fasting

Statistics generally support fasting as a method of increasing longevity and healthy ageing. Alternate-day fasting or intermittent fasting is also cited as being beneficial for longevity.[12] However, some scientific evidence suggests that fasting may be detrimental, particularly to our ability to detoxify.

Fasting can be anything from a total fast where nothing passes the lips to a variety of semi-fasts (for example, allowing intake of water and fruit juices or eating fruits and vegetables). *Except under expert advice, any fast must include a suitable amount of water intake.*

Fasting has the following benefits:
- It gives the mouth time to be properly rinsed naturally by saliva, which contains many antibodies and cleansing chemicals.
- The parietal cells of the stomach, which produce hydrochloric acid, can replenish.

- The pancreas is rested as it can make less insulin through the fasting period while less sugar is ingested.
- The muscle wall of the bowel does not have to contract as frequently, and any muscle functions better when it has had a period of rest.
- The colon is given time to evacuate the faeces that can build up and adhere to the large intestinal wall.
- The liver, the chemical factory of the body, can spend time cleaning the blood, rather than digesting new foods. Food restriction also decreases oxidative stress and free-radical production, and increases cellular repair.[13]
- The kidneys have time to filter out some of the longer-lasting toxins in the system.
- The fat stores containing some of the body's toxins can discharge some of these toxins into the bloodstream for removal from the body.
- Fasting itself results in weight loss if continued for more than 24 hours or so. (Simply missing a meal is not fasting and, in fact, is likely to lead to a 'starvation' response and the absorption of calories, thereby actually increasing weight.)

However, fasting is not without risks. The liver detoxifies in two phases as described in Chapter 4. Fasting increases Phase 1 detoxification, which may be a good thing, but it can also turn some toxins into more aggressive poisons. Removal of these depends on Phase 2, which relies on available nutrients – these may not be present during a fast.

So, we may increase toxic burden by fasting.

One study monitored long-term fasting and found that it caused the nervous system to alter hormonal production.[14] Another study showed that it led to decreased protein metabolism and increased the production of damaging free radicals.

Be aware also that the benefits of fasting decrease as we age.[15] If you are over the age of 65, keep the periods you spend fasting to a minimum – and never fast for more than 72 hours. Ideally, you should be monitored by your doctor and/or a nutritionist.

A semi-fast

There is no set fasting technique. Individuals with any tendency to hypo-glycaemia (low blood sugar) will not benefit from a complete fast. If you are unwell, undertake a fast only under the guidance of your doctor. Fasting may make a condition worse by increasing nutritional deficiencies.

A short time on a semi-fast diet may help you to feel generally better, and it can be a great pick-me-up if you are chronically tired. It is better to start the semi-fast on a day when you do not have to exert yourself physically.

Day 1
Drink freshly squeezed or pressed fruit and/or vegetable juice approximately every four hours. Quench your thirst with mineral water or herbal tea and make sure you drink at least 2 litres (4 pints) of fluid during the day. Some suggested juices are apple, orange, grape, pineapple, grapefruit, blackcurrant, mango, cranberry, carrot, beetroot or celery.

Day 2
As for Day 1, but add up to 500 g (1lb) of grapes and three bananas. Eat only as much of these as you feel like.

Day 3
Add raw and lightly cooked vegetables and fruit to anything you want from the previous days.

Day 4
Eat anything you want from the previous days, but add wholegrain cereals, nuts and seeds.

Day 5
As for Day 4, but add fish.

Day 6
As for Day 5, but add eggs, offal, poultry or game.

Day 7
Return to your normal diet, or if you are not sure that it is healthy, establish a new diet with a professional nutritionist.

Obesity

Obesity is a term used by health professionals to describe a level of weight that is likely to be detrimental to health. Although the word obesity is used colloquially as a derogatory term, medics are not passing judgement, so do not be offended if you hear them use it with reference to you.

Obesity can be defined through basal metabolic index (BMI), by waist-to-hip ratio or by the percentage of body fat.

Basal metabolic index (BMI)

BMI is calculated as your weight in kilograms divided by your height in metres squared. It is no longer as popular as it once was as large muscled bodies can produce high figures without being obese.

Important foods for healthy ageing

Make sure that you have a balanced diet. The following simple summary explains why certain foods from some of the major food groups are particularly important for healthy ageing.

Fibre-rich food

High-fibre foods are principally those that are difficult to digest because of their cellulose content. Found in most plants, cellulose or 'roughage' scrapes

---

OBESITY, DISEASE AND MORTALITY

The number of years a person is obese is directly associated with that person's mortality.

- Being overweight for 1–5 years increases the risk of dying by 51 per cent.
- Being overweight for 25 years increases that risk by 152 per cent.[16]
- Obesity accounts for 20 per cent of all female cancer deaths and 14 per cent of deaths in men.[17]
- Obesity is a cause of 25–30 per cent of cancers of the colon, breast and uterus.[18]
- Normal weight along with regular exercise and not smoking can substantially reduce premature death in women and men, perhaps by as much as 8 years in men and 15 years in women.[19]

Basal metabolic index (BMI)

Typical BMI ranges are:

BMI	Classification
< 18.5	Underweight
18.5-24.9	Normal weight
25.0-29.9	Overweight
30.0-34.9	Class I obesity
35.0-39.9	Class II obesity or severe obesity
≥ 40.0	Class III obesity or morbid obesity

Waist-to-hip ratio (WHR)

Waist-to-hip ratio is useful in predicting problems arising in the arteries and heart

Male	Female	Health risk based solely on WHR
0.95 or below	0.80 or below	Low risk
0.96 to 1.0	0.81 to 0.85	Moderate risk
1.0+	0.85+	High risk

Body fat percentage

Recommendations on acceptable ranges for body fat percentage varies worldwide, but the following are the recommended figures for the UK and USA:

Description	Women	Men
Essential fat	8-13%	3-5%
Body fat in athletes	14-20%	6-13%
Body fat in fit individuals	21-24%	14-17%
'Average' body fat	25-32%	18-24%
Excess fat	32%+	25%+

adhesive debris off the bowel wall and also acts like a sponge, absorbing many compounds that are detrimental to health, in particular excess fats and cholesterol. The human gut is not adept at breaking down cellulose, so it remains in the gut, acting as a cleanser and detoxifier.

Fibre gives bulk to the faeces, which allows the muscle wall of the colon (large intestine) to maintain its strength. This encourages the fast removal of waste products, and oxygenation to the bowel itself.

Foods that are high in fibre are:
- vegetables;
- fruit;
- wholegrains;
- nuts and seeds.

VEGETABLES
Try to eat a variety of different-coloured vegetables in the following proportions over the course of the week (keep a note of these when you go shopping for food):
- 5 parts *dark green* – spinach, kale, collard greens, broccoli;
- 4 parts *light green* – cabbage, leeks, lettuce;
- 3 parts *yellow* – carrots, swede, yams;
- 2 parts *white* – potatoes, parsnips;
- 1 part *red* – peppers and tomatoes (yes, I know they are really fruits!).

Aim at a 50:50 intake of cooked to raw. Lightly steamed and/or stir-fried vegetables can be considered a mix of both.

FRUIT
Balance is the order of the day here, but it is best to eat one type of fruit at a time to avoid competition in the absorption of different nutrients at the same receptors.

Although it is fine to enjoy an occasional apple pie or stewed prunes, generally try to eat your fruit raw as cooking it reduces some of its nutritional value.

There is plenty of discussion in the media surrounding so-called 'superfoods'. These tend to be expensive, and as their benefits become hyped by PR, they appear in shops and online as the 'must-have' nutrient. Most are, indeed, high in one or more vitamins and minerals, and provided they are not packed full of preservatives and pesticides, they will be beneficial to

FIVE A DAY

The 'five a day' slogan was started by a group of Californian famers paying a nutritionist to come up with an advertising slogan and has no specific scientific validity! In reality, most of us need more – perhaps closer to 9 or 10 portions – for optimum health and longevity.

Modern farming methods compromise the vitamin content of many fruits and vegetables. For this reason, many people, including those who eat the recommended five portions of fruits and vegetables a day (a portion fits in an open hand), are not getting enough nutrients.

health if eaten in the correct quantities. Such foods include 'exotic produce' (such as goji and acai berries, agave and pomegranate); simple foods such as cacao (from which chocolate is derived) and nuts (particularly Brazil, cashew and macadamia). The 'supergreen' foods such as spirulina, chlorella and barley greens are, if organic, packed with goodness. Availability can be a problem, but adding affordable amounts of these into a selection of meals, including smoothies, juices, soups and salads, is a worthwhile thing to do.

GRAINS AND 'CARBS'
Wholegrains include:
- wheat;
- oats;
- barley;
- rye;
- corn;
- brown or wild rice;
- myriad lesser-known but equally available complex carbohydrates such as millet, buckwheat and spelt;
- potatoes and other starchy vegetables.

Protein-rich food

Meat, fowl and fish are the best sources of protein, but your body finds animal protein harder to break down, digest and absorb than vegetable proteins.

Eating red meat shortens life expectancy, so eat it only in moderation – not more than once or twice a week. Make sure it is as organic as possible and do not char it as this leads to the formation of cancer-causing substances.[20]

Beans, lentils, soya products and nuts are all high-protein foods and provide easily available amino acids, the building-blocks of protein.

Other animal products such as yoghurt and cheese fall halfway between the two types of protein above as far as ease of absorption is concerned.

Water

Without good hydration, all other nutritional advice arguably becomes pointless. No biochemical process works without water. Ignore any claims you may hear that water does not hydrate you!

Water has special properties that are still not fully explained by modern physics – in the future, we may even find that the 'unscientific' effects and successes of homoeopathy are down to the unique properties of the electrons within the water molecules.[21]

Aim to drink 250ml (approximately ½ pint) of water per 30cm (1ft) of your height daily and increase this amount to compensate for any excess sweating. Water in herbal teas counts toward this quota. Caffeine in large amounts dehydrates your body. An occasional coffee or cola will probably not have a substantial effect in an otherwise well-hydrated body receiving a balanced diet, but it certainly does not do any harm to have an additional glass of water with any such drink.[22]

Alcohol also dehydrates you by stimulating a hormone from the pituitary gland known as anti-diuretic hormone (ADH), so if you enjoy the occasional tipple, make sure you drink some water as well.

We rarely have access to natural sources of water and most people in Western societies are now drinking water that may have been recycled up to 15 times and that contains industrial or toxic waste. Many doctors are particularly concerned by the levels in our water supply of synthetic hormones (derived from the contraceptive pill), heavy metals and their breakdown products.[23]

Water *should* arrive in a pure state from the skies to fill our lakes and reservoirs, but, of course, air pollution is having a negative effect on that.

DEFICIENCIES CAUSED BY ALCOHOL AND CAFFEINE

- Alcohol removes vitamins A, B1, B2, B3, folic acid and magnesium from the body.
- Caffeine removes vitamin B1, potassium and zinc and inhibits the assimilation of other minerals and vitamins into the body.

Atomic fall-out, pesticides, insecticides and other agrochemicals are filling our soil and finding their way into our drinking water.[24]

Bottled water has its critics, but is probably safer than most tap water. However, be wary of heated plastic bottles as heating releases oestrogen-like compounds found in plastic into the water inside. For this reason, buy water in glass bottles whenever possible. Human cells are occasionally found in bottled water samples, but I dare say that these would be found in tap water, too. One arguable criticism of bottled water is its mineral content. While the body does need minerals, the absorption of these is energy-consuming, and water that actually tastes salty is probably best avoided. All bottles are now labelled, so avoid anything with a sodium content over 5mg/l.

You might also consider installing a filtration system under the kitchen sink. Built-in filters, particularly reverse-osmosis filters, certainly remove a lot of the contaminants in tap water, making it safer for you to drink.

Your specific nutritional plan

When creating your own eating plan, it is most important to follow one that you enjoy; otherwise, you simply will not stick to the programme for long.

I have already stated my belief that we need to eat by instinct as far as possible and that this should lead to a healthy diet that is suited to individual requirements. However, there are a couple of methods for testing which foods you should base a nutritional life plan around:
- Metabolic typing
- Blood group typing

Metabolic typing
Strictly speaking, this is more of a theory than a scientifically established format for designing an optimum diet. My own experience and that of several leading nutritionists from whom I have learned a lot lead me to believe that metabolic typing should be considered as a method of dietetic planning. The nutritional programme is designed around a specific questionnaire created by William Donald Kelley, a dentist, in the 1960s. According to his theory, certain foods either stimulate or relax the nervous system, or more specifically the sympathetic or parasympathetic systems. A health practitioner advises the individual of the food groups – protein, carbohydrate or other – that most suit his or her body type. Self-testing is available online although my preference is always to consult practitioners that specialize in the area. A leading book in this field is *Metabolic Typing* by William L Wolcott.[26]

COOKING UTENSILS

Avoid using pans that contribute chemicals to the water or fats used in cooking. Aluminium is the most notorious and is associated with neurological conditions, particularly Alzheimer's disease and Parkinson's. You should also avoid cooking in tin pans – stainless steel is safer – as tin, like any heavy metal, can attach to DNA and alter cell function. Non-stick surfaces on cookware are safe, provided they are intact. Check such utensils regularly and replace them immediately if you notice any wear and tear. Finally, a word of warning about washing your dishes: detergents are known to be potentially carcinogenic.[25] Therefore, ensure adequate rinsing and do not add a 'rinse' compound to your dishwasher to make utensils more shiny.

Blood-type diet

Dr Peter D'Adamo brought this hypothesis to the public in his book *Eat Right 4 Your Type*.[27] His premise is that particular poisons developed by plants to protect themselves from being eaten react with different blood group types (A, AB, B and O) and other blood-type gene activity. As the human species evolved out of central Africa, different blood types enhanced survival in different geographical areas. Hunters tended to have blood group O, agrarians or cultivators had blood group A, wanderers or nomads had blood group B as they ate a variety of different foods, and AB (a blood group that has been around only for about 1,000 years) is a hybrid of A and B. There is scientific scepticism surrounding this theory, but, in practice, many people who follow D'Adamo's guidelines in establishing a preferential diet seem to do well on it. You can be tested for your blood group at most health clinics or medical laboratories.

It is my opinion, apart from restricting calories (or at least ensuring you have the appropriate calorific intake for the amount of calories you expend), following one of the two diet concepts below is likely to enhance healthy ageing and longevity:
1. The modified Mediterranean diet
2. Food group separation programmes – less accurately, but more commonly referred to as 'food combining'

The modified Mediterranean diet

The traditional Mediterranean diet meets most of the important criteria for a healthy diet and is associated with longer survival and fewer age-related diseases.

The consumption of olive oil, vegetables and fruits providing food-state antioxidants provides a plausible explanation for this diet's apparent benefits. Very high quantities of nutrients known as flavonoids in the diet, including those found in red wine and/or black tea, are also important.[28]

The modified Mediterranean diet is based on a pyramid of nutritional content and is expanded by specific daily and weekly guidelines. Original versions of the diet are too heavy on carbohydrates as they were based on the more active life we used to lead in the fields, on the dockside and doing other physical work. My modifications, which are now adopted by many nutritionists, increase the percentage of fruits and vegetables and reduce the carbohydrate intake (see diagram on the following page).

This diet works well in rural or seaside communities where exercise is a predominant part of lifestyle. It is not suitable for those who have a mainly sedentary lifestyle or do not exercise. It also does not work if the carbohydrates (grains and cereals) are not wholegrain. In most developed societies, we are confronted by an abundance of refined carbohydrates (white bread, white pasta, white flour, white rice), and these products, devoid of important nutrients, cannot be considered to be a healthy part of an otherwise statistically effective diet programme.

Where physical activity is not part of the lifestyle and wholegrains are absent, the Mediterranean diet needs to be modified by reducing the carbohydrate intake in favour of vegetables, fruit and protein.

Use your instinct. In the earlier part of this chapter I have stressed the importance of individualization. If you are not feeling energized, if you have specific symptoms (such as headaches or dizzy spells) or if you are unable to concentrate and are losing enthusiasm for physical activity after a few days on restricted carbohydrates, then your body type is telling you to increase the carbs. *These must be wholegrain*, and you must actively avoid the refined, overly sweet, easily available foods that we tend to crave.

Food group separation. Dr William Hay devised this concept in the 1920s. He hypothesized that because the human race developed as both hunters and gatherers, it was unlikely that we would eat animal protein and carbohydrates together. He further suggested that the stomach and digestive tract were geared toward digesting one type of food at a time. Food-combining – better termed as 'food non-combining' – regimes have developed from this

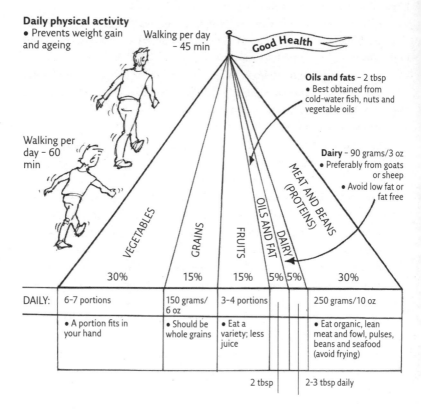

Daily physical activity
• Prevents weight gain and ageing

Walking per day – 45 min

Good Health

Oils and fats – 2 tbsp
• Best obtained from cold-water fish, nuts and vegetable oils

Walking per day – 60 min

Dairy – 90 grams/3 oz
• Preferably from goats or sheep
• Avoid low fat or fat free

	VEGETABLES	GRAINS	FRUITS	OILS AND FAT	DAIRY	MEAT AND BEANS (PROTEINS)
	30%	15%	15%	5%	5%	30%
DAILY:	6–7 portions	150 grams/6 oz	3–4 portions			250 grams/10 oz
	• A portion fits in your hand	• Should be whole grains	• Eat a variety; less juice			• Eat organic, lean meat and fowl, pulses, beans and seafood (avoid frying)
				2 tbsp		2–3 tbsp daily

Figure 2: **Dr Sharma's food pyramid**

Standard Mediterranean diet recommendations

A portion should be considered as an amount that fits into an open palm.

Daily
8 portions* *grains*
6 portions *vegetables*
3 portions *fruit*
2 portions *dairy products*
4 tablespoons *olive oil*
1–2 glasses *red wine*

Weekly
6 portions *fish*
4 portions *poultry*
4 portions *other proteins* such as eggs, pulses, nuts
3 portions *starchy vegetables* such as potatoes
1 portion *red meat*

You can enjoy treats such as *sweet desserts or chocolates* up to three times per week.

hypothesis. Protein takes longer to digest and is kept in the stomach acid for longer than other food groups. If starch is kept in the stomach for too long, the carbohydrate is reduced to glucose in greater quantities, leading to it being absorbed at a much more rapid rate once it enters the small intestine. This, in turn, causes greater insulin production, leading to a rapid drop in blood sugar levels, and causing tiredness and other biochemical changes that influence arterial health and the risk of diabetes.

The format for food group separation is really quite simple:

- Protein foods should not be eaten at the same meal or within two hours of any carbohydrate.
- Carbohydrates, likewise, should not be eaten with proteins.
- Vegetables may be mixed with either group as they contain slow-release carbohydrate and vegetable proteins.
- Separate the consumption of fruit from other foods by at least one hour as fruit has a higher immediately available sugar content than carbohydrates.

A fruit or vegetable meal encourages alkalinity, and this aspect of food separation allows the body to detox effectively. Consider having a day or two per week where you eat only fruit and vegetables – as part of an intermittent fasting regimen – and for the rest of the week aim to eat:

- one predominantly protein meal a day;
- one mainly starch meal a day;
- one meal comprising vegetarian food or fruit a day.

Choosing and using ingredients

You will find countless recipe books to help you if your own culinary skills and common sense do not allow you to formulate menus and enjoyable meals. Here are some guidelines for choosing and preparing delicious dishes.

Animal protein

- Red meat (such as beef, lamb) – should be organic, lean and cooked without burning or charring. Venison is a particularly good meat.
- Fowl (such as chicken, duck, turkey or partridge) – avoid too much skin and subcutaneous fat where chemicals and toxins settle, particularly in non-organic produce.
- White meat such as pork as well as rosé veal (red meat from a high-welfare young beef calf; avoid white veal from animals reared in veal

crates) do not present cholesterol issues if eaten once a week.

- Fish should preferably come from non-polluted waters or be farm-reared with some certification that it is organic or untreated. Fish from polluted waters, particularly that caught in rivers in or around industrial cities, may provide you with an unwanted daily dose of toxins such as oestrogens or mercury (these are also quite high in large, predatory saltwater fish such as tuna, mahi-mahi and swordfish caught close to industrial countries). However, all fish do contain beneficial proteins and essential fatty acids.
- Nuts and seeds and sprouting greens such as alfalfa, watercress and beanshoots are all high in easily digestible protein. Mycoproteins, or fungal proteins, are now readily available and used as meat substitutes in vegetarian dishes – but be wary of additives and preservatives.

Dairy produce

- Milk, cheese, yoghurt, and so on, all provide protein, but come with health warnings (discussed later in the chapter). However, I do recommend cottage cheese from an organic source and organic yoghurts, preferably from goats or sheep.
- Eggs are a particularly good source of protein and do not carry a cholesterol-raising risk. Eating one or two eggs a day provides many other nutrients such as amino acids, vitamins (particularly A, D and E) and minerals (including selenium and zinc) as well as useful and healthy fats.

Starches – grains and cereals

Many people consider themselves sensitive, intolerant or even allergic to grains. At worst, coeliac disease (an intolerance of gluten and glyadin proteins) can lead to fatigue, anaemia and illness. Adverse reactions are not always obvious, but some people report symptoms of bloating, diarrhoea, abdominal pains and constipation. Each individual has to recognize his or her own reaction and also note that the same grain from different sources may create a different response, possibly as a result of the chemicals used in its manufacture.

Those grains least likely to cause a reaction are:

- maize or corn;
- millet;
- quinoa;

- rice;
- sorghum;
- tapioca.

Other common starches include:
- barley;
- buckwheat;
- oats;
- rye;
- spelt;
- wheat.

Try to get used to the flavours and textures of wholegrains rather than refined versions as wholegrains have a higher protein content and help your body digest, absorb and utilize nutrients.

Fruit and vegetables

I am sure I do not need to provide a list of fruit and vegetables here! Fruit is generally best enjoyed raw as cooking destroys many of the nutrients. To enjoy vegetables in all their variety, you only have to look in a vegetarian recipe book. Most good cookbooks will remind you of the need to eat organic where possible, or at least to buy produce from local farmers' markets, as this might contain less pesticide than produce grown in collaboration with large supermarkets. Wash any fruit or vegetables thoroughly – a rinse in a colander is not enough to remove the adhesive chemicals used to fend off insects or make fruit shiny, and even organic produce may be cross-contaminated by chemicals. Be careful also to remove all traces of soil as this can contain harmful bacteria.

A rule of thumb is to go with 75 per cent cooked vegetables and 25 per cent raw in winter and reverse these proportions in warmer weather. It is a good idea to steam vegetables until just tender as cooking to a point of softening may denature (break down) some nutrients. However, cooking to softer levels may have the benefit of allowing more of the nutrients out of the cells and demand less activity from the digestive acids and enzymes. The rule here is: the harder the vegetable, the softer when cooked and the better (suede, parsnips and turnips, for example, are probably most nutritious when mashed). Potatoes have much of their goodness in the skins, so eat them unpeeled when possible.

SOUP RECIPES

Add ingredients of your choice (such as mushrooms and tomatoes) to the basic onion and stock mixture. Here are two of my favourites:

GREEN SOUP

1 tsp olive oil
1 red onion, finely chopped
1 sweet potato, diced
240 ml (½ pint) vegetable stock
Approximately 150 g (5oz) each of organic watercress, rocket and spinach
Black pepper

1. Heat the oil in a large saucepan. Sweat the onion and sweet potato for 4–5 minutes. Add the stock, cover with a lid and simmer for 10 minutes.
2. Add the watercress, rocket and spinach and simmer for a further 5 minutes.
3. Season with black pepper to taste. Remove from the heat, blend with a hand-held blender and serve.

YELLOW SOUP

1 tsp olive oil
1 red onion, finely chopped
1 sweet potato, diced
½ butternut squash, diced
240 ml (½ pint) vegetable stock
Black pepper

1. Heat the oil in a large saucepan. Sweat the onion and sweet potato for 4–5 minutes. Add the stock, cover with a lid and simmer for 10 minutes.
2. Season with black pepper to taste. Remove from the heat, blend with a hand-held blender and serve.

Another 75–25 per cent rule, to avoid excess fruit sugars that may encourage diabetes and feed cancer cells, is to have three portions of vegetable to every one portion of fruit daily.

Remember, vegetables should make up one of your meals per day and, of course, must not include any addition or topping that might be unhealthy, such as cheese sauce, although a small amount of nuts and seeds, olive oil and non-fat dressing is allowed.

JUICE AND SMOOTHIE RECIPE
Juice two apples or half a pineapple and then add one orange and one Conference pear (or other fruit of your choice). Pour over ice and serve.

For a smoothie, add a tablespoon of yoghurt and a banana or avocado to the juice recipe and blend.

Pulses

Pulses (such as lentils and kidney, azuki, mung, lima and butter beans) form a separate category. They are protein rich, yet predominantly starch/carbohydrate. Eaten by themselves or with vegetables, they can be considered either a protein or a starch meal.

Vitamins and minerals

Vitamins are a group of organic compounds that are present in variable and minute quantities in natural foodstuffs. As a rule, the human body is unable to manufacture (synthesize) vitamins, and as they are required for normal growth and maintenance of life, 'vital' became part of the name ('vital-amine').

Generally, we need vitamins only in small amounts. They have no calorific value, but they are essential for transforming nutrition into energy and for the regulation of most, if not all, biochemical processes in the body (see 'Vitamins and their actions' table, pp 44–5).

Are you getting enough?

You may think that you can get all the vitamins and minerals you need from a healthy, balanced diet – but according to the Journal of the American Medical Association (2002), this is not the case. It states that 30 years of research show that deficiencies raise the risk of chronic disease and that we should all be taking a multivitamin every day. There are few complete natural packages containing all we need when it comes to vitamins and

FOOD FARMING AND PROCESSING

Owing to intensive farming methods, fewer minerals are returned to the soil than taken out. We have suffered declining mineral values in farm and rangeland soils over the last 100 years, with depletion levels as follows:

North America	85 per cent
South America	76 per cent
Europe	72 per cent
Asia	76 per cent
Africa	74 per cent
Australia	55 per cent

(Source: Earth Summit Report, 1992)

Many fruits and vegetables are now grown hydroponically (that is, using mineral nutrient solutions, in water, without soil and under artificial lights) and so are likely to lack trace elements provided by nature, while others are plucked before ripening – all of which may influence the plant's nutritional value.[30]

Pesticides and insecticides further upset the natural probiotic ecobalance in the soil. Food processing methods can also dramatically reduce the mineral content of food – between 20 per cent and 80 per cent, depending upon the processing method and food involved.

Preserved food has its place, but bear in mind the simple science behind preservation. Preservatives kill life – they kill bugs that might rot food. Can you be sure that your digestive juices have destroyed all the preservatives you eat before they manage to devour your good bowel bacteria? You carry 100 trillion bacteria in your gut that are essential to life. As far as possible, avoid anything with preservatives that might destroy them.

minerals. Some foods have a more complete vitamin content than others: for example, the so-called 'superfoods' mentioned earlier and, perhaps, eggs come *close* to providing vitamins, minerals, amino acids and fats – but are by no means perfect. As with most things, it is about mix and balance. The Anarem Report by the US Department of Agriculture surveyed 21,500 people in 1982 and found *not one* of them consumed 100 per cent of the recommended daily allowance (RDA) of vitamins and minerals. According to Carol Bellamy, Executive Director of UNICEF (1995–2005): 'It is no longer a question of treating severe deficiency in individuals. It is a question of reaching out to whole populations to protect them against the devastating consequence of even moderate forms of vitamin and mineral deficiency.'

There is nothing new about this. Back in 1936, the USA Senate saw increasing problems with farming and nutrition. Here is a quote from the 74th Congress, Second Session:

> *The alarming fact is that foods (fruits, vegetables and grains), [are] now being raised on millions of acres of land that no longer contain enough of certain minerals, [and] are starving us – no matter how much of them we eat. No man of today can eat enough fruits and vegetables to supply his system with the minerals he requires for perfect health because his stomach isn't big enough to hold them.*

Another document from the US Senate Committee Report (1936) states: 'Ninety-nine per cent of the world population are mineral deficient.'

I too have concerns about the nutritional quality of food in general. We encourage everyone to eat organic food as much as possible, but even organic fruits and vegetables may lack certain minerals and vitamins as a result of overfarming and the leaching of nutrients from the soil.[29]

Supplementation

There is a vast range of supplements available on the shelves of chemists, drugstores and health food shops. However, we need to pay attention to the potential dangers of these pharmaceutical-grade vitamins and minerals. Since 2007, there has been a steady flow of studies showing the health risks involved in taking them. The European Court of Justice upheld a ban on vitamins and supplements in July 2007. This was based primarily on the research of The Cochrane Database of Systematic Reviews (2008, Issue 3) and the Journal of the American Medical Association (2007), which gave rise to the statement 'Supplements raise death rate by 5 per cent' (*The Times*, London, 29 February 2008).

However, the fact of the matter is:
- This study applies only to synthetic forms of vitamins (as produced by the pharmaceutical industry).
- It does not assess antioxidant supplements for the treatment of specific diseases (tertiary prevention).
- It does not highlight antioxidant supplements for patients with demonstrated specific needs of antioxidants.

Vitamins and their actions

Vitamins	Needed for	Good vitamin sources
Vitamin A	Membranes; eyes; skin health; arterial health; immune system	Orange and yellow vegetables and fruits (such as carrots, yams, sweet potatoes, pumpkin, suede, mangoes, papaya); dark green vegetables (such as spinach); dairy products; liver has particularly high levels.
Vitamin B1 (Thiamine)	Energy production and breakdown of carbohydrates; muscle contraction (including smooth heart and artery muscle); nervous system	Wholegrains (particularly oats and the germ of grains); most seeds (especially high levels in sesame); nuts; most meats
Vitamin B2 (Riboflavin)	Essential for the metabolism of carbohydrates, fats and proteins; mitochondrial function	Mushrooms; brewer's yeast; leafy green vegetables; wholegrain cereals; dairy produce; eggs; almonds
Vitamin B3 (Niacin)	Essential for the metabolism of carbohydrates, fats and proteins; mitochondrial function; nervous system; the control of cholesterol levels; stabilization of blood sugar; helping the body process fats	Mostly animal sources (such as beef, chicken, tuna, liver); peanut butter; barley, wheat bran, wholegrain rice
Vitamin B5 (Pantothenic acid)	Essential for the metabolism of carbohydrates, fats and fatty acids and proteins; cholesterol processing; joint health	Egg yolk; legumes; wholegrains; liver and kidney; fish; avocados, mushrooms
Vitamin B6 (Pyridoxine)	Essential for the metabolism of carbohydrates and amino acids; nervous system function; production of red blood cells; hormone receptor function	Bananas; mackerel, salmon, tuna; meat; liver; hazelnuts, walnuts; brown rice; sunflower and sesame seeds

I therefore suggest that this research has no relevance to natural sources of vitamins and minerals or antioxidants sourced from plants (such as flavonoids, anthocyanins, sulforaphanes, salvestrols/resveratrol, and so on).

The problem with most supplements is that they lose much of their effectiveness through the manufacturing process and that is if they ever saw a fruit or vegetable in the first place! Most supplements are now manufactured as byproducts of other industrial processes or are made up through chemical pathways in laboratories and factories (*see* 'The Manufacture of Vitamin C and Vitamin B1' box on page 48).

Vitamins and their actions (cont).

Vitamins	Needed for	Good vitamin sources
Vitamin B12 (Cobalamin)	Nervous system function; production of red blood cells; energy and mitochondrial production	Most meat and some seafood (particularly oily fish, mussels, oyster and crab); liver, offal; dairy produce; eggs; soya; vegans should eat fortified foods such as cereals and meat substitutes.
Folic acid	Energy production; detoxification; RNA and DNA production; foetal development	Legumes (particularly lentils, chickpeas, kidney beans); green leafy vegetables (particularly broccoli); citrus fruits; nuts; liver
Vitamin C	Skin health and collagen production; membrane health (especially gums and arteries); bones; immune system; tissue repair	Citrus fruits (particularly oranges and lemons), papaya, kiwi; green leafy vegetables; spices (such as capsicum and chilli)
Vitamin D	Calcium and phosphorus absorption for bones and teeth; blood sugar control and avoidance of diabetes; cancer prevention; immune stimulation; skin health	Dairy produce; oily fish (such as tuna, sardines, mackerel, salmon); egg yolk; sunflower seeds
Vitamin E	Arterial health; skin health; cancer prevention; immune system	Safflower, peanut and sunflower seed oil; seeds; almonds and other nuts; olive oil; green vegetables
Vitamin K	Blood clotting; cancer prevention; immune system	Dairy produce; liver; green vegetables (especially spring onions, Brussels sprouts, broccoli, asparagus, cabbage); prunes; wholegrain wheat

Nutrient depletion

Not only is our soil depleted, but modern lifestyles deplete nutrients in the body and increase the numbers of pollutants that enter out bodies. The list is extensive, but let me cite some basic examples:

- Non-steroidal anti-inflammatory drugs (ibuprofen, and so on) that are commonly used for mild ailments such as headaches remove folic acid and iron from the body.
- Alcohol removes vitamins A, B1, B2, B3, folic acid and magnesium.
- Caffeine removes vitamin B1, potassium and zinc, and inhibits the assimilation of other minerals and vitamins.
- Oral contraceptives can lead to deficiency in vitamins C, B2, B6, B12

VITAMINS – DOSAGE AND TOXICITY

Vitamin	Maximum recommended dosage before possible toxicity	Toxic signs and symptoms
Vitamin A	Infants 10,000iu Adults 50,000iu	Appetite loss, headache, blurred vision, unusually dry or cracked skin, loss of hair, muscular stiffness and pain
Vitamin B group (see individual compounds below)		
Thiamin (B1)	100mg	No toxic effects
Riboflavin (B2)	25mg	No toxic effects
Niacin (B3) or Niacinamide	100mg	Flushing, headaches, cramps, nausea, vomiting, burning or itching skin
Pantothenic acid (vitamin B5)	Not tested so follow the instructions given on label or by practitioner.	Occasional diarrhoea
Pyridoxine (B6)	200mg	Numbness, tingling and other sensory nerve effects
Biotin (B7)	30mcg	No toxic effects reported
Folic acid (B9)	15mg	Abdominal distension, appetite loss, nausea, vivid dreams
Vitamin B12	Oral dosage in supplements should be around 2.5mcg, but oral and nasal supplementation vary, so read the label.	No toxic effects
Beta-carotene – the inactive precursor to Vitamin A found in nature	60mg	No toxic effects recorded up to 250mg per day
Vitamin C	10g per day, except under supervision	Nausea, diarrhoea
Vitamin D	Minimally 1,000iu daily and discuss with practitioner up to 5,000iu daily.	Excess of 10,000iu per day: nausea, vomiting, appetite loss, diarrhoea, headache, excessive urination, constipation, pallor
Vitamin E	800iu	Weakness and fatigue; may worsen hypertension
Vitamin K	100mcg	No toxic effects if taken orally

and vitamin E. Folic acid, magnesium and zinc are also depleted when taking the Pill.
- Smoking causes depletion of vitamins B1, C and folic acid.
- Antibiotics interfere with bowel flora, which reduces digestive capacity and can interfere with absorption of all and any nutrients.
- Toxic elements such as aluminium and mercury interfere with the absorption of the minerals calcium, iron and selenium and also vitamin C, among others.

In this book, I mention how specific drugs remove minerals and vitamins from the body. Various mechanisms make this happen, so I strongly recommend that you review what nutrients you should take if you are placed on any medication at all.

To find out what to take, I recommend reading *Drug Muggers* by Suzy Cohen, a licensed pharmacist in the USA.[31]

Intravenous (IV) nutrient therapy

Scientific literature has highlighted the benefits of IV nutrient therapy for over 20 years. Throughout the 1950s, John Myers MD, a physician from Baltimore, Maryland, USA, one of the therapy's best-known pioneers, developed the 'Myers' Cocktail', which mostly contains vitamins C and B-complex, magnesium and calcium, but doctors add in other nutrients based on the patient's case history and the results of investigations.

The use of IV nutrient therapy supplementation does not have to be related to specific illness and can be used for the following:
- fatigue and unexplained tiredness
- helping achieve optimum performance both mentally and physically

The Myer's Cocktail has been found to be effective against:
- acute asthma attacks;
- migraine;
- fatigue;
- fibromyalgia;
- acute muscle spasm;
- upper respiratory tract infections;
- chronic sinusitis;
- seasonal allergic rhinitis;
- cardiovascular disease.[32]

THE MANUFACTURE OF VITAMIN C AND VITAMIN B1

Vitamin C

World production of synthesized vitamin C is currently estimated at approximately 110,000 tonnes annually. Main producers have been BASF/DSM, Merck and the China Pharmaceutical Group Ltd.

The Reichstein process was developed in the early 1930s and uses chemical processing: glucose > sorbitol + fermentation > sorbose > diacetone-sorbose > keto-gulonic acid > keto-gulonic acid methylester > ascorbic acid.

An improved method using a two-step fermentation process was developed in China in the 1960s: glucose > sorbitol + fermentation > sorbose + fermentation > keto-gluconic acid > ascorbic acid.

Both processes use acetone – a compound that is highly toxic to humans.

Vitamin B1

Coal tar + hydrochloric acid + fermentation + chemical treatment, then heated and cooled > 'natural' Vitamin B1.

The term 'natural' can be used – even though it never saw the sun, soil or any other natural product – as it is identical to the vitamin B1 found in plants, except that there are no co-factors. (Many nutrients need co-factors, which occur in plant-derived vitamins in order to function properly at a cellular level. Vitamin C has eight co-factors: ascorbinogen, bioflavonoids, rutin, tyrosinase, Factor J, Factor K, Factor P and ascorbic acid.)

I always recommend supplements that are either in natural food state or manufactured to encompass co-factors such as citrates, which is how many minerals are presented at a cellular level after digestion.

Such products are extracts from natural foods or almost identical to what the body would recognize as natural. This means that the body absorbs them more efficiently and is better able to process and benefit from the vitamins and minerals they contain.

Furthermore, IV nutrient therapy using vitamin C is cited by the Linus Pauling Institute and other authorities as being effective in cancer treatment.

A growing number of centres use a technique known as phospholipid exchange (PLX) – the use of intravenous essential fatty acids. The technique may be used for neurological damage and disease (such as motor neurone disease, multiple sclerosis, Parkinson's disease and the effects of stroke). It is also being considered in the treatment of dementia and in cases where cell damage might have occurred (such as in the inner lining of arteries in arteriosclerosis – blocked arteries).

Therapeutic diets

When a health issue requires attention, the saying accredited to Hippocrates, the father of medicine, is well worth repeating: 'Let food be thy medicine and medicine be thy food.'

I would draw your attention to the following diets for specific health-related issues. I humbly mention that you can find summaries of the following in my book *The Element Family Encyclopedia of Health*; the Internet is also a good source of information.[33]

Anti-candida/yeast diet

This diet is for those with yeast overgrowth in the bowel. Such anti-fermentation diets are based on removing the sugars that survive the process of the yeast eating sugar in fermentation and cause alcohol release into the system. Anti-yeast diets contain high roughage and prebiotics to encourage normal bowel flora growth.

The Budwig, Gerson or Plaskett Therapy diets

These are designed to support anti-cancer therapy. They all revolve around a theme of strict vegetarianism, high doses of specific nutrients and detoxification.

Detox diets

Many authors and practitioners use the term 'detox diet' when referring to the intake of less-contaminated or non-contaminated foods that have high levels of nutrients and roughage and are easy to digest. These diets encourage us to drink 3 litres (6–7 pints) or more of water a day – twice as much as is generally recommended – thereby reducing the amount of toxins in the body and giving a rest to the organs responsible for their breakdown and removal.

Hypoglycaemia diets

These control sugar levels by avoiding high glycaemic index foods (that is, foods that discharge sugar rapidly into the bowel and bloodstream). Complex carbohydrates are encouraged in small amounts among plenty of vegetables and proteins.

Macrobiotic diets

These are popular for controlling blood pressure, cholesterol levels and oestrogen balance. They focus on simple, organically grown vegetables, lightly cooked and steamed foods, low-carbohydrate foods and very little animal produce.

The Ornish diet

Developed by Dean Ornish, a cardiologist from San Francisco, this is a strictly vegetarian diet that provides fewer than 2,000 calories a day – mostly from carbohydrates and fewer than 10 per cent from fat. It is recommended for those with cardiovascular disease, particularly angina (heart pain), raised cholesterol and arterial occlusion.

The Pritikin diet

Named after Nathan Pritikin, this is a vegetarian, complex-carbohydrate and high-fibre diet that is specifically low in cholesterol and fat. It is prescribed in association with 45 minutes of daily walking and benefits patients with cardiovascular problems and non-insulin-dependent diabetes, provided that it is initiated early on in the diagnosis.

Vegan diet

This excludes all products of animal origin and requires a good knowledge of how to obtain adequate amounts of protein from vegetable sources. Many vitamins such as vitamin B12 are found predominantly in animal products and deficiencies are common in poorly informed vegans. The choice of becoming an educated vegan is up to the individual, but I think that this diet is more suited to people who have a smaller bone and muscle structure (such as Asians).

Acid-alkaline diet

Patients being treated for cancer may benefit from their body tissues being alkaline for as much of the time as possible and are therefore advised to focus on alkaline-forming foods in this diet. Designing specific diets around

ACID AND ALKALINE LEVELS IN THE BODY

- The body starts to fail if the bloodstream is not maintained at a steady pH (the measurement of acid/alkaline levels) of 7.35–7.45. Most enzyme and metabolic systems do not function outside of this narrow range, and the kidneys will be damaged as they try to control any imbalance.
- A food is not judged to be alkaline by its own pH but by the effect that it has on the body.
- A common misconception is that milk is alkaline. If it is unpasteurized, it has a neutral quality, but generally the alkalinity in the milk itself causes the stomach to produce more acid and therefore makes the system acidic.
- Acid production is dependent upon how much we eat: the less we fill ourselves, the less acidic we are.
- Not mixing foods – as in the Hay diet or other 'non-food-combining' disciplines – generally moves food out of the stomach more quickly, thereby reducing acid production and creating a tendency toward alkalinity.

Acid and Alkaline Foods

Acid-forming foods	Alkaline-forming foods
Animal protein	Most vegetables
Most grains	Most fruits
Most nuts	Salty fish
Plant seeds	Soya
Sugar	Almonds
Honey	Brazil nuts
Coffee	Millet and buckwheat
Dairy products	
Most berries and tomatoes	

the foods in the list above is best done with a specialist. There is actually no health benefit from being too acidic, and although acid foods carry nutrients (particularly certain essential amino acids) not found in abundance in alkaline foods, you could argue that avoiding acid foods generally is a good thing.

What's in your shopping basket?

There are a number of foodstuffs that many of us consume on a regular basis. Below are some important facts about what you may be putting into your body that may make you decide to change some of your lifestyle and eating habits.

Probiotics for health and longevity

Acidophilus, probifidus and *bifidobacteria* and some *E. coli* species encourage and promote the growth of the human bowel flora, in particular, *escherichia coli*. However, there are some bad *E. coli*, and if an infection is known to have been caused by one of these, probotics should not be taken until the infection has cleared.

Although probiotics are commonly found in yoghurt, for therapeutic effect you would need to consume about 1 litre (1¾ pints) of yoghurt a day. A more sensible way to take probiotics is as a supplement in capsule or powder form. Choose a brand that uses acid-resistant capsules or mixes the formula with an alkalining agent. Probiotics are best taken before bedtime when stomach acid and digestive enzyme production is likely to be reduced. *Acidophilus* and other beneficial flora are quite delicate. If probiotics do not get past the acid in a healthy stomach, they will die off before offering their health benefits.

Alcohol

Fun and with some potentially good implications for health, alcohol is nonetheless not nutritious and is harmful when taken in excess. It may relax the nervous system and muscles, and there is an association with reduction in arterial and heart disease. However, it is probably not the alcohol itself that is protective but the nutrients that it contains, such as resveratrol which exists in grape skin.

It is hard to define a safe level of alcohol consumption, but, as a rule of thumb, if you do not feel the effects psychologically, then the body is probably dealing with the amount you have drunk. Statistics suggest that up to 14 units a week for a woman and 21 for a man may actually have health benefits – or at least no harmful effects. However, there is some controversy here. No alcohol is probably better in general for the liver, gut and detoxification, but a little of the right stuff (red wine particularly) as part of a healthy diet may offer benefits to the heart and arteries and reduce the effects of stress hormones.

Such crude analysis cannot take into account personal variation and should be considered only a rough guide. Learn to recognize your own tolerance levels and have four or five days a week without alcohol as often as possible. If you exceed your tolerance level, note that it takes the liver approximately two days to recover from being tipsy or drunk. Try to give the liver that amount of time between alcohol binges and never drink to a point where your coordination is affected – a sure sign of neurological toxicity.

Free radicals and antioxidants

Free radicals are often positively charged particles, lacking an electron, that are known to affect many metabolic pathways, damage cell walls and arterial lining. They also damage the DNA genetic memory and cell organization within the cells. This can trigger potentially cancerous change.

Antioxidants donate an electron to free radicals, thereby neutralizing them and rendering them no longer harmful.

Free radicals are found in animal products, fried foods and any fat exposed to heat, oxygen and light. Barbecued and smoked products are particularly full of free radicals. Anything that produces smoke such as tobacco and engine fuel provides free radicals.

The common antioxidants are vitamins A, C and E, selenium, coenzyme Q10 and, to a lesser extent, magnesium and zinc. There are many other compounds such as the hormone melatonin and the plant extract astaxanthin. Lots of different plant extracts contain some or all of these antioxidants.

Artificial sweeteners

As a general rule, I advocate avoiding artificial sweeteners. This is because:
• artificial sweeteners have been linked with cancer.

HEALTHY BOWEL FLORA

Bowel flora break down indigestible foods and so are partly responsible for the release of nutrients from cells. They also provide vitamins and trace elements as byproducts of their own metabolism: for example, the body is dependent upon bowel bacteria for the production of vitamin B12.

Bifidobacteria attach to the bowel wall providing a barrier and stimulating the production of a vital first-line defence, secretory immunoglobulin A (sIgA). This is thought to help protect us from allergies and all their associated conditions (such as arthritis) and chronic conditions (such as cancer) as we age.

- they can have mild effects on the nervous system and may cause a hangover effect.
- large amounts of the common sweetener aspartame can cause seizures as well as rashes and itching.
- aspartame is over a thousand times sweeter than sugar and may trigger insulin production via a reflex caused by recognition of sweetness by the taste buds.

Caffeine

Found in abundance in coffee, tea, many 'soft' drinks, chocolate and other cocoa products as well as a myriad of over-the-counter drugs used for anything from a common cold to stomach upsets, caffeine is a powerful nervous-system stimulant.

Initially, caffeine gives a 'buzz' by increasing energy, improving concentration and creating a sense of euphoria, acting like an adrenaline compound and raising blood sugar levels, giving a short-term supply of available energy.

Decaffeinated coffee is rarely completely free of caffeine. Moreover, the chemicals used to remove the caffeine may themselves be stimulating and are potentially carcinogenic (cancer-causing). It is also worth remembering that most coffee-making countries treat their coffee plants with pesticides and insecticides, which will also enter your system.

Milk

I do not think that milk is good for us. I do not recommend that it is fed to infants or children, I doubt that it has value for adults, and I suspect that

COFFEE CONSUMPTION – THE HIGHS AND LOWS

- Caffeine may be associated with miscarriage, diabetes and hypertension.
- Coffee causes certain types of cancer. There is a clear association between caffeine and cancer of the pancreas and bladder.
- In one study, 1–2 cups of coffee drunk daily by post-menopausal women reduced breast cancer. [34]
- Coffee has been found to reduce prostate cancer in men if drunk at a level of 1–2 cups per day. [35]
- Coffee aggravates dementia in women. [36]

CALCIUM

Calcium is found throughout the body, either as a structural or biochemical necessity. Calcium is the main component of teeth and bones and enables muscles to contract. It is very difficult to become calcium deficient through poor diet because calcium is found in all kinds of foods that we eat. However, menopause and vitamin-D deficiency are known to interfere with normal calcium deposition and storage. Calcium-rich foods include sesame seeds, kelp, almonds, meat, poultry, fish (especially salmon) and most deep-green leafy vegetables.

it is dangerous to us all as we age. The proteins casein, lactalbumin and lactoglobulin found in milk are known to cause allergies and are not easily broken down by the human gut. If a protein is not well broken down, it can be absorbed in its entirety and the body will consider it to be a potential virus or bacteria and produce an antibody response. If the partially broken-down protein resembles the proteins within our body, then this immune system response may well attack our own cells. This is known as 'molecular mimicry'.

Milk sugar, lactose, is not well tolerated by many races. 90 per cent of Filipinos, 50 per cent of Indians and approximately 8 per cent of the populations in the UK and USA do not have the necessary enzyme to break down lactose. This makes the sugar, by ranging degrees, useless as an energy source and encourages fluids to stay in the bowel, leading to dehydration.

Homogenization, a process used to sterilize milk to ensure that it is safe to drink leads to the production of a chemical called xanthine oxidase in the body, which destroys a compound in the blood called plasmogen. This, in turn, leads to the loss of a protective factor in the arterial walls, which then encourages atheroma (the clogging up of arteries by calcium, special defence cells called platelets and fatty deposits, including cholesterol).

Milk is considered to be a major source of calcium – indeed, the calcium content of milk is very high and well absorbed into the bloodstream. The problem is that such large amounts stimulate bone-forming cells (osteoblasts) to work harder and so they wear out sooner. According to Riggs *et al* (1987), there is no evidence that high-calcium diets enhance bone health.[37]

In fact, the opposite may be true: according to author Russell Eaton, long-term epidemiological studies show that countries where people drink more milk have higher rates of osteoporosis (thinning of the bones).[38]

Health campaigner Dr Justine Butler notes that milk has been related to myriad symptoms and conditions, including problems associated with mucus (such as respiratory infections, ear, nose and throat problems, sinus congestion and asthma), colitis, diabetes, acne and eczema, arthritis, heartburn, ulcers and even cancer.[39]

Milk raises Insulin growth factor IGF-1 and contains oestrogen-like hormones and prolactin, any of which can cause cellular growth in the breast. There are grounds to believe that milk may promote cancer in the colon, prostate and bladder as well as breast cancer.[40]

NUT MILK

You can prepare 'milk' from a variety of nuts and seeds (such as almonds, cashews, hazelnuts, sesame, pumpkin or sunflower seeds) by following these simple instructions:

1. Soak the nut or seed mixture overnight in enough water to cover by at least 1 cm (½ in).
2. The next morning, pour the soaked nuts or seeds and water into a blender and pulverize. (Discard the overnight water that the nuts or seeds have been in as the taste is unpleasant.) If the solution is too thick, add more fresh water.
3. If the flavour is not to your taste, add a spoonful of honey or some raisins to the blender and mix.

Cholesterol-containing and cholesterol-forming foods

Cholesterol is not the only nor arguably the main cause of arterial and cardiovascular disease. Certain facts highlight this: 50 per cent of heart attacks occur in people who do not have raised cholesterol; 80 per cent of arterial disease or coronary heart disease (CHD) occurs in those with normal cholesterol.

Cholesterol levels are not predominantly dependent upon cholesterol-containing foods, but, more importantly, they rise with high carbohydrate intake. Good carbs such as wholegrain foods are not an issue: it is the refined sugars and foods such as white bread, white pasta and the hidden sugars in things like alcohol that tend to cause problems.

Conversion of carbohydrates to cholesterol

There are many sizes of cholesterol – cholesterol is mainly an issue if it is of small particulate size, which tends to be 'sticky' and attaches to arterial walls if these are damaged or inflamed by sugars and inflammatory compounds

EGGS

Although egg yolks have a high cholesterol content, eggs actually promote a rise in HDL. In any case, during digestion in the acid environment of the stomach cholesterol binds with lecithin (found in the egg white), with the result that the cholesterol is not easily absorbed.

in the bloodstream. LDL and HDL are not different types of cholesterol, but refer to the complex molecules that transport it around the bloodstream.

I strongly recommend reading Justin Smith's *$29 Billion Reasons to Lie About Cholesterol* or visit the associated website.[41] He explains all you need to know about cholesterol, including the fact that there is little evidence to support the benefits of statins (cholesterol-lowering drugs) for women and men between the ages of 40 and 60 – other than those with cardiovascular disease – that is not markedly skewed by the pharmaceutical companies.

Cholesterol is required for the cell membranes of nearly all the tissues in the body and is also required for the production of adrenal hormones, which govern our stress and water balance, for coating the nerves to allow correct conduction and for all the sex hormones.

Raised cholesterol by itself does not suggest danger because the amount of protective HDL is the relevant factor. The ratio of HDL to total cholesterol indicated as a percentage is usually a predictive marker of whether there is an issue – above 20 per cent is a good sign.

Cholesterol needs only to be considered dangerous when other factors are considered, such as deficiencies in certain vitamins, minerals and amino acids, and where inflammation is prominent.

Along with refined carbohydrates, you might consider reducing the following foods, not only because of their cholesterol content, but mainly because they can form free radicals, which are probably much more likely to cause arteriosclerosis, heart attacks and strokes.

Foods containing high cholesterol include:
- red meats;
- offal – especially kidney and liver;
- cheese;
- dairy produce (except specially prepared low-fat produce);
- prawns and shrimps;
- pork.

Fats

Fats are good for you – in fact, they are essential for your well-being. Fats are made up of fatty acids, which are principally carbon, hydrogen and oxygen molecules joined together in a variety of combinations. Fats have strong and weak bonds and fall into the following categories.

SATURATED, UNSATURATED and POLYUNSATURATED FATS

Saturated fats are carbon molecules joined by a single connection or bond that is difficult to break. Saturated fats are harder to utilize for the body and have been considered unhealthy fats thought to settle into blood vessels and organs; they are the main form to build up fat tissue. However, many authorities are now suggesting we have been misled about the potential dangers of small and even moderate amounts of saturated fat. These have important functions, which include being stable, and are not easily broken down when used to pad bony surfaces such as the palms, soles and the bones we sit on. Saturated fats also cushion vital organs such as the heart, kidneys and intestines. There are more saturated fats in animal proteins than in vegetable fats. Animal fats are typically solid at room temperature.

The double bonds of unsaturated fats are individually weaker than single bonds and are more easily broken down. There may be one or more of these double bonds in a fat molecule. If there are many, the fat is known as 'polyunsaturated'. Unsaturated fats (such as vegetable oil) are generally liquid at room temperature unless they have been hydrogenated.

We derive energy from saturated fat, which is our body fat store. The saturated fats stearic acid and palmitic acid are the preferred source of energy for the heart.

Coconut oil and palm kernel oil are both abundant sources of medium-chain fatty acids, particularly lauric acid, which is a fast energy source and used in structure and function.

Cooking at high temperatures damages fats and oils, making them dangerous. This is especially the case with unsaturated and polyunsaturated fats, which are the most unstable. Cooking oxidizes and forms free radicals that are highly damaging to cells. Free-radical damage from polyunsaturated fats is now considered to be the main contributor to atherosclerosis and therefore heart disease. So the polyunsaturated vegetable oils that have been touted as healthy, including soybean oil, safflower oil and corn oil, are not if used in cooking. Furthermore, these are what we get in the manufacturing of processed foods.

Use butter and coconut oil to cook with. These contain fats that are stable

MORE FACTS ON FAT

'Good fats' – these are the sort we can utilize. They are associated with fat-soluble vitamins, particularly vitamins A, D, E and K.

Essential fatty acids (EFAs) – these are fats that humans cannot synthesize and must therefore obtain through their diet. They are found in meats, oily fish, green vegetables, nuts and seeds, and some fruits.

Triglycerides (TGs) – these are three fatty acids joined together and vary in their length and carbon-to-hydrogen ratio. Dietary fat is mostly composed of triglycerides. They are found in both animal fats and vegetables. Cooking fats are high in triglycerides, as are butter and vegetable spreads. They are not good to have in too high a level in the bloodstream.

Phospholipids and glycolipids – these are triglycerides that contain phosphorus and other molecules. They are important constituents of biological membranes, blood plasma and most cell walls. Nervous tissue is made up of a type of phospholipid known as sphingomyelin and cannot function without it.

Cholesterol and its derivatives – cholesterol is the starting point for hormones of the adrenal glands and sex glands, vitamin D and the bile acids, all of which are essential to life.

Omega fats – these are best in a ratio of 4:1 Omega-6 – Omega-3 oils. They include docosahexaenoic acid (DHA) and eicosapentaenoic acid (EPA). In a Western diet, we consume too many Omega-6 oils without enough Omega-3 oils.

Hydrogenated fat – this has had additional hydrogen ions added to it, usually by being exposed to heat, oxygen or light. This process alters the natural structure of the fat and 'improves' its shelf-life or consistency (such as in the semisolid vegetable oils for spreading or baking). An otherwise 'good-for-you' polyunsaturated fat may become harmful through this type of food processing.

Trans-fatty acids – these are forms of EFAs that have been altered by exposure to heat and oxygen during processing. Trans-fatty acids cannot be used by the body and interfere with the biochemistry of one of the body's protective compounds known as prostaglandin E1. Check the labels on processed food and avoid these where possible.

and are highly nutritious as they carry the fat-soluble vitamins A, D and K2 – important to boost the immunity and for direct antimicrobial effects.

Saturated fat makes up more than half of most cell membranes, is essential to bone formation, helps lung elasticity and barrier protection and is needed by bowel flora for their growth.

The body must have fats to survive, so although you should keep fat in your diet to a minimum, do not avoid it totally: fat is only likely to be a problem if it exceeds more than 15 per cent of your dietary intake. Each type of fat has its place and function in human health, but be careful to include each type in appropriate amounts to avoid the risk of disease. It is best to include more polyunsaturated and unsaturated fat and less saturated fat in your diet. Use 'virgin' oils as much as possible (this refers to the process of a single, simple pressing of the olive, which reduces the risk of breaking down the oil excessively). 'Cold-pressed' is a marketing term, but it is important that oils are not heated as this too breaks down the oil structure. 'Extra' and 'fine' refer to the taste and are not related to health benefits.

Food additives

We have no evolutionary capabilities to deal with the many artificial compounds used to enhance the appearance, flavour and shelf life of pre-prepared foods. We are finding increasing levels of additives as well as preservatives, insecticides, pesticides, household chemicals and airborne pollutants stuck to our cell membranes and DNA. Wherever possible, do not eat them!

Fruit juice

Fruits are nature's abundant suppliers of vitamins. Fruit juice, freshly extracted and immediately drunk, is one of the best forms of nutrition – it contains a variety of vitamins, nutrients, minerals and even proteins. In juiced form, these are easily digested and transferred across the bowel membrane. Drinking 120 ml (4fl oz) of freshly pressed organic apple juice twice daily may help slow down the development or even delay the onset of Alzheimer's Disease.[42]

Juices that are processed and packaged are possibly harmful. Without many exceptions they have added sugar. Even those that claim 'no added sugar' may have up to 6 teaspoonfuls of refined glucose added on the basis that the manufacturing process removes sugar that would otherwise be present. Adding sugar back in not always as natural fructose claims to be replacing the fruits' own stores, but usually with refined, unhealty sugars.

Many vitamins are altered through the juice-manufacturing process. The addition of artificial vitamins at a later stage is the food industry's answer, but our bodies do not absorb these as well because processing causes an imbalance in the proportion of co-factors needed to help absorption.

Mass-produced juices generally contain some form of preservative. The fruits themselves are mass-produced, often hydroponically, and are usually encouraged to grow larger by means of chemicals. The latter are also added to remove the unpleasant flavour of the skin and pips (seeds) that are all pulverized in the juice-making process. One of these chemicals is formaldehyde, a chemical used for preserving bodies in the anatomy lab!

Genetically modified (GM) food

Over the last three decades, the enormously powerful food industry and its political lobbyists have been researching, producing and promoting genetically altered food. Scientists have methods of altering the genes in the nucleus of the cells of food crops. This has the advantage of faster growth, yeast and fungus resistance and even insect repellence.

Lauded as the first step toward eliminating worldwide food shortage (an untruth as there is plenty of food – it is just not distributed as it should be), in principle the technique is a good idea. The problem lies in the inability of the scientific world to assure us that the techniques (chemicals and radiation) used to alter the food genes will not carry on their effect within the human body. There is also the fear that the genetically altered genes may, in some way, incorporate themselves into our own cells and alter their function.

For now, where possible, avoid genetically modified foods.

Gluten and gliadin (grain proteins)

These two proteins are found predominantly in wheat, but also in varying amounts in other grains. They are accepted as the main causes of coeliac disease (*see* page 60) as well as allergic, intolerant or inflammatory responses in the human body. These problems often result from introducing wheat too early in an infant's life or because a large quantity of grain is eaten.

If you have any sense of intolerance or a recognized coeliac disease, you should avoid foods containing these proteins and consider consulting a nutritionist who will help you maintain a varied diet and avoid deficiencies.

Nitrates and other additives and preservatives

Avoid these if at all possible. It seems that the hundreds of food preservatives, colourings and flavourings are poorly tested for safety and some are downright dangerous. I am particularly worried by the fact that some countries still allow certain E numbers that have been banned in other parts of the world.[43]

Of all additives and preservatives, the most common ones found in our food are nitrates. These are used to colour and preserve foods, especially meats. It has been found that these destabilize the body's oxygen supply, with potentially fatal results if eaten in sufficient quantities.[44]

Blackouts are uncommon, but can occur because of a drop in blood pressure owing to nitrate ingestion. Beware and avoid any foods containing nitrates E249–252.

Salt

The sodium component in salt controls a multitude of biochemical processes in the body, including the bloodstream and tissue fluidity, blood pressure, hydration and permeability of cells. Salt is essential.

There is an abundance of salt in many processed foods, and there lies the danger in our shopping bags. Avoid adding extra salt to cooking or at the table. It may take up to two weeks to get used to, but a diet with no added salt will soon satisfy your taste buds.

Soya

There is a lot of discussion around soya, the bean originally grown in the East. Soya contains enzyme inhibitors, phytoestrogens and other chemicals, all or any of which may act as anti-cancer and anti-atheroma compounds.

Phytoestrogens help in the production of oestradiol, one of the active forms of oestrogen, and occupy oestrogenic receptor sites, providing potentially beneficial effects. It is suggested that soya's natural oestrogens, genistein and daidzein, combine with oestrogen receptors in the body and prevent oestrogen from affecting the growth rate of particular

SALT GENES

As we evolved from the plains of central Africa to the coastal areas, we came across abundant salt from fish and sea produce. Up in the mountains and plains, where less salt was readily available, we had genes that absorbed and stored salt. By the sea, that was not a good thing, so the genes died out due to natural selection. Now some of us have salt-storing genes and others do not. For some people, salt is a danger, but for others less so.

GM SOYA

Soya has been the main vegetable crop to be experimented on using gene-altering or genetic-tampering techniques. Ensure that any products containing soya come from a natural, organic source and do not contain genetically modified substances.

oestrogen-sensitive cancer cells. A paradox occurs because we use soya for its oestrogen-like effect in menopause, but use it as an oestrogen blocker to help prevent cancer. Until clearer evidence is available, enjoy soya as a food, but do not consume it in excessive quantities, particularly if you are at risk of oestrogen-sensitive cancer (breast or prostate). Soya is also associated with hypothyroidism, so avoid eating large amounts if there is any suggestion of low thyroxine levels.

Sugar

All carbohydrates break down into sugar. In its natural form as glucose or fructose (fruit sugar), sugar is an excellent source of energy.

In nature, sugar is always found in association with a variety of other nutrients: it is bound up with larger molecules so that the body is taking in useful building blocks as well and does not absorb it too quickly.

Refined sugar, on the other hand, such as in cakes, has been separated from other nutrients. The body absorbs it rapidly, creating a fast insulin response, which, in turn, leads to dramatic low blood sugar levels, potentially causing hypoglycaemia symptoms. This can cause symptoms of fatigue, depression, irritability, muscle weakness, shakiness, headaches and even asthma. Diabetes is encouraged, arteriosclerosis (hardening of the arteries as a result of atheroma) is propagated and blood pressure is elevated.

Sugar requires vitamins and minerals to be utilized; high doses of refined sugar keep the metabolism going, but, without a nutrient supply, deficiencies will arise.

Worst of all, refined sugar makes us fat and increases our cholesterol levels – even more so than eating cholesterol-containing foods.

Investigations and tests

The better investigations and tests give broad indications of deficiencies both at cellular level as well as in the bloodstream. This is important, as a 'healthy

SENSITIVITY, ALLERGY AND INTOLERANCE

Sensitivity occurs when white blood cells produce inflammatory or other compounds that arm or prepare the immune system for activity.

Allergy is a blood response forming immunoglobulins (Igs) to a foreign substance that may be a food.

Intolerance is less well defined by the orthodox world, but holistically would be considered to be a substance to which the body responds with symptoms such as nausea or vomiting, headaches, abdominal pains, skin rash, diarrhoea or frequent urination.

It may be an 'energetic confrontation'. All cells in the body resonate at a particular frequency, and any foreign molecule whose electrons resonate in such a way as to inhibit or block the body's natural resonance is capable of creating an intolerance reaction.

Allergies and intolerances are not about the causative agent, but are reflections of our immune system's reaction, which is affected by lifestyle and habits.

meal' eaten in the hours before a nutritional study can skew the results if only blood levels are reviewed.

Food sensitivity, intolerance and allergy tests are performed using a number of techniques:

Antigen leukocyte cellular antibody test (ALCAT)
This was developed in the USA and is my preferred food sensitivity test. It looks at white-blood-cell responses to foods, herbs and common drugs.

Patch testing or skin-prick testing
These are the preferred food-allergy testing methods in the UK and USA. Of the available blood tests, those looking for IgE antibodies – known as immunoglobulins and responsible for a potentially lethal allergic reaction (anaphylaxis) – are the main and conventionally accepted method of registering allergic responses that lead to serious reactions (such as asthma, hives and anaphylaxis).

Applied kinesiology (muscle testing) and bioresonance computers and techniques
These test for intolerance, not allergy, and have less scientific credibility. Nevertheless, they seem to work well for many people.

Hair analysis
Hair samples are often tested in the alternative world by the unproven techniques of a swinging pendulum or radionics. They only show levels of compounds that have been eliminated and therefore suggest an intolerance within the system.

Chapter 3

Exercise

We are constantly told that we should exercise, and there is no doubt that this is wise advice. From the time humans evolved from apes until the Industrial Revolution in the 19th century, the majority of us walked or ran approximately 30 km (19 miles) per day and generally lifted over seven tonnes in weight during the week. People built their own shelters, farmed land and controlled animals. They worked on or by the sea and transported food and goods over great distances. They survived or earned a living by hunting animals or by foraging, which required moving from one area to another looking for fruits and vegetables. The sedentary few were supported mostly by the manual labour of others.

With the advent of the Industrial Revolution came machines and, later, computers, which have led to fewer of us burning off calories and getting rid of stress chemicals through physical activity. Furthermore, we have a ready supply of calories in the food that lines our cupboards and fridges, and convenience and fast food is generally easily available to those who live or work in an urban environment.

As you read this book, you will see how exercise influences every part of the body and its systems, and, indeed, any other book or article you might read on longevity will talk about a decrease in 'all-cause mortality' for those who exercise – in other words, exercise reduces the likelihood of all causes of death, even accidental.

You even might consider paying no attention to any other factor other than exercise when thinking about longevity.

Let me highlight how important exercise is simply by listing the regions in the body affected by it:
- Libido (sex drive)
- The immune system's fight against infections and cancer
- Bones

GLOSSARY OF TERMS

Glycogen, a compound manufactured by the body, allows the body to store glucose.

Mitochondria are small chemical factories within most cells, converting oxygen and sugars into energy in the form of electrons. They are abundant in muscles, and the more we exercise, the more mitochondria we make and the more active they become. This applies not only to muscles that are in use – through hormones and electrical information, mitochondria are transmitted throughout the body. *Myoglobin* is a protein found in muscle and has oxygen bound to it, providing an extra reserve of oxygen so that the muscle can maintain a high level of activity for a longer period of time.

- Joints and muscles
- The digestive system
- The cardiovascular system, arteries and heart
- The nervous system

Muscles

In order to fully appreciate the importance of exercise, it is useful to have some understanding of the muscles in the human body.

There are three types: skeletal (voluntary), smooth and cardiac (both involuntary).

Skeletal muscle

Skeletal muscle is so called because this muscle type is attached to bones. Its tissue can be made to contract or relax voluntarily through conscious control. Not all skeletal muscle tissue behaves in the same way: different types contract at different speeds and start to get tired at different times.

Skeletal muscle is divided into three types:

Type I fibres
The body uses this type of skeletal muscle to maintain posture (sitting, standing) and slow actions such as strolling. Type I fibres, also called 'slow-twitch fibres', contain large amounts of *myoglobin* and *mitochondria* (*see*

'Glossary of terms' box on page 67) and have an ample blood supply from many tiny blood capillaries. Type I fibres contract more slowly than other fibres and are resistant to fatigue, but are relatively weak. They have a high capacity to generate energy (using ATP, the 'energy molecule').

There are also other type 1-like intermediate fibres that come into play before we use the 'fast-twitch' ones.

Type II B fibres

These are powerful 'fast-twitch' muscles used for high-demand, strong movements. They account for 60 per cent of the muscles in the body and contract five times faster than the others, but fatigue easily. They contain a small amount of myoglobin, large amounts of glycogen (*see* 'Glossary of terms' box on page 67) and relatively few mitochondria and blood capillaries.

Power exercise makes more Type II B fibres, which bulk up the muscle. This encourages the release of muscle growth-like hormone, which speeds up repair. Endurance exercise transforms Type II B fibres into Type II A fibres.

Type II A fibres

These make up a low percentage of the muscles in the body, but are more active than Type II B fibres. They are also 'fast twitch' and come into play at times of extreme exertion such as sprinting. They have more mitochondria and better blood supply and are overall good stuff!

Smooth muscle

This type of muscle is found in the walls of hollow internal structures such as blood vessels, the stomach, intestines and the urinary bladder. Smooth muscle fibres are usually involuntary (that is, not under conscious control). Smooth muscle, like skeletal and cardiac muscle tissue, can grow bigger, narrowing the space or tubes it surrounds.

Cardiac muscle

This forms the bulk of the wall of the heart. It has some characteristics of skeletal muscle, but its contraction is usually involuntary.

How does exercise influence longevity?

By following 1,200 pairs of twins, one study has shown that those who take moderate or higher levels of exercise for 180 minutes per week can have a physical age up to nine years younger.[1] This is because exercise modulates the body's metabolic activities and organ performance in a number of different ways:

Cellular effect
The more we exercise, the more the body's cells – particularly muscles – demand energy. This is derived from mitochondria.

Cardiovascular activity
The cellular demand for energy and the release of hormones and neurological reflexes at the start of exercise all combine to speed up heart rate, optimize blood pressure and, together, increase blood flow. All organs in the body benefit from this increased cardiovascular activity, and the heart itself strengthens through the development of more mitochondria. In the average person, heart muscle fibres generally contain 2,000 to 3,000 mitochondria per cell, while an elite athlete's may have up to 10,000.

Exercise has been found to encourage the self-destruction of old dysfunctional cells (autophagy) and a particular biochemical process that directly influences arterial stiffness and inner artery health – the aptly named *NO/ONOO* (pronounced No, Oh No!) cycle reaction.[2]

Hormonal influence
The glands of the body increase their production in the bodies of those who exercise more because healthier arteries and an increased heart rate improve blood flow throughout the body. More hormones generally means better-functioning cells. We can consider the chemicals within the nervous system also to be a type of hormone (a neurohormone), and these too benefit the function of the nervous system, muscles, the immune system and the health of the cardiovascular system, particularly heart rate and blood pressure.

Endorphins and encephalins are hormones similar to plant-based opiates (opium and heroin), which enhance general mood and the feeling of well-being. Exercise increases production of these 'fun' hormones, while also reducing the presence of excess catecholamines (adrenalin and other excitatory hormones). Optimum levels of exercise stimulate the stress-coping hormone cortisol.

Detoxification

Exercise increases heart rate and optimizes blood pressure. This increases the rate of blood flow through the liver and kidneys, encouraging detoxification and the removal of waste.

The faster heart rate and increased muscular activity during exercise requires energy, which is produced through a process that releases heat. Muscular contraction itself also causes body temperature to rise. The body then has to be cooled – predominantly through sweating. Sweat carries water-soluble toxins out of the body and has a similar composition to urine – effectively making the skin a third kidney as far as the excretion of waste is concerned.

Digestion

As the body demands more sugar and other nutrients owing to increased usage, neurohormonal changes increase gastric acid secretion, pancreatic digestive enzymes and absorption from the gut. Exercise increases oxygen demand, which leads to an increased contraction of the diaphragm (the muscle at the base of our rib cage that contracts causing air to be drawn into the lungs). The contraction pushes down on the abdominal contents, thereby massaging the digestive organs, including the stomach, pancreas and liver, all of which respond by having increased blood flow. (I should point out that intense activity temporarily slows down intestinal traction because blood is diverted from the intestines to active muscles, but, overall, exercise enhances digestive activity.)

DNA

Exercise also appears to switch on a part of our DNA that helps detoxify cells through one particular pathway known as methylation.[3]

Cancer prevention and survival

The National Cancer Institute cites 50 studies on colon cancer and 60 studies on breast cancer that show decreased rates of cancer in those who exercise. They also cite increased survival rates within these studies. There are an additional 20 studies each on uterine and lung cancer, and 36 studies on prostate cancer, which confirm the benefits of exercise for improved mortality.[4] Exercise was found to reduce the growth rate of prostate cancer by 30 per cent.[5]

CALCULATING VO2 MAX

The simplest calculation is based on peddling a stationary cycle at a set upward grade of stiffness of the wheels until your heart rate no longer increases, and measuring your heart rate:

- *VO2 Max = Heart rate at maximum intensity of exercise divided by heart rate at rest, then multiply that number by 15.*
- Other, more detailed methods of calculating VO2 Max include taking your age, weight and height into account.
- It all gets rather complicated and unless you 'hit the gym', you are unlikely to be governed by such measurements.

VO2 Max ratings (ml/kg/min) MEN

Age	Very low level of fitness	Low level of fitness	Average level of fitness	High level of fitness	Very high level of fitness
20-29	38	39-43	44-51	52-56	57
30-39	34	35-39	40-47	48-51	52
40-49	30	31-35	36-43	44-47	48
50-59	25	26-31	32-39	40-43	44
60-69	21	22-26	27-35	36-39	40

VO2 Max ratings (ml/kg/min) WOMEN

Age	Very low level of fitness	Low level of fitness	Average level of fitness	High level of fitness	Very high level of fitness
20-29	28	29-34	35-43	44-48	49
30-39	27	28-33	34-41	42-47	48
40-49	25	26-31	32-40	41-45	46
50-59	21	22-28	29-36	37-41	42

What kind of exercise do you need?

How do you go about exercising at an optimum level, practically? If you research online, you might come across the 117,000 articles on this topic – and that's just scholarly articles! While there is a general consensus that exercise is beneficial, the quantity and intensity required is clearly in dispute. Different studies from different authorities have certainly muddied the waters, but I hope I can simplify matters for you here.

First, it is necessary to have different types of exercise to optimize health and longevity. According to Singh,[6] there are four main areas to focus on:
1. *Aerobic exercise* – improves the efficiency of the body's cardiovascular system in absorbing and transporting oxygen.
2. *Resistance exercise* – strengthens the muscles and increases muscle mass.
3. *Balance* – reduces risks of falls and reduces anxiety about rapid movement.
4. *Flexibility* – encourages joint health and blood flow.

All of these areas are covered by Eastern philosophies such as yoga, tai chi and martial arts. Everyone should try to have a go by seeing if there are classes available locally or by purchasing a self-help exercise DVD. If you do some research, you will find that there are hundreds of different avenues to explore and you are bound to find something that you enjoy. Even simple activities such as gardening can give you quite a workout.

How much exercise should you do?

This question needs to be broken down into:
A. What intensity of exercise is best?
B. What is the optimum exercise duration?
C. How often or what exercise frequency is best for me?

Each of us has an individual requirement. The retiring Ms Jones, 64 years of age and with a history of angina, will need a different protocol from 50-year-old Mr Smith, active farmer. How to calculate what is ideal for each person is best done through individualized assessment by an exercise specialist or by personal design with some understanding of what you need. However, if you're the kind of person who is never going to go out and find a personal trainer, let me help you to make some informed decisions.

Heart rate increase according to level of exercise

Level of exercise	Heart rate increase	Example of beats/minute (bpm)
Sedentary	Resting heart rate	72bpm
Light	Increase of 25 per cent	90bpm
Moderate	Increase of 50 per cent	108bpm
Vigorous	Increase of 75 per cent	126bpm
Strenuous	Increase of up to 90 per cent	137bpm
Excessive	Increase greater than 90 per cent	137+bpm

Most guidelines seem to require a calculation based on VO2 Max (*maximal oxygen consumption*), which is the maximum capacity of an individual's body to transport and use oxygen during a test over about 10 minutes where the person increases the intensity of activity. This reflects physical fitness very accurately – but not strength, balance or flexibility. Blood pressure has been shown to drop after four weeks when exercising up to three times per week above 70 per cent VO2 Max, but no further benefit is gleaned above that (*see* page 74).

What we know for sure is that health and longevity derive benefit from activity that is of moderate intensity; they are optimized by vigorous activity. Mild exercise, while better than none in some aspects of health, is of no consequence in longevity or avoiding incapacity as we age.[7]

What is meant by intensity?

What exactly do the experts mean by light, medium/moderate, vigorous, strenuous, optimal and excessive? (These are the words constantly bandied around.) It is really not clear, and I believe if I drew in a collective of specialists, they would probably each come up with different criteria for each category of intensity.

To simplify:
Light exercise
Walking, household chores, keeping up with the grandchildren, and so on, all fall into this category of light exercise. I look at this level as being possible to do while holding a conversation without interrupting the flow.

Moderate exercise
More than 30 minutes of brisk walking, light gardening or heavy but short bursts of household chores constitute moderate exercise. You can hold a conversation throughout these activities, but would struggle to keep up with a song on the radio without having to take in a breath (thereby missing the beat!). 'Brisk' might be best calculated by walking at 100 steps per minute.[8]

Vigorous exercise
This might be 20 minutes or more of jogging, uninterrupted heavy gardening, light gym work, non-competitive or non-timed swimming. Your conversation is now broken by increased respiration and you are missing every other line of your song.

Strenuous exercise
This includes 20 minutes or more of running, maximum gym workout, competitive sports. You cannot hold a conversation and cannot complete a mental task as efficiently or swiftly as you might at rest.

Optimal exercise
This varies enormously according to the individual. The closest definition is 'the level of exercise you can perform to the best of your ability without injury or stress'.

Excessive exercise
You hurt or are incapacitated to a point that the process cannot be repeated when you could reasonably expect to do so.

I quite like the American College of Sport Medicine's categorization from 2003, to which I have added some minor adjustments to make it more broad. For this, you simply need to establish your heart's resting rate (*see* page 76).

Overall, it appears that intensity of exercise is more relevant than the duration. A study in 1995 demonstrated an inverse relationship between vigorous activity and longevity. Non-vigorous activities extend your life. However, exercising strenuously will keep you healthier while you age, but may not necessarily affect longevity. As usual, a compromise is the answer.

Optimum duration
Some studies suggest that duration does not make a whole lot of difference in the outcome of weight loss and fitness as long as the exercise was more than moderate in intensity.[9]

OPTIMIZING EXERCISE

As long as you are not injuring yourself, you will be fine – provided you do not have medical conditions requiring specific advice. Sadly, you will not get that from most doctors who have little or no training in how to advise on optimizing exercise – it is best to try and find a physiotherapist or personal trainer.

Vary your routine: mixing sports with walking/running, visiting the gym, digging the garden one day and mowing the lawn the next are likely to keep you fit.

Tests have shown that people on a treadmill need only about 10 minutes to get to a level where their cardiopulmonary levels are at a peak,[10] suggesting that anything over that is likely to be beneficial. Therefore, aerobically speaking, 20 minutes up to a point of failing (that is, you just cannot take another step) is where the benefit lies.

Muscle building, an important part of optimum fitness, is best kept to short bursts of eight repetitive cycles repeated eight times, but the whole workout should be less than 45 minutes. After that, the body is likely to be releasing levels of cortisol, the stress-coping hormone, which will break down muscle – catabolic as opposed to anabolic – and nullify the benefits.

Optimum frequency

Anyone without health issues, particularly heart or artery disease, is going to gain some benefit from exercise. A vitally important exception is when a long period of inactivity is followed by a sudden extended burst of moderate or strenuous exercise. This presents a risk of sudden death, and you need to consider this when commencing an exercise programme.

I agree with the research suggesting that men aged over 40 should aim at 30 minutes a day, six days a week, for the best benefit; below that age, add on 15–30 minutes a day to the regimen.[11] There seems to be less research about optimum frequency for women, and also more variation in the advice given, but the 30-minute mark remains standard, although the frequency can be reduced to four days a week at the very least. Daily is best.

Women, more than men, develop thin bones (osteoporosis). It is well documented that this condition benefits from weight-bearing exercise – being on your feet as opposed to swimming, rowing or floor exercises. One study suggested that daily hopping exercises increased femoral neck density in premenopausal women, but less frequent hopping exercise was not effective. (My wife pointed out that this research was probably done by a man who had not had children! Pelvic floor exercises may be needed prior to such an activity.)

Brief, high-impact exercise such as running has a role in reducing hip fragility, but needs to be performed frequently (at least four times a week) for optimal results. An eight-year study of 400,000 people in Taiwan[12] came up with some other conclusions. This paper from the most prestigious of journals suggested that low-intensity exercise of just 15 minutes per day would increase life expectancy by three years.

This level of exercise decreased all-cause mortality by 14 per cent and specifically over eight years reduced the incidence of cancer by 10 per cent. The paper then went on to suggest that a further 15 minutes of exercise per day would decrease overall mortality by a further 4 per cent and cancer by 1 per cent. In short, the more you do and the higher the frequency, the better.

Conclusion

The best way to exercise for healthy longevity is:
- Perform moderate- to high-intensity aerobic exercise.
- Do short, repeated spells of muscle-building activity at least five times a week.
- Exercise aerobically for at least 20 minutes for a minimum of five days a week.
- Do 50 hops on each leg daily if you do not do weight-bearing (on your feet) exercise.
- Walk on uneven surfaces whenever possible or get a wobble board to enhance balance.

How can I personalize my requirements?

The conclusions relating to optimum exercise programmes are conflicting, so try to find a routine that suits you personally by following this advice:
1. Sit down and relax. Give yourself five minutes of meditating and take your pulse at your wrist. Do this on three or four occasions over a week or so, making sure you have not had caffeine or alcohol in the previous six hours and have not eaten in the previous three. This should give you, by taking an average, your *resting pulse* (RP). Those of you with less patience can simply take your pulse now.
2. Next, build up to what you consider to be the maximum amount of exercise (running, rowing, swimming) you are comfortable

with and after 10 minutes take your pulse. This is your *maximum intensity heart rate*. Use this calculation for VO2 Max (*see* page 71) and look on the chart to establish the level you are at.
3. Do some exercise – neither your health nor your longevity will have any hope without it. However, doing too much may be detrimental for two reasons: first, if the exercise is too strenuous, you may hurt yourself; second, as 'too much' is rather subjective, if you are doing more than you enjoy, you will probably stop.

There is no evidence to suggest that the phrase 'no pain, no gain' is accurate, except when the pain is short-lived and you recover quickly.

May I have a regimen, please?

I believe that we all fit into one of three groups when it comes to addressing an exercise programme – those that say:
1. "There is no time!"
2. "I'll fit it in."
3. "I'm off to the gym."

We are either too busy or just do not like exercise; we will try to place exercise into an otherwise busy existence; or, at the other end of the scale, we will fit our work life around our sporting activities. I think that if you have reached a point where you do not like exercising, you have either a memory of discomfort from activity and sports or you have never been introduced to something that you might enjoy. You need to address and consider your personal history, your current work and your social life when choosing an exercise plan.

"THERE IS NO TIME!"

There is, of course, always time, but not enjoying exercise usually allows us to fill the healthy parts of the day with something less strenuous. If your life is such that you are up so early and home so late owing to commitments, whether these are pleasurable or otherwise, your body will be under stress. If you are at such a place, you are probably not getting enough sleep, your mental activity has lost its connection with your physical being, and I need to warn you that there is no scientific evidence that suggests you will live healthily or long.

You are not in a good place, so *find the time*! If you are sleeping enough, then get up half an hour earlier and fit in some exercise. I hope I have helped establish that as little as 15–30 minutes of moderate exercise (brisk walking) will influence health and longevity. If you can up that to vigorous or even strenuous exercise, it will make a profound difference.

Kettle bells are becoming popular and web pages abound on both short and long exercise programmes using these. If you do not enjoy using equipment or simply do not have space in your home for a treadmill or rowing machine, then go for 6–10 sessions of tai chi, pilates or yoga and pick up a life plan from the teacher for a 15- to 30-minute/daily programme.

A recent body of research has led to the design of a 12-minute/per week programme by Dr Doug McGuff and John Little. Their *Body by Science* book, 'a research-based programmeme for strength training, body building and complete fitness in 12 minutes a week', might be the answer for the 'There is no time!' brigade. This programme is based on some scientific evidence and suggests that exercising a muscle group to the point of failure (the muscle just cannot repeat the action) may act in place of the more established programmes as highlighted in this chapter. Apparently, this 'straining' of a muscle group builds up mitochondria not only in the muscle group that is worked but also in other places – the heart in particular. This provides the muscle mass strength in those muscles worked as well as cardiovascular fitness. However, it will not deal with any balance and flexibility issues. Furthermore, it is not suitable for all body types and genetic makeups, but those with good sugar control and insulin resistance and those with low cardiovascular risk will be fine with it. Genetic testing, while not yet shown to be accurate in longer-term studies, can differentiate those of us who can do these short-burst programmes.

"I'LL FIT IT IN"
Find what you enjoy. This may be a brisk walk in a healthy environment, competitive sport such as tennis, badminton or even a game of frisbee in the park. Do not forget that gardening is rarely further than your back door or allotment or a visit to a grateful friend.

Aim at the moderate levels as described in this chapter with regard to intensity.

The minimum time spent exercising, both aerobically and using weights, or floor exercises to strengthen muscle should be 30 minutes for men and 20 minutes for women.

Eight repetitions, eight times using one particular set of muscles should not take more than five minutes, and rotating the following exercises through the week using specific muscle groups should fit into a daily timetable (or at

least four to five times per week):
- bicep curls;
- triceps contractions;
- lateral deltoid extensions;
- push-ups;
- abdominal curls;
- squats or thrusts.

You can find examples and demonstrations of these simple exercises on the Internet and in most basic exercise books. The purchase of handheld weights of 2 to 3kg (4 to 7lb) should suffice for those of you who are not bodybuilders.

"I'M OFF TO THE GYM"

Many of us enjoy vigorous or strenuous exercise. The evidence suggests that the more we do, provided we do not injure ourselves, the less likely we are to develop illnesses and the longer we will live.

We have to balance this enthusiasm with good nutrition and tailor-made programmes as there is a fine line between achieving elite athletic prowess and developing conditions such as being tired all the time (TATT) and chronic fatigue syndrome (CFS). One of the most common groups to struggle with CFS includes those who are most athletic.

It is not in the remit of this book to help design vigorous exercise programmes, and such individualized systems are best put together by a qualified personal trainer.

What tests are worth doing?

Tests for exercise are not generally considered necessary, but the concept of differentiating between those of us who need longer, more aerobic exercise and those who can benefit from short-burst, high-intensity exercises may now be entertained.

One large and long-term study, the *Heritage Family Study,* led to over 120 papers being published between 1997 and 2004. Among the many interesting facts gleaned from the study was one that stated that of 1,000 people who exercised four hours a week for 20 weeks, only 15 per cent of them made a marked impact on their aerobic fitness (VO2 Max increased and they were labelled 'super-responders'), whereas 20 per cent showed no real improvement at all ('non-responders'). Knowing whether you are a responder or not makes a difference to how you should exercise.

There are now gene tests performed from simple swabs from inside the mouth that can advise which type of exercise and level of intensity is likely to be optimum for you. We have genes that help select sport style, motivation to exercise (perhaps not a test that is needed) muscle and cardio-vascular capacity and ability to expend energy. Such reports tell us whether we would benefit or not from endurance exercise, our risk of creating heart problems from over-exercising and whether we should be aiming at muscular body building or not.

Chapter 4

Detoxification

If you want to make conventional doctors raise their eyes to the ceiling and sigh with frustration, tell them you feel 'toxic' and ask how best to detoxify! The term 'detoxification' seems to be abandoned after most students finish their biochemistry and basic physiology courses at medical school. This is a shame as it is so important to rid ourselves of toxic build-up. Particularly as we age, the waste product inside our bodies, commonly referred to as 'junk' by gerontologists, is primarily responsible for the faltering systems that lead to age-related problems.

The more holistic or broader-minded health professional will recognize that detoxification is the foundation for ensuring longevity and good health, along with good nutritional intake and controlled psycho-emotional well-being.

The removal of toxins is fundamental to good health – from the Greco-Roman and Western perspective as well as in Eastern traditions. If we look at the humours (blood, yellow bile, black bile or phlegm) or the element theories from Eastern philosophy (earth, fire, water and air), we infer or get a sense of how the production of fluids and heat influence the movement of toxins out of the body. We detoxify by breathing out and passing wind (air), sweating and urinating (water), passing stool (earth), and metabolizing and burning waste product (fire).

Why does it matter if I am toxic?

Toxins interfere with intracellular and extracellular structure and function, which, in turn, leads to organ and system dysfunction.

Intracellular toxicity

When toxins build up around cells in tissue, on cell walls and within the cells themselves, we lose the ability to control what enters the cell and how cells then function. Compounds adhere to receptors and the small parts within cells known as organelles that carry out the function and cleansing of the cell, including the energy-producing mitochondria.

Pieces of DNA that have toxic compounds adhering to them are called adducts. This state of affairs directly alters the command system for cellular function. Blockage of the part of the cell that cleans the DNA may be affected along with the mitochondria, and many receptors become blocked, reducing the number free to receive nutrients and hormone instructions. A failure in this intracellular detoxification leads to a build-up of free radicals (*see* Chapter 6), which causes a process known as oxidation leading directly to cell damage and upsetting the normal processing of fatty acids and sugar metabolism. When this happens, a compound known as lipofuscin builds up. Lipofuscin is frequently associated with dementia, but can halt normal function of any cell or tissue, not just the cells of the brain.

Extracellular toxicity

Toxic build-up in the space outside the cells can lead to free-radical damage, directly influence receptors on the outside of cells and lead to the build-up of protein chains that cause blood supply to diminish. It also blocks the waste drainage (through the lymphatic system). When this happens, protein complexes known as crosslinks and amyloid build up (another cause of dementia if this occurs in the brain), and tissues are obstructed as if they were caught in a fine mesh of net.

Sugars trapped in this net heat up because of the body's temperature and effectively 'caramelize'. If you think of the fine, needle-like projections that form in a frying pan when food is caramelized or of the hard crisp nature of a toffee apple, you can imagine how the formation of such crystals can damage tissue.

This intracellular and extracellular damage not only overtly causes disease, but effectively forms the basis of a major theory of ageing by being a part of the eventual dysfunction of systems and organs.

Toxic build-up influences the nervous and cardiovascular systems directly and damages the barrier-protective mechanisms of the skin and inner lining of the body (the epithelial layer), which, in turn, allows organisms and more toxins to invade.

The liver, kidney and skin (through sweating) are the main organs of elimination or detoxification. Damage to their tissue by a build-up of toxins creates a vicious circle leading to further damage and less ability to detoxify.

How do toxins cause dysfunction?

A toxin interferes with the function of cells and tissues and causes damage at different levels.

A toxin coming into contact with the skin either by direct application or exposure to contaminated air will potentially cause damage. A breakdown of the skin barrier will allow more toxins in. As we age, more and more toxin damage accumulates, which is exacerbated by the fact that the lower hormone levels associated with ageing slow the repair process. The combination leads to a dysfunctional outer barrier. Keeping the skin healthy is therefore of prime importance in supporting detoxification.

The same can be said for the internal barriers. Our airways are lined by little hairs known as cilia, which are extremely sensitive to the noxious compounds that we inhale. One puff on a cigarette can stop cilia working for several hours. The cilia are supposed to constantly flick out any debris we inhale, and this, in combination with mucus production, reduces the rate at which toxins settle on the cells and block absorption. The morning cough of a smoker is partly the result of the resurrection of cilia function through the hours of non-smoking – sleep allows particle-laden mucus to be pushed toward the upper respiratory tract, which triggers the cough reflex.

Ingested toxins, interfering with the bowel bacteria that line the bowel wall, diminish a first layer of defence. Toxins landing on the bowel epithelium (gut lining) can damage the cell surface. Receptors have evolved for specific food molecules and are required to help the larger molecules we need cross the membrane into the bloodstream. Toxins damage these and lead to deficiencies despite a healthy intake of nutrients.

The loss of bowel wall integrity owing to damage and inflammation can lead to a loss of the full effectiveness of the barrier between the bowel and the bloodstream. Waste products, bacteria, viruses, yeasts and fungi and any environmental toxins that we have ingested or that have been recycled by the liver have the potential to enter the bloodstream. A permeable bowel is often not taken seriously enough. In medical terms it is known as increased intestinal permeability or, more colloquially, as leaky gut syndrome.

Where does detoxification take place?

Good health requires the liver to break down the majority of poisons that have entered the bloodstream from the gut. The liver changes the molecular structure of toxins and, after binding them to compounds known as conjugates, passes them back via the bile into the gut, from where they can be expelled. Liver toxins that pass into the bloodstream and the lymphatic system are eliminated from the body via the kidneys in the urine, via the lungs in the breath and via the skin in sweat.

Detoxification also takes place at a cellular level. Zinc and other minerals activate an enzyme system known as superoxide dismutase (SODase). This is one of the most important intra- and extracellular antioxidants along with glutathione (also made in the body, predominantly in the liver). Tissues bathed in SODase and other antioxidants such as vitamin C protect cell membranes and the smaller blood vessels from free-radical damage.

Once inside the cell, DNA adducts and mitochondrial toxic attachments are dependent on zinc/copper SODase as well as manganese SODase. Special little chemical detoxification factories known as lysosomes are sacks full of enzymes geared toward destroying unwanted compounds – proteins in particular. A build-up of toxins within the cells can inhibit these, leading to further toxic build-up.

Which toxins adversely affect healthy ageing?

Unfortunately, everything is potentially toxic if it is in our system for too long or at too high a level, if we are too frequently exposed to it or if the toxin's potency is so high that even a small amount bothers us. These factors are not only dependent upon the intake of the poison but also on the efficiency and speed of our ability to remove it.

Our body also has to recognize that there is a toxin present. There are obvious symptoms of toxicity such as:
- nausea and vomiting;
- sweating;
- diarrhoea;
- increased urination;
- skin rashes (irritation of a toxin excreted through the skin).

Less obvious signs of toxicity include:
- being tired all the time (TATT);
- poor concentration/memory;
- sleep disturbance;
- abdominal symptoms;
- neurological signs (tingling), numbness, loss of function;
- muscular weakness;
- visual disturbance;
- illnesses such as asthma and eczema, which may eventually occur.

EVERYDAY EXPOSURE TO TOXINS

Of 2.5 million tonnes of pesticides used each year, only 0.1 per cent is taken up by insects; 99.9 per cent of pesticides enter our water supply and food chain.[2]

Pesticides are also found in all these materials and we are constantly breathing in fumes from the detergents and the dry-cleaning chemicals used on our clothes and bedlinen.

Household toxins include chlorinated and brominated compounds (PCPs, PBPs and PCBs) found in carpets, curtains, chairs and sofas, mattresses, and so on, as fire retardants.

Volatile oxidative compounds (VOCs) is a broad term for chemicals that are formed from heated chemicals and plastics. It can include anything from artificial compounds to natural heavy metals. Computers are a major source of VOCs. The inside of a computer can reach very high temperatures, causing very high levels of exposure to the emission of components of metals and plastics.

Sources of toxins

Toxins effectively accumulate in the system either from within or without. Those that we are exposed to in our environment are found in the air we breathe and the food and water we ingest. Direct contact is another source.

Toxins that form internally accumulate due to poor excretion of normal cellular metabolism, absorption of toxins from the gut (including micro-organisms) and the outcome of our attempts to detoxify, which lead to the accumulation of free radicals.

Environmental toxins

The following are the main types of toxins found in our environment:

Air
- Cigarettes
- Petrochemicals
- Industrial chemicals
- Heavy metals
- Volatile oxidative compounds
- Household pollutants

Water
- All of the above
- Medication or its metabolites enter our bodies via our drinking water supply as the water purification process does not filter out all of these chemicals. Traces of the oral contraceptive pill, taken by millions of women worldwide, are particularly evident in drinking water. The Pill is associated with the triggering of autoimmunity through its toxic effects.[1]

Food
- All the pollutants found in air
- Additives
- Preservatives
- Pesticides
- Foods causing allergy or intolerance
- Excess caffeine, sugars, fats and alcohol (all act as toxins)

Nutrition

I have listed above a few of the nutrients your body needs to activate detoxi-fication. Frankly, it needs most of the major minerals, vitamins and essential fatty acids and a variety of amino acids to detoxify effectively. The inter-action is not only directly with the toxins or the enzymes breaking them down, but also directly with genes such as the *MTHFR* gene with a control of methylation (Phase II).

Magnesium and B vitamins are important in glucuronidation and folic acid in methylation.

Fresh fruits and vegetables contain plenty of glutathione for glutathione conjugation, which is why so many detoxification diets recommend these foods in abundance.

Garlic and onions, most legumes and wholegrains are rich in sulphur

VISCERAL OBESITY

Visceral fat is that surrounding the abdominal organs and tends to manifest itself as abdominal weight. We also have subcutaneous fat under our skin, our breasts and our thighs. Visceral obesity is dangerous as toxins harboured in fat close to vital organs are more likely to damage them.

HOW TO IMPROVE DETOXIFICATION

Nutrition, dietetics, exercise, lifestyle changes, supplementation and certain therapies can all influence detoxification. To help you understand how nutrition and supplementation helps, I would like to give a little background on the detoxification pathways found in the liver. It is here that the majority of fat-soluble toxins and many water-soluble toxins are dealt with.

There are two main detoxification pathways in the liver – Phase I and Phase II.

Phase I

A group of enzymes known as cytochrome P450 control Phase I. These enzymes alter the nuclear structure of toxins as they enter the liver in an attempt to make the toxins less harmful. In some cases, this process has the opposite effect, making a more toxic 'intermediate metabolite'. To get rid of this, the liver enters Phase II.

The cytochrome P450 enzymes attempt to change the molecular structure of the toxin in the following ways:
- Oxidation – removing an electron
- Reduction – removing oxygen
- Hydrolysis – interacting with a water molecule
- Hydration – adding of a water molecule
- Other specific chemical reactions

Phase II

This is known as the conjugation (joining together) pathway. There are six main conjugates. These are:
- sulphation – requiring a sulphur molecule;
- glucuronidation – requiring glucuronic acid;
- glutathione conjugation – requiring glutathione made in the body from glutamic acid cysteine and glycine (all ingested as proteins);
- acetylation – requiring vitamins B1, B5 and C;
- amino acid conjugation – requiring predominately glycine and glutamine but also other ingested proteins;
- methylation – the addition of a methyl group (CH_3) requiring folic acid, vitamin B12 and several other nutrients.

as are the brassica (broccoli, spinach, kale) family; the sulphur found in asparagus causes the strong smell in urine.

High water intake is extremely important to ensure the dilution of toxins and Phase I hydration as well as providing the necessary hydration for all the body's chemical reactions to take place.

Exercise

Exercise heats the body and sweating cools it down. Sweat is one of the main ways in which the body detoxifies, making exercise an important part of the detoxification process.

Exercise increases circulation throughout the body, and muscles pump the lymphatic system to drain toxins back to the liver. Exercise increases oxygen intake, which encourages Phase I oxidation processes, and has direct effects on certain genes, increasing the stimulation of detoxification.

Lifestyle

Do not smoke! The risks to health for those who smoke are well established, and I don't feel I need to list all of them here. The number of chemicals in cigarettes may be as high as 4,000, many blocking metabolic pathways, and more than 50 are cancer-causing.[3]

Reducing your exposure to toxins is as much about common sense as consulting facts. Think about what toxins may be present in your environment (including hidden dangers) and take the least toxic options whenever possible. For example, if there is a computer in the room, try to keep a window open or the room well ventilated. Consider getting an ionizer or an ozone generator – both remove electrically charged particles from the air.

Volatile Organic Compounds (VOCs) are chemical compounds present in many new soft furnishings. If you are having new carpets or new furniture in your house, install them in the spring or summer, when you can open windows and doors to let the worst of the VOCs escape from the air inside the house.

Ensure that you open your bowel once, if not twice, daily. Get the toxins that are recycled by the liver or rejected by the absorptive processes out of the body as often as it asks you to!

Drop your weight. Fat-soluble vitamins do not dissolve in water (and so are not excreted in sweat; *see* page 89), which means that they are absorbed into your fat stores. Compounds that bind in these stores can sit there only to be released years later or slowly over time. Of more concern as we age is that our detoxification processes weaken, and so if decades of fat-soluble toxins are suddenly released, we increasingly do not have the processes in place to get rid of them.

Dr Sharma's Programmes

I have mentioned a few of the nutrients needed to activate detoxification in the liver and intracellular and extracellular detoxification. The high level of toxicity that we encounter in our polluted lives means we have to have an available source of many different nutrients to ensure we are detoxifying at an optimum level. I believe that the following are therefore a prerequisite for healthy ageing and longevity in addition to a healthy diet and lifestyle.

Dr Sharma's Maintenance Programme
This is a basic programme to detoxify the body's systems. Many of these nutrients can be found in the same tablet or capsule as multivitamin and multimineral complexes.

MINERALS
• *Multiminerals* – your multimineral tablet must include calcium, zinc, magnesium, manganese, copper and sulphur.

VITAMINS
• *B complex* – take twice daily.
• *Folic acid* – preferably this should be in the active form of 5-methyltetrahydrofolate (5-MTHF).
• *Vitamins A, C, and E* – antioxidants.
• *Vitamin D3* – minimally 1000iu daily, but discuss the option of up to 5,000iu with a practitioner.

ESSENTIAL FATTY ACIDS
• *Omega 6 and 3* – in a ratio of 4:1.

AMINO ACIDS
A protein-rich diet should cover the proteins required for detoxification. If you are a vegetarian, please look at Dr Sharma's Advanced Programme recommendations, on the following pages.

OTHER NUTRIENTS

Probiotics – maintaining bowel flora health is a prerequisite for encouraging bowel detoxification. I recommend you take probiotics nightly.

Far infrared sauna therapy (FIRST)

Along with exercise to encourage sweating and other detoxification pathways, I think every household should have a Far Infrared Sauna.

Albert Szent-Gyorgi, discoverer of vitamin C and a Nobel Prize winner, has shown how sunlight may benefit many aspects of health. One wavelength of light, known as 'far infrared' light, is warming and penetrates about 3cm (1in) below the skin (it is the same wavelength that feels warm on a subzero mountain top or cold day). Human cells also generate far infrared wavelengths. The penetrating rays heat up the cells and subcutaneous tissues causing a shaking of cell membranes, inner cell organelles and DNA. This breaks bonds that form adducts, making the removal of toxins easier. Heating cells also encourages the activity of lysozymes, and heat generally speeds up metabolic pathways including detoxification processes. Far infrared penetrates fat stores breaking bonds of the fat-soluble toxins. In FIRST therapy, special sleeping bags, known as cocoons, small tents, lamps and arc/tunnel-shaped devices generate far infrared waves to the whole or part of a body. Cardiovascular studies suggest that lower cholesterol and other fat-related benefits are seen when using FIRST and ongoing research supports this.[3]

Although there are many benefits to FIRST therapy, it is important that, as with any detoxification process, you are careful that toxins are not released into your system too rapidly, which could lead to acute poisoning and even kidney damage. Always consult a qualified practitioner and insist on seeing credentials, and ensure that the equipment used is up to date and well-maintained.

Dr Sharma's Advanced Programme

This programme is for those with symptoms of toxicity or with particularly toxic lifestyles (smokers, drug-takers or those with a high alcohol intake) or professions, and also for vegetarians who may fall short of their intake of certain amino acids (generally, though, although a vegetarian's protein-intake may be low, avoiding meat is a good lifestyle choice for minimizing toxicity). Discuss with your healthcare provider how adding the following supplements to your daily intake might boost your health.

VITAMINS AND MINERALS
- As for Dr Sharma's Maintenance Programme.

AMINO ACIDS
- *A broad spectrum supplement* – preferably whey or a vegan equivalent taken daily.
- *N-acetyl cysteine (NAC)* – activates Phase I and Phase II pathways.

OTHER NUTRIENTS
- *Milk thistle* – take daily to support Phase I.
- *Alpha lipoic acid* – a naturally occurring compound that crosses the blood-brain barrier and acts as an antioxidant.

OTHER WAYS TO DETOX
Even if we lead a generally healthy lifestyle and follow my programmes of detoxification supplements, there will be times when we need a detox boost following a short period of excess. Infrequent alcohol binges, over-eating and under-exercising all lead to my recommending the use of the following as additional detoxification aids.

Ionizers
As you read this book, you will recognize that much damage to the body that leads to disease and advances the ageing process occurs as a result of free radicals. These are the positively charged molecules produced by artificial chemicals and manufacturing processes. Appliances called ionizers 'neutralize' these particles because they electrically charge air molecules with a net negative charge and disperse the negative ions throughout a room.

Regular sauna
If you suffer with heart problems, I do not recommend sauna as a treatment method. Otherwise, however, sauna is great for reducing toxicity levels. Although some people do not tolerate heat well, being in a hot environment (conventional saunas can reach 110°C/230°F) removes toxins. (FIRST reaches only around 54°C/130°F and is better tolerated.)

Liver detox
This popular detoxification technique involves drinking olive oil and lemon juice. The linoleic acid in the oil binds with the citric acid to form semi-solid, green, slimy, peanut-sized globules – these, in fact, are *not* gallstones, which

would be extremely painful were you to start passing one, let alone masses of them! However, the process may have some benefit as the Omega-6 fatty acid in cold-pressed, organic olive oil is good for you; citric acid and other components of lemons may also be beneficial; certainly the vitamin C alone will help to improve your health.

Colonic irrigation

This is the technique of flushing the bowel (an enema) with water or, on occasions, a dilute solution of herbs or even caffeine. Versions such as the Gerson and Plaskett therapies use caffeine enemas to encourage venous blood flow from the bowel to the liver, thereby enhancing detoxification. The process is generally preceded by fasting and the use of laxatives to give the bowel an initial cleanse.

If you decide to try colonic irrigation, use probiotics to enhance bowel bacteria activity. Ensure you have a good fluid and fibre intake to ensure that you regularly pass stool. Although many people avoid colonic irrigation because they do not like the idea of having a tube inserted into their anus and a bag of fluid flushed through their large intestine, it can be a good way to quickly rid the bowel of toxins. It is not essential, but it certainly has its place in the detoxification process.

Skin brushing

The skin is a vitally important barrier to toxic overload and an organ of detoxification in itself, so it is important to keep it in a healthy condition. If you use moisturizers and other skin lotions, your pores are likely to become clogged up as much by these as by pollutants in the air. That is not to say that you should not use them to keep your skin supple. However, bathe or take a shower twice a day and use a skin brush or coarse flannel to scrub away dead skin cells and ensure that your pores are open.

Investigations and tests

Try not to wait until you show signs of toxicity before you investigate what is going on in your body – think pre-emptively. Your first investigations need to establish whether your barrier membranes – the skin and inner linings of the gut and respiratory tract – are intact. Then, look into how your liver is functioning. If you are unwell, you may find it helpful to look into your intracellular detoxification functioning.

First-line investigations

Use the following investigations if you are looking for a baseline understanding of your levels of toxicity.

BLOOD TESTS
Enzyme testing
The liver manufactures an enzyme called glutathione-S-transferase (G-S-T), levels of which rise when your liver has to work harder to break down toxins in your system. Ask your medical practitioner for a G-S-T test to see if your current lifestyle is proving to be a burden to your liver, and note that a G-S-T test will show liver burden long before a conventional 'liver function test' reveals liver damage.

Cheek cell swab for genomic testing
Specific genes govern Phase I and Phase II detoxification. Slight changes in the gene pattern (polymorphisms or single neucleotide polymorphisms) can increase or decrease the production and the activity of these detoxification genes. Cheek cell swabs can detect activity levels. The tests measure gene expression of:
- cytochrome P-450 (Phase I);
- methylation (Phase II);
- acetylation;
- glutathione conjugation;
- oxidative protection (cellular ability to make SODase).

Genomic testing does not predict a definite toxic state or inability to detoxify, but it can indicate whether we are a 'good' or a 'weak' detoxifier and therefore help us make more informed choices about diet and lifestyle.

Second-line investigations

If you already show signs of having health issues related to your levels of toxicity, or if you just want a fuller picture of your levels of toxicity, try the following tests.

BLOOD TESTS
Bile acid profile
Some laboratories are able to ascertain levels of bile acid production. This is another method of establishing how active the liver is. If the liver is overrun by toxins, then bile acid levels will fall.

White-blood-cell (leucocyte) sensitivity
This is not a widely available test, but it is one that I think is invaluable. As soon as your body's cells recognize invasion by a toxin, your immune system launches an army of white blood cells to neutralize the attack. Measuring white-blood-cell activity can tell us if toxins are present at potentially harmful levels. Furthermore, it can tell us which pollutants cause the defence systems to move to action. Testing for metals is perhaps a sensible investigation for all of us, but certain professions might warrant a broader test: for example, those working in the petrochemical industry might look for sensitivity to common industrial chemicals. Individuals working in hair salons might look for sensitivity to hair products; cleaners might choose to test for sensitivity to household compounds and solvents. With the potential to detect toxicity from a wide range of chemical and metal pollutants, the test can be expensive, which often puts people off taking it.

URINE TESTS
Phase I and II detoxification profile
This test involves taking a small amount of aspirin, paracetamol, acetaminophen and caffeine on an otherwise empty stomach. The liver uses different pathways (as discussed previously) to detoxify these compounds. Urinalysis (analysis of the urine sample) detects breakdown products (metabolites) of these compounds and the low, normal or high levels of any one of them indicate detoxification ability.

Intestinal permeability or 'leaky gut' test
In various guises, all leaky gut tests involve swallowing a drink containing molecules that should not be found in the urine, because they are too large to pass through a healthy bowel wall. If the bowel membrane has increased permeability, a subsequent urine sample will detect the molecules in the drink, indicating leaky gut syndrome.

Advanced investigations
Although it is much better to preempt problems caused by toxicity and undergo preventative testing, as described so far, there are also certain tests that I recommend to people who already show signs of toxic overload.

Toxic metals screen
Metals (either individually or as part of industrialized chemical pollutants) are frequently found to be an underlying toxic cause of disease. Accumulation

as we age is a problem, and I strongly recommend establishing toxic metal levels as soon as health conditions arise, or if any of the aforementioned tests suggests toxicity. Toxic metal screening has flaws, as metals can remain in body tissues or fat stores or inside cells from where they are not necessarily picked up in tests. However, challenge tests are available in which you would be asked to drink compounds (such as dimercaptosuccinic acid – DMSA) that bind to metals in your system and draw them out in your urine. Tests on your urine then reveal the levels of metal toxicity in your system.

Hair analysis
This popular test tells you only about the levels of metal outside your body in the 'waste material' that is your hair. High metal levels in your hair do not necessarily reflect high levels of metals in your bloody – just that you have had metal toxicity at some stage. I recommend the toxic metals screen as the more efficient and accurate testing method.

Intracellular/Serum nutrient evaluation
Specialized laboratories have methods of looking at how much of zinc, magnesium and manganese you have in your body at the intracellular level. In the absence of certain minerals, our SODase and other cellular detoxification pathways do not work well and allow DNA and mitochondrial adducts to interfere with cellular functions.

Chapter 5

Minerals – Cell Function, Organs and Bones

Directly or indirectly, minerals affect every structure and every functional process in the body. Broadly divided into major and trace minerals, differentiated by the amount we need, all minerals have important roles in healthy body function, and therefore ageing.

In this chapter I will briefly explain the importance of minerals, what they do and how best to obtain them, and I will focus attention particularly on the areas of health that are dependent upon a good supply.

What minerals do

The table on the following pages shows the minerals found in the body and their role in bodily functions. We all have many other minerals inside of us, too, which are probably ingested as part of food, but these minerals do not have actions or necessarily beneficial effects in the human body.

There are several kilograms of the major minerals in the body – calcium and magnesium in particular. The recommended daily allowance (RDA), as set by conventional nutritional standards, suggests we need to take in about 200mg of these per day. We need less of the trace elements: perhaps only a few milligrams each day in our diet is sufficient.

The RDA provides a level that avoids the presentation of acute disease such as rickets (a lack of calcium in the bones). The methodology of setting these standards is controversial, and I have been unable to find any evidence of scientific experimentation by which scientists reached the supposed RDA of minerals. In reality, if we do not take in more than the RDA, a lot of the illnesses we struggle with as we age will develop more swiftly.

MINERAL T = Trace M = Major		ACTION
Boron	T	Influences bone structure.
Calcium	M	Major component of bone and teeth structure; has multiple roles in many metabolic pathways; essential for muscle contraction.
Chlorine	M	Helps body fluid balance and energy production; regulates blood pressure and acidity/alkalinity or pH balance.
Cobalt	T	Found as part of vitamin B12, which is important in many pathways and metabolic functions, including the production of red blood cells.
Copper	T	Important in red-blood-cell function, muscular contraction/relaxation, detoxification processes and other metabolic pathways; also important for HDL/LDL cholesterol balance.
Flourine	T	Important in hardening teeth enamel.
Iodine	T	Needed for the production of thyroxin.
Iron	T	Primarily important in the production of haemoglobin to carry oxygen around the body; important for immune system function; of importance in protein structure in muscles.
Lithium	T	Influences brain activity, particularly enhancing mood.
Magnesium	M	Important in the building and function of bones and teeth structure; has multiple roles in metabolic pathways; this is the mineral responsible for muscle relaxation including arterial wall muscle thereby regulating blood pressure; also important in energy production and DNA cleansing; influences susceptibility to asthma, diabetes, depression, painful periods, epilepsy, gum disease and multiple sclerosis.
Manganese	T	Helps balance calcium and iron intake; important in preventing dementia, diabetes, epilepsy, Parkinson's disease, schizophrenia, other neurological conditions and rheumatoid arthritis.
Molybdenum	T	Influences iron uptake and utilization, and several enzyme pathways.
Nickel	T	Important in some enzyme activities.
Phosphorus	M	Influences bone structure, metabolic pathways and formation of DNA.
Potassium	M	Affects multiple metabolic pathways; involved in the movement of nutrients in and out of cells; directly involved in the production of energy; important in maintaining blood pressure and heart muscle contraction.
Selenium	T	Protects the arteries; powerful antioxidant; involved in energy production.
Sodium	M	Vital component of multiple metabolic pathways, involved in the movement of nutrients in and out of cells; directly involved in the production of energy; important in maintaining blood pressure and heart muscle contraction.
Sulphur	M	Important in helping to bind proteins in hair and nails; is of structural importance to hair, nails, muscle, skin and bones; vital in detoxification pathways and other metabolic functions.
Vanadium	T	Function is uncertain, but is involved in the control of blood sugar.
Zinc	T	Active in multiple metabolic pathways, cleaning DNA, prostate health, function of the immune system.

Age-related conditions associated with mineral deficiency

Let me list the *main* conditions associated with deficiency in minerals and you will clearly see how important these nutrients are.

- *Osteoarthritis* – calcium, magnesium, selenium, sulphur and boron
- *Rheumatoid arthritis* – zinc, copper, selenium, silicon
- *Arterial disease* – selenium, magnesium, chromium, manganese and potassium
- *Diabetes* – chromium, magnesium, zinc, copper, manganese and vanadium
- *Asthma* – magnesium, potassium and molybdenum
- *Osteoporosis* – calcium, manganese, boron, silicon, magnesium and strontium
- *Depression* – lithium
- *Fatigue syndromes* – magnesium
- *Poor general immunity* – zinc, iron, iodine
- *Weak immunity against cancer* – selenium, zinc and magnesium
- *Hypertension (high blood pressure)* – magnesium and selenium
- *Prostatism (enlarged prostate)* – zinc
- *Cataract* – zinc, selenium
- *Macular degeneration* – zinc, selenium
- *Erectile dysfunction* – zinc
- *Tinnitus* – zinc

Another way to look at the problem of mineral deficiencies is to define which parts of our body and which systems fail in the absence of these nutrients. Below is a list of the most studied minerals:

- *Calcium* – rickets, muscular cramps, osteopenia (thin bones), osteoporosis (bones at risk of fracture), hypertension and colon cancer
- *Chromium* – poor sugar control and possibly diabetes, cardiovascular disease, poor stress response
- *Iron* – anaemia, immune deficiency, hair and nail growth problems
- *Magnesium* – muscular weakness and spasm, high blood pressure, cardiovascular disease, increased risk of heart failure and heart attacks, depression
- *Manganese* – thin bones, poor connective tissue growth, poor sugar control and fat metabolism, dry skin and hair, allergies and behavioural problems

- *Molybdenum* – detoxification problems, iron-balance issues
- *Potassium* – problems with cell membrane function, heart failure, heart arrhythmia
- *Selenium* – cardiovascular disease, thyroid dysfunction and poor antioxidant activity leading to free-radical damage (cancer and arterial disease)
- *Sodium* – loss of water balance control, hypertension issues, poor cell-membrane function
- *Zinc* – free-radical concerns, loss of smell and taste, lack of stomach acid production, vision problems, immune dysfunction, poor wound healing, tiredness, energy issues

HOW TO AVOID MINERAL DEFICIENCY

I talk at length in Chapter 2 about a lack of nutrients in both our agricultural and animal food supply. Mineral deficiency is a particular concern and was highlighted by the 1992 Earth Summit Report. This found mineral depletion of soil to be as much as 76 per cent in Europe, 80 per cent in the USA and over 50 per cent in other parts of the world compared with 100 years ago. The inference is that intensive farming in particular, with the addition of specific farming processes, pesticides and other chemical additives, has contributed to the problem.

Nowadays, more of our food is developed hydroponically (grown in nutrient-rich fluids rather than soil). This process depends upon scientists matching nature's expertise. Quite frankly, as we are uncertain about the necessity in the human body of a few minerals (vanadium is an example), we are unlikely to get everything right. Furthermore, much of today's nutritional science is based on RDAs, which are geared only toward avoiding acute diseases rather than maintaining long-term health. Furthermore, the nutrients in hydroponically grown foods are often pharmaceutical grade, which means that they do not have the necessary co-factors to make them available to us once we ingest them.

We could argue that most diseases and many age-related issues can be linked to mineral deficiencies, which is why I think it is so important to understand the main causes of mineral deficiency. The reasons for deficiency fall into the following categories:

- Inadequate nutrient levels in food
- Poor nutritional intake

- Poor digestive capabilities – reduced stomach acid and pancreatic enzymes owing to stress levels
- Poor availability of nutrients (owing to reduced efficiency of bowel bacteria as a result of antibiotic use or ingesting food preservatives/ additives)
- Poor absorption at a cellular level owing to pharmaceutical-grade nutrients
- Increased excretions of minerals owing to the use of medications and drugs
- Toxic metal and pollutants blocking receptors

Using nutrition to improve your mineral levels

Consider increasing your intake of mineral-rich foods if you have any of the problems mentioned at the beginning of this chapter or if tests have defined a mineral deficiency.

Where to find the most important minerals

Fruits, vegetables and meat can provide us with most of the trace minerals that we need for good health. The major or trace minerals that have particularly important roles in body function are listed below.

Calcium
Found in most meat, poultry and vegetables, calcium occurs in particularly high levels in nuts and seeds. Just two tablespoonfuls of sesame seeds each day gives more than the required minimum calcium intake. The following are also rich in calcium: almonds, broccoli, halibut, kale, oatmeal, oranges, rhubarb, salmon, spinach and tofu. (The body needs adequate levels of vitamin D in order to properly absorb and use calcium. Try to get at least 30 minutes of sunlight a day, as this helps the body to manufacture vitamin D.)

Chromium
Wheatgerm, chicken, clams and liver all provide high levels of chromium.

Copper
Found in liver, oysters, beans (there is a higher concentration in dried varieties), peas, wholewheat, prunes, offal (organ meats), shrimp and most other seafood, copper is the third most abundant trace mineral in the body after zinc and selenium.

DAIRY PRODUCE

Despite prominent advertising, milk is not a good source of calcium. Our body needs to produce stomach acid and certain digestive enzymes in order to absorb nutrients from cow and dairy produce. Although humans frequently achieve high blood calcium levels, it is more often deposited in general tissue, rather than in bones and teeth or muscles, where we need it most.

Iodine
Fresh fish (haddock in particular) has reasonable iodine content. Iodine is also found in cheddar cheese, eggs, fish and crustaceans, kelp, seaweed and non-refined sea salt.

Iron
The best natural sources of iron are offal, meat and egg yolks. For vegetarians, bran and wheatgerm are good sources as are the better-known vegetable sources such as spinach, broccoli, kale, leafy green vegetables, cabbage, asparagus, beetroot and capsicum. Dried peaches, most nuts, legumes, oatmeal, dates, almonds, and fresh orange juice contain quite high levels. Herbs and spices such as thyme, rosemary, cinnamon and the Indian spice combination garam masala are rich in iron.

Magnesium
Dark green vegetables, bananas, nuts (especially almonds), figs and seeds of all sorts are good sources of this mineral. Magnesium is a main component in muscle and is therefore found in meats.

Manganese
Manganese is found in wholegrain cereals, nuts, green leafy vegetables and particularly peas.

Molybdenum
The best sources of molybdenum are pulses and legumes, but this mineral also occurs in whole grains and dark green, leafy vegetables.

Medication/drug	Nutrient deficiency
Alcohol	Vitamins A, B1, B2, B15, biotin, choline, niacin, folic acid; magnesium
Antacids	Vitamins A and B-complex
Antibiotics in general	Vitamin B12; essential fatty acids
Anticoagulants	Vitamins A and K
Antihistamines	Vitamin C
Aspirin	Vitamins A, B-complex, folic acid and C; calcium, potassium, Co-Q10 and iron
Diabetic drugs (including insulin)	Vitamin B12
Diethylstilbestrol (in the contraceptive pill)	Vitamin B6
Diuretics	Vitamin B-complex; potassium, magnesium and zinc
Flourides	Vitamin C
Gout drugs	Beta carotene, vitamin B12; potassium
Indomethacin	Vitamins B1 and C
Isoniazid	Vitamin B6
Laxatives	All vitamins and minerals
Methotrexate	Folic acid
Nitrofurantoin	Folic acid
Non-steroidal anti-inflammatory drugs (NSAIDs)	Folic acid; iron
Oral contraceptives	Vitamins B2, B6, B12, folic acid, C and E; magnesium and zinc
Penicillamine	Vitamin B6
Penicillin	Vitamins B6, niacin and K
Phenytoin	Folic acid and vitamin D
Prednisone	Vitamins B6, D and C; potassium and zinc
Pyrimethamine	Folic acid
Sulfonamides	Vitamins B2, folic acid and K
Tetracyclines	Vitamin K; calcium, magnesium and iron
Tobacco	Vitamins B1, folic acid and C
Topical and systemic steroids	Vitamins B12, folic acid and K

Toxic element	Element antagonistic to uptake/retention/accumulation
Aluminium	Iron, calcium and vitamin C
Antimony	Magnesium, selenium and methionine
Arsenic	Selenium and iodine
Cadmium	Zinc, calcium, magnesium and copper
Lead	Calcium, zinc and phytates
Mercury	Selenium
Nickel	Manganese, zinc and copper
Thallium	Potassium and selenium
Tin zinc	Iron and copper
Uranium	Calcium and iron

Potassium
The best natural sources of potassium are citrus fruits, apricots, cantaloupe melon, currants, sultanas, raisins, figs, most nuts, bran, sardines and pilchards. Rosé veal, tomatoes, all green, leafy vegetables, bananas, potato skins and water cress make this a difficult mineral to avoid!

Selenium
Found in meat, fish and offal, selenium occurs in particularly high levels in Brazil nuts. You should avoid eating more than four or five Brazil nuts on any one day. Selenium also occurs in wholewheat foods, but levels vary depending on the soil in which the wheat is grown.

Zinc
Zinc can be found in meat, seafood, whole grains (particularly wheat and wheatgerm), eggs and pumpkin seeds.

Avoiding mineral depletion

There are a number of mineral deficiencies associated with specific drugs. For example, diuretic drugs prescribed to adjust levels of sodium and potassium in the body (for example, in the treatment of hypertension) also cause the loss of large amounts of magnesium (in the urine, via the kidneys). Alcoholic and caffeine-containing drinks also have a diuretic effect and therefore encourage mineral depletion. High levels of insulin, injected by Type-I diabetics or by obese people with reduced insulin resistance, also eliminate magnesium. I list a few more deficiencies associated with specific drugs below, but you can find a more comprehensive list and a fuller explanation of the causes and effects in *Drug Muggers* by Suzy Cohen.[1]

In addition to losing minderals, we are also at risk of having mineral intake blocked. Toxic metals block the receptors for specific minerals, preventing absorption. These toxic elements are found more and more in our environment, food chain, water supply and polluted air.

Osteoporosis and osteopenia

Osteoporosis is the medical term for bones that have demineralized (predominantly losing calcium, but also losing other minerals), thereby increasing the risk of fracture. *Osteopenia* is the term given to a bone that is less dense than expected for its age, but is not yet at a risk of fracture.

Many factors increase risk of osteoporotic fractures. These include:
- genetics and heredity – a parent who has had a fracture; being small or too thin;
- being Caucasian or Asian, as opposed to of African descent;
- obesity;
- diseases such as diabetes;
- deficiency in vitamin D, and calcium and other minerals;
- low levels of thyroid hormone and the sex hormones;
- smoking;
- previous trauma;
- lack of balance and neurological disease;
- sight issues leading to increased risk of falls;
- certain medications.

Life expectancy

The average life expectancy after a hip fracture is under six years for both men and women although men fare slightly worse. The range is from 1.5 years to about 11 years.[2] This is partly because of a drop in time spent exercising, which itself is partly a result of fear of falling. Depression from isolation contributes if people are fearful of venturing outside. Not being exposed to the sun leads to vitamin-D deficiency, and this is a major factor in

OSTEOPOROSIS FACTS AND FIGURES

- Three million people have osteoporosis in the UK. This results in 230,000 fractures each year. There are 10 million osteoporotics in the USA.[3]
- In the USA, 45 per cent of post-menopausal women have low bone density.
- Although predominantly 70 per cent of people with osteoporosis/osteopenia are women, these are not conditions that men escape. Over the age of 50, there is a 5- to 8-fold increased risk for all-cause mortality during the first three months after hip fracture and mortality persists over time for both women and men.[4]
- The lifetime risk of a fracture of the hip, spine or forearm is 40 per cent in Caucasian women and 30 per cent in Caucasian men. African-Americans have fewer fractures than many other races.
- There is a higher risk of hip fracture if:
    - your parents had a fracture;
    - you use steroids;
    - you smoke;
    - you have a high intake of alcohol;
    - you have rheumatoid arthritis.[5]
- Hip fractures in women leap up from 250 per 100,000 women at the age of 70 to 2,500 per 100,000 women at the age of 85.[6]
- Vertebral fractures tend to rise more slowly after the age of around 75.

mortality rates as the ability of your bones to absorb calcium depends upon good levels of vitamin D. Osteoporosis is yet another sign of poor mineral absorption, which this chapter has highlighted as an influence in so many other areas of health.

Investigations and tests for bone health

Unfortunately, diagnosis of osteoporosis is often made only after a fall leads to a fracture and X-rays indicate that the bone is thin. However, with earlier testing you can minimize the risk of experiencing a break.

Urinary free deoxypyridinoline (DPD)

The most easily available and common test for osteoporosis is the urine test known as DPD urinalysis. DPD increases in the urine when bone is breaking down more quickly than it is able to be built up. There is strong evidence that this sort of testing, especially if combined with bone mineral density (BMD) scanning (*see* below), can predict risk of fracture even in premenopausal women.[7]

Osteogenomic profiling

There are now investigations, known as genomic tests, based on cheek-cell sampling. Through an analysis of gene makeup these can indicate who might be at genetic risk of osteoporosis and what dietetic, environmental and lifestyle changes might help each individual keep osteoporosis at bay. Osteogenomic test results need to be interpreted by a doctor in light of the individual patient and their medical and family history.

Bone mineral density (BMD) scanning

Regular X-rays cannot actually assess bone mineral density in a quantative way. Rather, a specialized low-dose X-ray, known as dual-energy X-ray

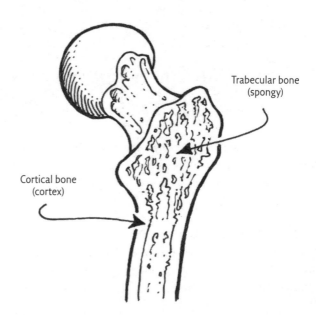

Figure 3: **Cross-section of a bone**

absorptiometry (DXA), previously known as a DEXA scan or quantitative ultrasound (QUS), show how dense bone really is.

Considered the gold standard in identifying fracture risk, through only low-dose radiation the DXA test also has good precision and accuracy. Two X-ray beams of different low intensity are aimed usually at the top of the femur (leg bone), at the hip and also at the lower spine (lumbar) vertebrae. The computer takes into account the tissue density of the leg and determines the density of the bone from the amount of X-ray that the bone absorbs. The results are compared to the expected density for a healthy individual of the same age.

DXA is the most widely used and most thoroughly studied bone-density technology. Statistically, 68 per cent of repeat scans fall within what is known as one-standard deviation, which can be the difference between normality, osteopenia or osteoporosis. Scanning machines vary from centre to centre, and even within the same centre the same machine may show a marked variation on the same patient. We also know that exercise increases bone density and so having a DXA scan performed after, say, a 3–5 km (5–8 mile) walk could lead to variability and influence accuracy.

One major disadvantage of DXA is that it does not differentiate between cortical (outer) and trabecular (inner) bone, so a thin and therefore weak inner bone may be hidden by a thicker, less structurally supportive outer. Also, previously fractured bone or spinal deformities (showing up in a spine scan) may give inaccurate results.

The QUS has the advantage of being portable, is low cost and results in no radiation exposure. It is useful as a fracture risk assessment tool and to screen for osteoporosis. However, changes in bone mass density of the heel (the area generally measured) revealed by QUS may not reflect changes in BMD at the spine or hip, although there is some evidence to the contrary.[8]

QUS, in addition to BMD evaluation by DXA, may give a better estimate of fracture risk than DXA scanning alone.[9]

There are other techniques performed in specialist centres, such as:
- single photon absorptiometry (SPA);
- quantitative computed tomography (QCT);
- radiographic absorptiometry (RA).

According to Ann Larkin, Physicist at St James's Hospital, Dublin, these techniques are less precise than DXA, tend to be more expensive and deliver a larger radiation exposure.[10]

OTHER TESTS

There are a number of blood tests that indicate increased bone 'turnover' or loss. This summary list of bone formation markers would be considered by your doctor:

- Serum total alkaline phosphatise
- Serum bone-specific alkaline phosphatise
- Serum osteocalcin
- Serum type 1 procollagen (C-terminal/N-terminal)
- Urinary hydroxyproline
- Urinary total pyridinoline (PYD)
- Urinary collagen type 1 cross-linked N-telopeptide (NTX)
- Urinary or serum collagen type 1 cross-linked C-telopeptide (CTX)
- Bone sialoprotein (BSP)
- Tartrate-resistant acid phosphatase 5b

Treatment

CONVENTIONAL MEDICINE

Conventional treatment principally uses drugs known as biphosphonates. These are often given in combination with pharmaceutical-grade calcium and vitamin D.

Some doctors recommend special hormone replacement therapy drugs, called selective oestrogen receptor modulators (SERMs). These have been shown to pinpoint their activity on bones (as opposed to other tissues where HRT may have an influence, such as the tissues of the breast, skin, ovaries, and so on). The mineral strontium is also used in certain pharmaceutical drugs, as this can help rebuild bone.

All of these medications, unfortunately, have potential side effects. In the case of the biphosphonates, these can be serious – particularly the development of jawbone necrosis (death of tissue).[11] Nor are biphosphonates popular with dentists or women (statistically, women seem not to take the optimum amount of these drugs).[12] I doubt that biphosphonates will continue to be widely prescribed as more information comes to light about other potential risks. Among those other side effects are stomach ulcers, atrial fibrillation and fractures in unusual sites.[13]

Despite all the potential dangers, the approach in conventional medicine appears to be that the potential benefits of taking medication to improve bone density far outweighs the risks. I personally recommend the use of biphosphonates only as a last resort when other options are failing.

VITAMINS AND MINERALS

Calcium

Although it seems obvious that taking a pharmaceutical calcium supplement could improve osteoporotic conditions, the situation is not that straight-forward. Calcium binds to phosphates in the bone. If our blood calcium levels become too high as a result of supplementation, the body will try to draw calcium out of the body. The calcium that we lose may therefore take phosphates with it, weaking the bone and potentially worsening an osteo-porotic situation. More worryingly, calcium carbonate, the usual form of conventional supplementation, has been shown to increase heart attacks.[14]

The situation is better, though, for natural calcium, which is generally a combination of calcium and phosphate molecules. It enters into bones easily because we have evolved receptors for this task. Blood levels aren't artificially high, and the calcium and phosphates can improve bone strength.

A 1,000-kg (157-stone) elephant needs up to 9 g of calcium a day.[15] This generally comes from food such as leaves and bark. Our osteoporotic population (predominantly women over 60) weigh generally one-twentieth of the weight of an elephant and so should aim at 450 mg daily. Doctors generally prescribe between 1,200–2,000 mg daily. Accepting that we are not necessarily metabolizing in the same way as an elephant, it still seems odd that the bones of an elephant apparently require proportionately far less calcium dosage than that of a woman. Perhaps calcium supplements do not get to the bones?

Vitamin D

Healthy bones need vitamin D. Although our vitamin-D receptors appear to receive natural food sources of vitamin D well (they may not receive pharmaceutical-grade vitamin D), the best source is via sunlight. Vitamin-D deficiency has become more widespead since we have become more worried about spending time with our skin in the sun. While it is essential to ensure that the skin does not turn pink, redden or burn, it is important to expose the skin safely to the sun as much as possible. Note that osteoporosis demands levels of 2000iu or more vitamin D every day – dosages of pharmaceutical supplements are often well below this level.

Vitamin K

Bone assimilation requires vitamin K as well as certain amino acids (proteins) that we need to make the mesh upon which calcium, boron, strontium and other required minerals sit.

BIOIDENTICAL HORMONE REPLACEMENT THERAPY

Oestrogen is considered by many to stabilize bone density, while progesterone actually promotes bone regrowth.[16] As women go through menopause, levels of oestrogen and progesterone fall. The orthodox medical world is able to produce oestrogens from pharmaceutical sources that are accepted by the body without too many side effects and risks. The same cannot be said for artificial progesterone, which is not well tolerated at high doses. Therefore, artificial oestrogen is often prescribed as a treatment for osteoporosis, but progesterone is not.

Natural progesterone from the wild yam may be of benefit, but has to be prescribed by a physician or herbalist. Taken in pill form, it generally does not work as it gets destroyed in the stomach acid and needs to be taken transdermally (through the skin). However, one authority, Dr Ellen Grant, considers any form of progesterone to be potentially dangerous,[17] and as we are now aware of progesterone-sensitive tumours, we need to try to keep up to date with all pieces of new research.

Artificial oestrogens can interfere with oestrogen receptors on the bone and work in the opposite way to that intended by pharmaceutical-grade HRT and our own naturally produced oestrogen. With so many women taking the contraceptive pill, exposure to harmful oestrogens is higher than ever before for all of us because they are urinated into our water supply. Furthermore, many industrial processes also release harmful artificial oestrogens not only into the water supply but into our food (through the soil) and into the atmosphere. One of the worst sources of oestrogens is heated plastics. Therefore, tap water (unless travelling through a reverse osmosis purifier) and water contained in hot plastic bottles provide small doses of potentially harmful oestrogens that can accumulate in the body and may increase our risks of developing osteoporosis.

Some researchers suggest that the highest levels of osteoporosis are found in developed countries where greater numbers of the population drink cows' milk, thus unwittingly ingesting more oestrogens.[18] This may be a result of the pasteurization process rather than the milk itself. Pasteurization (and homogenization) break down protein, change the chemical structure of nutrients in the milk and make fats rancid; they are also able to form free radicals, which are harmful.[19]

Fat tissue makes oestrogens, and thinner post-menopausal women have a slightly higher tendency toward osteoporosis than those with a certain amount of fat. One of the most important ways to increase bone density is to undertake weight-bearing exercise. Walking – ideally around 30 minutes

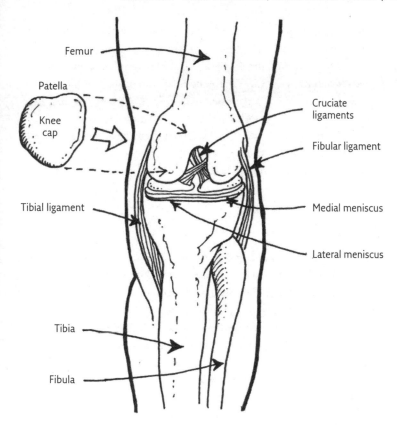

Figure 4: **The knee joint**

Joints are fluid-filled areas of cartilage-covered bone where flexion and extension occur. Joints themselves are dependent upon muscles straddling the joint to allow movement and upon ligaments joining bone to bone.

a day – is all that you need to do, although if you are very keen, you can wear a backpack weighing 5–10 kg (11–22 lb) placed as high up your back as possible to enhance the positive effects.

RECOMMENDED SUPPLEMENTATION

As well as the joint and bone formulae that contain the main minerals and vitamins essential to bone, health consider taking the following specific supplements:

- *Spring horsetail* – the aerial part of the spring horsetail plant (*Equisetum arvense*) is a rich, natural source of silica. For the best effects, take it with specific marine oil extract and flavinoids to enhance a better cell-membrane penetration.

- *Amino acids* – found in whey or other natural products, amino acids help build structures in the body. However, stay away from the artificial pharmaceutically produced powders.
- *Vitamin D* – consider taking up to 10,000 iu under the supervision of a physician. This strength is much higher than supplements you can buy over the counter.
- *Vitamin K* – women should take around 90 mcg and men up to 120 mcg daily.

Arthritis

Medically defined as the inflammation of a joint, arthritis is divided into acute and chronic, depending upon the longevity of the discomfort. Arthritic pain may be a dull ache or a sharp and severe pain. The joints may be inflamed and deformed or show no external changes at all. Rheumatoid arthritis and osteoarthritis are the most common forms.

Rheumatoid arthritis (RA) is an autoimmune disease in which the body attacks its own joints (I touch upon possible causes and treatment in Chapter 9) and is not strictly an age-related disease.

Osteoarthritis (OA) is commonly down to the ageing process and is created by wear and tear on joints. All joints will have evidence of osteoarthritis as we age and will show some stiffness, usually owing to wear and tear on our ligaments and tendons rather than any underlying problem in the joints themselves. OA is more common among those individuals who have led particularly sporting and active lives because high activity levels cause more impact on the joints and so more repeated small injuries. OA can therefore occur at a young age in sportsmen and -women.

Arthritis is less common in women who wear gold. It appears that gold blocks the release of the inflammatory molecule HMGB1, which is released from the nucleus of cells and has a particular sensitivity in joints.[20] Studies have also shown that smoking worsens arthritis – yet another reason to quit!

Investigations and tests

Diagnosis of arthritis often requires:

Radiological investigation – to confirm the condition and also gauge the severity. You may also want to consider these tests:

- *Measuring serum and red cell copper levels*
- *ALCAT food-sensitivity testing*
- *FACT food-allergy testing*

Acute arthritis

Acute (short-term) arthritic conditions are triggered by viral and bacterial infections, as well as invasion by other pathogens. Certain drugs and injuries can all cause an acute attack, too. To ease the symptoms, try the following.

- To reduce the inflammation temporarily without influencing the healing ability of the body, wrap some ice in a flannel and apply it to the affected area. If ice does not ease the discomfort, try a heated application instead.
- As a general rule, rest the joint until there is a marked improvement.
- Acupuncture can be instantly relieving.
- Try homoeopathic remedies, including arnica, if the joint is better for resting (you could apply warm applications of water with arnica fluid extract), or *Rhus toxicodendron* if the joint feels better when you move it around.
- Apply an arnica cream to the affected joint several times a day.
- Try painkillers with low anti-inflammatory effects, such as paracetamol and acetominophen, to reduce the pain. If this and the naturopathic recommendations are not working, consider using anti-inflammatories (*see* below).
- If the discomfort persists, visit a complementary practitioner with knowledge of osteopathy or chiropractic.
- Avoid anti-inflammatories and cortisone injections until all else fails. These remove pain, but allow movement, which, in turn, can increase damage in the joint. Anti-inflammatory treatment can also prevent healing from taking place.

Chronic arthritis

Chronic arthritis is when the pain in the joint or joints persists for more than three months. The causes can be loosely divided into: persistence of injury or infection, RA, other autoimmune diseases and OA. In addition, food allergies or intolerances may also cause chronic arthritis – make sure your doctor tests you for them.

GENERAL TREATMENT ADVICE FOR OA

- Try wearing a copper bracelet if you have low levels of copper in your bloodstream. Your doctor can arrange a test to find your levels.

Copper supplements can help, too.
- Wear gold jewellery where it will make good contact with your skin (such as a ring or a tight bangle).
- Try reflexology, especially in conjunction with massage.
- Try yoga and qigong, which can provide relief from pain, while tai chi has been shown to relieve the symptoms of arthritis, especially in the winter months.

NUTRITIONAL ADVICE FOR OA
- Chicken cartilage is a Russian folk treatment. The cartilage from a chicken carcass should be eaten once a day. This includes the mobile part of the breastbone and the cartilage of the wing and leg joints. There is currently no preparation of this, so approach a friendly butcher or chicken farmer.
- An avocado a day (juiced or eaten whole) may protect your bones.

SUPPLEMENTS
Consider discussing with a nutritional expert the following safe dosages of nutrients:
- *Selenium* – at least 100 mcg each day
- *Vitamin C* – 1 g taken 2–3 times a day
- *Vitamin E* – 200 mg taken 1–2 times a day
- *Evening primrose oil* – 1–2 g taken with every meal
- *Vitamins B5 and B3* – 25 mg per day taken well away from bedtime (if you take them shortly before you go to bed, they may disturb your sleep)
- *Carnosine* – taken according to the packet instructions

HOMOEOPATHIC TREATMENT
A homoeopath is likely to recommend the following remedies:
- *Rhus toxicodendron*
- *Bryonia*
- *Apis*
- *Pulsatilla*

NATURAL EXTRACTS
- *Rosemary and chamomile essential oils* – add six drops of each to a bath or apply directly to the skin if mixed into almond oil.
- *Sesame oil* – rub this oil into the skin around the sore joints.

Adding cayenne or ginger may make it even more effective.
- *Aphanizomenon flos-aquae* – a form of blue-green algae, this treatment may enhance stem-cell activity, helping repair damaged tissue.
- *Green-lipped mussel extract* – take 100 mg twice daily.
- *Collagen* supplementation – ask a qualified naturopath to advise you on products that get past the stomach acid and digestive processes.
- *Glucosamine sulphate* – take 500 mg with each meal.
- *Chondroitin sulphate* – take 500 mg with each meal. Do not use chondroitin if you are at risk of prostate cancer.
- *Methyl-sulphonylmethane (MSM)* – this potent antioxidant and high-sulphur-containing compound has been shown to be beneficial in arthritis.

ORTHODOX TREATMENT
- Alongside naturopathic treatment, use painkillers with low anti-inflammatory effects (such as paracetamol and acetaminophen) to ease any pain.
- *Regeneresen* – keep an eye out for this anti-ageing 'designer drug'. It is extracted from placenta, pancreas, testes and other tissues and may stimulate protein biosynthesis in degenerative conditions.
- *Stem-cell therapy* – keep an eye on the development of stem-cell therapy in the treatment of arthritis, too.
- Avoid anti-inflammatory drugs as much as possible and use cortisone injections only when all else fails. The problem is that these remedies ease the pain, but allow movement, which can increase the damage. Anti-inflammatory treatment can actually delay healing.

Gout

When crystals of uric acid form within joint fluid, the joint itself suffers damage and becomes inflamed. This is gout, a painful disease that affects men more than women and generally appears after the age of 40. If you have a high-protein diet or drink excessive amounts of alcohol, uric acid can accumulate in the blood. Gout is also associated with a genetic inability to deal with proteins through other metabolic pathways and to remove uric acid from the system. Moreover, there are links with excess sugar in the diet, obesity, blood-pressure medication (diuretics) and anything that damages the kidneys.

Treatment for gout

NUTRITION

- *Avoid certain foods.* Restrict your intake of animal protein, particularly from meat but also from fish and fowl. Go vegetarian as much as possible. Avoid refined carbohydrates and artificial sweeteners, as these seem to have some correlation with gout – perhaps through the control of sugar levels. Sardines, mussels, anchovies, asparagus and alcohol are all high in uric acid or inhibit the removal of it – so avoid these, too.
- *Eat the following foods*, which may inhibit xanthine oxidase, an enzyme involved with the formation of gout: beetroot, celery seeds, cherries – 250 g (8 oz) per day if having an attack – blackcurrants, bilberries (blueberries), carrots, goat's milk, live yoghurt.

SUPPLEMENTATION

- *Anthocyanidin and pro-anthocyanadins* – these are found in bilberries (blueberries) and cherries.
- *Multivitamin/Mineral supplements* – take these in high doses with added antioxidants.
- *Bromelain* – for its anti-inflammatory effects, take the maximum dosage your doctor recommends.
- *Vitamin C* – you need to discuss the high doses needed with an expert.
- *Folic acid* – taken with vitamin C, this reduces serum uric acid by inhibiting xanthine oxidase activity.

Chapter 6

The Heart and Arteries

Blood is our life source, but without a pump – the heart – to move it around the body, cells would be starved of oxygen and, within a few minutes, would die. Death occurs when the heart permanently stops beating, but faulty or dysfunctional movements within the heart or circulation system can lead to many problems. These are described by the term 'heart failure', differentiating them from 'heart attack' (where the heart stops). If the brain is deprived of oxygen, the white and grey matter starts to dissolve within a few minutes. Blocked arteries prevent blood reaching the organs, and depending on which organs are affected, disease or death may occur within a matter of hours or days. Less dramatically, but no less importantly, age-related conditions such as loss of eyesight through macular degeneration, ageing skin and renal and other organ failure all benefit from keeping the heart healthy and the arteries open.

The structure of circulation

The heart is a four-chambered muscle built for stamina. It will beat more than three billion times in an average lifetime, and while the heart is a common cause of distress as we age and its failure is our most common cause of death, I cannot think of anything a human has ever built that could do something that many times without encountering a lot of problems en route!

The capabilities of the heart and its individual muscle fibres are pre-dominantly down to the high number of mitochondria, the 'batteries' and energy-providers for cell function found within most mammalian cells, and the integrity and efficiency of the muscle cell wall or membrane. The most common cause of mitochondrial and cell-membrane dysfunction is a lack of nutrients and oxygen reaching the cells, so keeping the arteries open needs to be the primary focus when maintaining a healthy heart as we age.

Many of the problems associated with or attributed to the heart (medically referred to as 'cardiac') are really a result of clogged-up arteries, depriving the heart muscle of oxygen and nutrients. The majority of heart attacks, known as myocardial infarction (MI), are really heart artery blockages. Artery blockage is commonly termed coronary artery disease (CAD) or coronary vascular disease (CVD).

The arteries

Understanding the anatomy of the arteries themselves helps us understand the different processes involved in the ageing of arteries.

Arteries are multilayered tubes. They are made up of an outer sheath known as the adventitia, consisting of connective tissue and elastic fibres. This covers a middle layer of muscle called smooth muscle. Smooth muscle is controlled by a part of the nervous system known as the autonomic nervous system (ANS), which is particularly responsive to stress hormones. These muscles lie over more layers of elastic fibres. Lining the artery tube or lumen is the innermost layer, which is known as the endothelium (*see* illustration on page 120).

Endothelium

You might be tempted to think of the inner lining of our arteries as nothing more than a barrier layer such as we might find inside a juice or milk carton. Not so! The endothelium is a very active layer:

1. It allows gases and nutrients to cross the arterial wall from the blood.
2. It produces a multitude of active chemicals, and many metabolic and chemical processes take place within the endothelial cells.
3. It not only has an important function as a barrier, but is involved in aspects of blood clotting and filtering, and has the ability to repair and grow.

The endothelium suffers a constant barrage by the contents of the blood itself. Red and white blood cells are designed not to have sharp edges, so are not a problem, but many much smaller components found in the bloodstream, some of molecular size, can cause damage. This is a rather complex area of biochemistry and beyond the scope of this book, but I think it is important to mention this in order to understand how to avoid age-related damage.

Arterial wall muscle

When the heart pumps, it does so to push blood out of its chambers into the pulmonary artery and the aorta (*see* illustration on page 124).

The pulmonary artery transports blood to the lungs to pick up oxygen and release waste carbon dioxide. The aorta receives oxygenated blood to be pushed around the rest of the body. These arteries have to expand to allow the blood to leave the heart. Once the heart has given a beat, it has to relax to allow itself to refill. The pulmonary artery and aorta, now filled, have to contract to push the blood along. It is the contraction of the smooth muscles in the artery wall that does this.

Like all muscles, the more the heart muscles are used, the thicker they grow. If the heart pumps very forcefully for too much of the time, the arteries have to thicken so that they do not rupture, and this can cause a thickening and strengthening of the arterial muscles. When we are stressed, we produce adrenalin and other stress-coping hormones, known as catecholamines, which are designed to increase strength and tension within muscles. These catecholamines also cause the heart to beat faster and more strongly, and the overall combination increases the tension in the arterial muscles.

THE MAIN CAUSES OF DEATH

The three leading causes of death in the developed world are:
- heart disease (38 per cent);
- cancer (17 per cent);
- stroke (10 per cent).

According to the British Heart Foundation's figures for the UK in 2012, one in three of all deaths were from cardiovascular disease (CVD) – 180,000 deaths; around one in five male deaths and one in eight female deaths were from coronary heart disease (CHD) – around 82,000 deaths; stroke caused over 49,000 deaths; CHD was the most common cause of death in the under 75s – 45,000 deaths; 17 per cent of premature deaths in men and 8 per cent of premature deaths in women were from CHD – 25,000 premature deaths.

Each year, more than 2 million Americans have a heart attack or stroke, and more than 800,000 of them die. Cardiovascular disease is the leading cause of death in the United States and the largest cause of lower life expectancy among the Black population. Related medical costs and productivity losses approach $450 billion annually, and inflation-adjusted direct medical costs are projected to triple over the next two decades if present trends continue.[1]

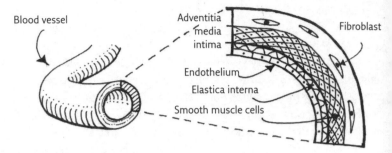

Figure 5: **The lumen**

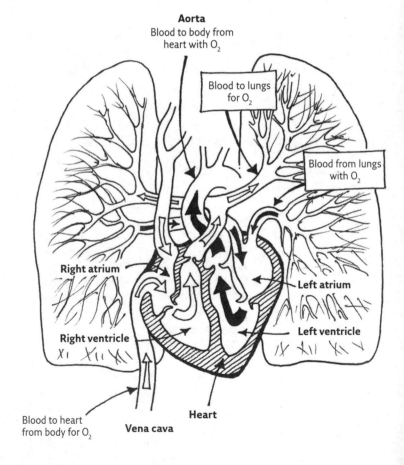

Figure 6: **The heart and lungs**

There are several other factors that add to arterial tension, but two of the more important ones are all too frequently found in the 'developed world'. The first is nutritional deficiency. Muscles contract under the influence of calcium and relax as a response to magnesium. There are many other vitamins and minerals involved in the heart's work, but these two are the most important. Calcium is abundant in our diet, whereas magnesium is not, because levels of it have fallen in overfarmed soil. Furthermore, magnesium is not easily absorbed nor is it easily taken into cells, whereas calcium seems to have an easier passage. As a result of a magnesium-deficient diet, there is a tendency for muscles to over-contract. Unopposed constriction of arteries causes high blood pressure.

The second factor is the build-up of calcium, fats, cholesterol and other blood components in the lining and wall of damaged arteries (known as atherosclerosis or arteriosclerosis). The occlusive material that builds up is called atheroma. Although our natural healing processes can remove atheroma, it is nonetheless the main cause of stiffening of the arteries, which, in turn, reduces the heart's supply of vital vitamins and minerals.

So, all these different physiological and pathological processes lead to changes that stiffen, harden and block our arteries. The heart loses its oxygen and nutritional supply, and if we are going to help avoid this, we need to focus on the main areas of maintaining health.

Blood components

Cholesterol

Let me start with an explanation of what cholesterol is and highlight some myths and misunderstandings.

Cholesterol is a molecule that is created when carbohydrate is converted into fats – a process that occurs mainly in the liver. This accounts for over 90 per cent of the cholesterol we find in the body, with the diet contributing less than 10 per cent. Importantly, this explains why fat in the diet plays only a small part in the provision of blood cholesterol levels.

A vital component in nearly every cell wall and membrane, cholesterol is an essential building block because without it, our cells would have no structural stability. It is also the starting point for many of our essential hormones. Crucially, there is no such thing as 'good' or 'bad' cholesterol.

Low-density lipoprotein (LDL) molecules are protein and fat complexes that transport a variety of useful nutrients around the body, including coenzyme Q10, vitamin E and beta-carotene, all of which are good for us, as well as acting as one of the transport mechanisms for cholesterol. LDL molecules are much larger than the smaller, high-density lipoprotein (HDL) molecules. To complicate matters further, there are also very low-density lipoproteins (VLDL), which have an even greater association with heart and arterial disease than LDLs.

Cholesterol itself is a good thing. The protein/fat molecules – the lipoproteins carrying cholesterol around – are neither good nor bad; they are just doing their job. Unfortunately, the larger molecules, VLDL and LDL, tend to be stickier and have a greater tendency to stick to damaged endothelium. However, these are, in effect, the molecules most responsible for repairing our systems. Unfortunately, being large and sticky, other things in the blood (such as calcium, cells involved in clotting and proteins) cling to them, causing the arteries to clog up more quickly. So, rather than blaming cholesterol or the LDL carriers, we need to focus on what is causing damage to the endothelium.

To get things into perspective, let me highlight two facts:
- More people who have died from heart disease had low cholesterol than high cholesterol.
- Most people who have a heart attack have an average cholesterol level.

STATINS – CHOLESTEROL-LOWERING DRUGS

In 2010, statistical analysis of studies into the life-lengthening effects of statins for those with high cholesterol showed that taking these cholesterol-lowering drugs had little effect on longevity at all – even in people whose cholesterol levels were thought to be dangerously high. Overall, it would appear that if you have cardiovascular disease and you are a male between the ages of 40 and 60, taking statins for 30 years may give you only a nine-month lenghtening of life. Statins appear to have no effect on the lifespan of women whatsoever.

This is highly controversial stuff, but considering what statins might do to other parts of the body, it may be worth listening to the experts that are sceptical about the benefits of taking these drugs!

Statins have the following effects:
- Statins lower LDL cholesterol, but may act on arterial health in other ways.
- Statins have a similar molecular shape in parts to vitamin D, which means that they influence vitamin-D receptors. Although the effects

of this may not all be bad, problems can arise when a vitamin-D receptor becomes blocked altogether. Cholesterol is the starting point for the synthesis of vitamin D.

- Statins block the production of coenzyme Q10.
- Statins cause muscular inflammation (myositis) as one of their recognized side effects. Severe myositis can be fatal if it inflames the heart or respiratory muscles.
- Reducing the body's production of cholesterol as a reslt of taking statins also has many effects:
  * It may influence its production of many hormones, particularly cortisol, testosterone, progesterone and oestrogen, and its ability to repair damaged cell walls and membranes.
  * It may lead to an increase in depression because cholesterol is a major component of the nervous system.
  * It may hinder the breakdown of fats because cholesterol is the building block for the production of bile acids that break down ingested fats in the liver.

I have summarized a topic of considerable controversy, and so I would like to draw everyone's attention to Justin Smith's *$29 Billion Reasons To Lie About Cholesterol* and the associated website (www.29billion.com). This book and the documentary *Statin Nation* expand on my comments above, and I am grateful to Justin for simplifying the matter so well. I would also recommend to those who want more information on cholesterol and statins *The Great Cholesterol Con* by Dr Malcolm Kendrick.[2]

Other blood components involved in arterial health

There are many other factors in the blood that may have equal, if not greater, relevance to arterial disease than cholesterol as they directly damage the endothelium or encourage clots and blockages. One of the most prominent is a protein called *homocysteine*, levels of which rise in the blood when we are deficient in vitamins B6 and B12 and folic acid.

Other components in our blood, such as *fibrinogen*, encourage clotting around damaged arteries. Doctors can measure markers such as highly sensitive c-reactive protein (hs-CRP) in the blood to determine the level of inflammation in the body – the inflammatory chemicals produced outside the arteries may actually damage the arteries' endothelium. I list other relevant markers that may have equal importance for determining choles-terol levels in my section on recommended tests on the following pages.

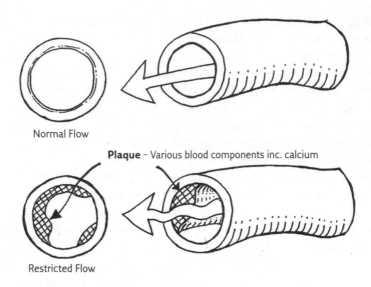

Normal Flow

Plaque – Various blood components inc. calcium

Restricted Flow

Figure 7: **The artery**

Be wary of fats. Many are good, but too many are not. One type found in the blood and generally measured in basic blood tests are triglycerides (TGs). These are made up from ingested and absorbed sugar, not – as many people think – from eating fats. I explain the perils of transfats and saturated fats in Chapter 2, but, in short, neither is good for the heart and arteries.

For the reasons given above, I believe that we need to be a little more sceptical about the importance and attention given to the use of statins.

FREE RADICALS

We have already encountered the term 'free radicals' in Chapter 2, but it is important to understand a little more about them.

Most cell walls have a positive or negative charge on the inside or outside (much like two poles of a magnet). These charges, caused by the active movement of minerals across the cell wall, repel similar charges and attract opposites. To put matters extremely simply, we have evolved to ensure that the charges on cell walls attract things that are good and repel things that are bad.

Free radicals are atoms or molecules that carry a positive charge as a result of losing an electron (electrons are negative particles that should be plentiful enough in number to make the substance that they are associated with neutral – that is, neither positive nor negative).

Lots of different processes produce free radicals. Smoking is a major factor, as are stress hormones. Chemical pollutants, fried foods, minor infections, heavy metals and even over-exercising trigger these damaging molecules.

If free radicals come into contact with negative charges on cell walls, they bind to the cell membrane. Unfortunately, this can cause damage directly to the cell membrane or the DNA in the cells. It is a bit like what would happen if you attached sticky tape to a painted wall: as the free radical is hit by other molecules in the bloodstream, it tears off the smooth endothelial surface, just as the tape would peel off the paint. Once the endothelium is damaged, it needs to be repaired. The body does this by providing its own 'plaster', which includes the sticky LDL cholesterol-carrying molecules.

As long as the right amount of cholesterol is in place and the damage is not too great, the body undertakes a simple repair process that maintains the integrity of the endothelial lining. If free radicals persist in damaging the vessel lining, the body uses more LDL cholesterol to plug the damage. Being 'sticky', the LDL cholesterol attracts other molecules, particularly calcium, which, in turn, can trigger further damage or inflammation. Thus, a cycle is set up allowing an increase in this calcium/cholesterol deposition. It is this that can make the arterial wall potentially brittle. If the build-up grows into the lumen of the artery, it causes occlusion (blockage; *see* diagram on page 124).

Molecules such as those of heavy metals (mercury, lead, aluminium, and so on) can cause direct damage, as can chemical pollutants, food particles that were not successfully broken down in the gut or the liver, and even compounds made up by the body such as uric acid (which can form sharp crystals). These all cause little tears in the endothelium.

Furthermore, any damage to any tissue triggers an immune response, which, consequently, causes inflammation. Then, inflammation encourages the endothelial cells to release other chemicals that further attract the repairing compounds in the bloodstream, such as LDL cholesterol, as well as compounds known as fibroblasts and specialized red blood cells involved in clotting called platelets. These then add to the calcium and cholesterol build-up, further stiffening and occluding the arteries.

What causes the heart and arteries to age?

There are many different conditions that can damage the heart and arteries. We have already seen the damage that toxic molecules and other components in the blood can cause. Other main causes of damage (and therefore ageing) are inflammation, inflexible arteries and nutritional deficiencies.

Inflammation

Many things inflame the endothelium. The most common culprits are smoking and infection (although sugars, stress hormones and free radicals play a part, too).

Smoking not only produces free radicals, but tobacco contains more than 3,000 different chemicals, and we do not fully understand what many of these do. There is evidence of many being carcinogenic (cancer causing), but they do not necessarily damage the arteries. However, heavy metals do, and tobacco contains high levels of cadmium. This, and other chemicals contained in tobacco, either directly or through free-radical activity, create an inflammatory response that the body tries to repair.

There is still lots of research going on into the relationship between infection and arterial disease. Statistics seem to suggest that infection with helicobacter pylori and chlamydia are particularly likely to increase or exacerbate susceptibility to heart conditions.

Helicobacter pylori is the bug commonly found in the stomach and is associated with gastritis and ulcers. Both of these inflammatory conditions increase the risks for stomach and oesophageal cancer. Chlamydia is most commonly thought of as a sexually transmitted disease, although that need not necessarily be the case. It may cause no symptoms whatsoever in most men and women, but its presence can lead to inflammation and scarring of the fallopian tubes, thereby leading to infertility. Quite why these bacteria that appear to live in the stomach and the genital tract influence the heart and arteries is not yet fully understood. Other infections have a direct effect on the heart, including streptococcus ('strep throat', which in rare instances is associated with damage to the arteries). Other infections can cause similar valvular damage.

Inflexible arteries

In the section on the arterial wall muscle, we learned that stress – through the production of catecholamines and stress-coping hormones – can lead to tension in the muscles within the arteries, creating a stiffness that may or may not be transient. Both psychological and physical stress (caused by too much alcohol, drug use, over- or under-exercising, or not enough sleep) all lead to stress responses that tighten the arterial walls. Atheroma causes the arteries to become more brittle and therefore more likely to crack and burst.

Nutritional deficiencies

I discuss the role of nutrition in cardiovascular health more fully later in this chapter. For now, it is enough to say that we know that arterial damage is much more prevalent in people with deficiencies in certain minerals such as magnesium, selenium and zinc; in those with deficiencies in vitamins A, C, E, D; and particularly in those deficient in vitamins B6, B12 and folic acid (owing to the build-up of homocysteine).

Perhaps one of the most important and frequently overlooked nutrients is coenzyme Q10, which is depleted by the use of statins (a drug frequently given to those with heart and arterial disease).

SLOWING DOWN THE AGEING PROCESS IN THE HEART AND ARTERIES

You can maintain the health of your heart, just as you can maintain the health of any body part, and perhaps even reverse cardiac damage, by reviewing your options in the following categories:
- Nutrition and dietetics
- Exercise
- Lifestyle changes
- Supplementation and medication
- Natural therapies

The essential information about maintaining an age-busting diet, exercise regime and lifestyle are covered in Chapters 1 and 2; the following advice is geared specifically toward the health of the heart and arteries.

Eating for a healthy heart

Fruit and vegetables

Research suggests that vegetarians and those whose diet predominantly comprise fresh, organic fruit and vegetables have much lower rates of cardio-vascular disease and therefore less risk of heart attacks, strokes, hypertension and other vascular-associated problems. This is mainly because fruit and

FIVE FOOD FACTS FOR A HEALTHY HEART

1. *One apple or a pear* a day may reduce stroke risk by half.[5]
2. *Beetroot*, probably owing to its high magnesium content but also due to several other, healthy nutrients, decreases blood pressure.[6] (To make your own beetroot juice: blend 2 apples, 2 carrots, ½ lime and 1 beetroot. For a smoothie: blend ½ avocado and add with ice to the juice mixture.)
3. *Peanut butter* (possibly owing to its high potassium levels) is not the evil we think it might be. According to research,[7] taking 5 teaspoonfuls weekly of organic and preferably fresh (unsalted) nut butter appears to have several benefits:
   - A 44 per cent decrease in cardiovascular disease and heart attacks
   - A decrease in sticky LDL cholesterol
   - An increase in endothelial function – so important to the health of the arteries
4. *Green leafy vegetables* contain magnesium and vitamin B-complex. Vitamins B6, B12 and folic acid all reduce the production of the protein known as homocysteine, one of the blood particles that damage the endothelium. Eat plenty of these! (*See* Chapter 2 for sources.)
5. *Citrus fruits are rich in vitamin C.* High blood levels of vitamin C are associated with lower CAD.[8]

vegetables are rich in antioxidants (which neutralize free radicals).[3]

Some of the minerals that are particularly good for the cardiovascular system are calcium, potassium, zinc, copper and selenium. Most healthy, well-balanced diets will provide all these minerals at optimum levels. Foods high in magnesium are especially good for the cardiovascular system. Try to eat some of the following daily: figs, almonds, most other nuts (but not more than four or five Brazil nuts daily to avoid selenium overdose), seeds of all sorts, dark green vegetables, bananas.

Remember that too much of a good thing may be harmful, Natural oestrogens, known as phytoestrogens, are found in many foods and have been cited as being good for the heart and arteries. However, in excess they may increase the risk of stroke. Enjoy, but *do not overdo* the following foods: soya or soya products, celery, peanuts, fennel and hops (including beer).[4]

I want to make a special mention of foods rich in vitamin E. The research around *natural* sources of vitamin E suggests that it reduces heart and artery problems. However, a few studies have suggested that *supplementation with pharmaceutical-grade vitamin E may actually be harmful*. Some Vitamin-E rich foods are: spinach, kale, collard greens, nuts (almonds are very rich in vitamin E), tropical fruits (such as papaya and kiwi), red bell peppers, broccoli, vegetable oils (such as olive oil) and wholewheat (especially wheatgerm).

High-fibre foods

There is plenty of evidence to suggest that having good amounts of fibre in your diet improves the balance and levels of healthy and unhealthy fats, triglycerides and cholesterol levels. Too much of anything is not good for us, but aiming at about 10 g (about 1/2 oz) per day of organic fibre has been shown to increase the beneficial HDL cholesterol.[9] Wheat fibre and oat bran both seem to have benefits, the latter reducing LDL cholesterol.[10]

Proteins

Proteins are good for us – they break down into amino acids, many of which have proven benefits for the cardiovascular system. Beneficial amino acids include: L-carnitine, L-arginine, L-taurine and a much underrated amino acid, L-carnosine, which happens to have the added bonus of being a good antioxidant. The foods containing these in high quantities are listed in the box below, and the recommended protein meals in Chapter 2, if eaten in rotation, will provide adequate levels.

According to many researchers, the Atkins diet – predominantly based on high animal protein intake – proved, paradoxically and contrary to expectations, to benefit cholesterol levels, reduce blood pressure, improve diabetic control and reduce the risk of CVD. The diet has its critics, but I think that a lower intake of carbohydrate as well as the higher intake of

SOURCES OF AMINO ACIDS IN FOOD

- *L-carnitine* is found in beef, pork and dairy. Lower levels occur in peanut butter, avocado, asparagus and wholegrain wheat, as well as in nuts, beans and seeds.
- *L-taurine and L-carnosine* are found in fish, chicken, milk and eggs. Neither are abundant in vegetarian protein sources.
- *L-arginine* is high in seeds and nuts. Sesame and pumpkin seeds are particularly high, as are hazelnuts and almonds.

protein will produce results. Taken with a high dosage of supplements, I think it could be of some benefit to heart health in the short term.

Processed meats are dangerous for the arteries as they release free radicals in the body. Depending on the method of cooking, the additives (mainly colorants and preservatives) cause harm. Eaten daily, processed meats can increase blood pressure and CVD by 42 per cent, and diabetes by 19 per cent.[11]

Contrary to some reports, eggs do not necessarily harm the heart. There is no correlation between blood levels of sticky LDL cholesterol and the consumption of one or two eggs a day.[12]

Fats

Coldwater fish have a high concentration of omega-3 fatty acids, which in balance with the vegetable-based omega-3, -6, -7, -9 and -12 oils offer protection for the arteries. The best sources of fish omega-3 fats are mackerel, herring and salmon, which you should aim to eat once or twice a week. (A restricted intake reduces exposure to heavy metals found in fish from polluted water.) Non-fish sources of healthy fats include flaxseeds (linseeds) and flaxseed oil, seaweed, soya beans, leeks, oat germ and wheatgerm.

Avoid fatty and fried foods, particularly burnt ones (those that are barbecued or over-grilled or -fried) as these build up trans- and saturated fats, which are large, sticky and harmful fat molecules.

Carbohydrates – sugars and 'carbs'

This food group is arguably the most relevant in cardiovascular health. Furthermore, the two most important things to understand when talking about carbohydrates are the glycaemic index (GI) and the fact that refined carbohydrates become artery-damaging cholesterol.

Sugars (which include carbohydrates) tend to be oxidized, causing free-radical production (*see* Chapter 2). Free radicals will damage the heart and arteries both directly and through inflammation of the endothelial lining of the arteries.

LOW GI DIET

The glycaemic index is a given value for every food that indicates the speed with which that food releases sugars into the bloodstream. Foods with a high glycaemic index release sugars quickly, giving a short, unsustained sugar 'hit'. Foods with a low glycaemic index release sugars slowly, sustaining our energy levels for longer and avoiding the energy peaks and troughs that

GOOD AND BAD CARBS

- High GI foods not only mess with our heart and arteries through sugars, inflammation, fat and so on; they also appear to trigger a body stress response, which, in turn, triggers inflammation in the endothelium that can last for hours after ingestion.[13]
- Maple syrup contains antioxidants and other compounds known as phenolic compounds that protect the cardiovascular system. A tablespoonful a day, while clearly in the high GI index range, may help cardiovascular health.[14]
- Chocolate is not always bad for you. Eating 6 g (a small piece) dark organic chocolate per day has been shown to reduce the incidence of heart attack and stroke, as well as lower blood pressure.[15]
- Eating buckwheat may lower cholesterol and inflammation.[16]

often send us reaching for sugary snacks. A low-GI diet focuses on foods that are slow releasing, making it healthier for your heart, arteries and general energy levels. Read this section and stick to the guidelines!

Avoid refined ('white') sugars, which are rapidly built up in the liver into blood fats called triglycerides. (These are large, sticky fat molecules, every bit as harmful as the ingested trans- and saturated fats, and the VLDL and LDL molecules that carry cholesterol.)

Nature provides carbohydrates such as whole grains in a complex with other molecules such as proteins, making them harder to digest. These are known as complex carbohydrates. All carbs are broken down into sugars, but complex carbohydrates slow down this process. Therefore, blood sugar levels do not rise as quickly as they do when we eat simple sugars, which, in turn, slows down the body's production of insulin.

SUCROSE

The most common sugar found in nature, sucrose is what we have on our table as white sugar.

- A high consumption of sucrose can increase the risk of abnormal blood clotting, atherosclerosis and heart disease – potentially leading to heart attack.
- Sucrose may contribute to an increase in blood pressure and may therefore contribute to the development of hypertension.

- A high consumption of sucrose may increase the risk of pre-eclampsia, a form of hypertension that can develop in pregnancy between the twentieth week and the first week after the baby's birth.

Fluids

WATER

Drink plenty of water to avoid dehydration. A lack of water causes cramps and tension in all muscles, including the smooth muscle in the arteries. Aim to drink about 1.5 litres (3 pints) a day (herbal tea also counts). Green tea is beneficial for the heart and arteries and may reduce atherosclerosis.[17]

Maintaining hydration dilutes the concentration of toxins in the bloodstream and free radicals and encourages the kidneys to flush these nasties out of the body.

MILK

There is evidence that the proteins casein, lactalbumin and lactogoleumin contained in milk can trigger allergies, which, in turn, cause inflammation that affects arterial health.

The process of homogenization (which, in effect, sterilizes milk to make it 'safe' for us to drink) leads to the production of a chemical called xanthine oxidase. This chemical destroys a blood compound known as plasminogen and dissolves the fibrinogen fibres that are involved in blood clots which are part of atheroma and the blocking-up of blood vessels.

Our cells do not find it easy to absorb the calcium in milk, which raises the levels of calcium in the bloodstream. This calcium gets caught in the lipoprotein used to repair damaged endothelium and speeds up the formation of atheroma.

Try weaning yourself and your children off cow's milk. Instead, use milk substitutes such as nut milk made from almonds, cashews, hazelnuts and others or rice milk. Soya milk is potentially good, but too much soya milk may cause problems (for the arteries, bowel and thyroid). Up to about 225 ml (½ pint) daily should be fine.

THE PROS OF ALTERNATIVE MILK PRODUCTS AND YOGURT

- Soya and milk protein supplementation may lower serum lipid levels.[18]
- Probiotics found in live yoghurt lower LDL and cholesterol levels.[19]

ALCOHOL

Most people gain no cardiovascular benefit from alcohol. This differs from much of the information in the popular press.

The bottom line is that one or two units of alcohol per day reduce the rate of CHD.[20] Two units per day have been shown to reduce stroke as well.[21]

Red wine in particular comes in for some good press. A bottle a week has been shown to reduce the incidence of heart disease, although one author suggests you should drink *to* the health of your heart, not *for* it![22]

There is quite a lot of talk about the benefits of a compound found in red grape skin known as resveratrol. Its presence in wine has been highlighted as being the component in red wine that actively benefits the cardiovascular system.

However, you would need to drink 170 litres (359 pints) of red wine *per day* to get near the resveratrol levels that have been found to be of benefit! Take the concentrated, high-dose supplement instead.

Too much alcohol will lead to hypertension and the introduction of too much sugar, which once processed by the body encourages insulin resistance and inflammation – so make sure you stick to the limits.

COFFEE

There are mixed messages about coffee both in the press and in scientific circles generally. Some authorities cast it is a drink of the devil (including myself in my *Encyclopaedia of Family Health*, published in 1999), but I have tempered my view as a result of more recent research. I think the evidence

CAFFEINE

We also now have the complication of having different strengths of coffee available to us. The easy availability and intense caffeine content of 'real' (not instant) coffee means that we may lose track of how much caffeine we are getting with each 'hit'.

Some processes simply wash the beans with hot water that is already full of other coffee bean chemicals, while other techniques convert the caffeine into harmless carbon dioxide. Some processes use chemicals, which, it could be argued, have been poorly studied. Methylene chloride continues to be used despite it having been found to be a cancer-causing agent in the 1980s. It is still used for decaffeinating, but within 'safe limits'. We had better hope the scientists are right.[26]

at the moment suggests that one or two cups of coffee a day reduces stroke risk[23] and that two to three cups a day decreases CVD generally.[24] There is also evidence from the mid-1980s and 1990s to suggest that five or more cups a day is liable to be harmful.[25]

Dr Sharma's Programmes

As stated many times throughout this book, a variety of factors leads to deficiencies in our diet and the draining of nutrients from our system. In the cardiovascular system, free-radical production, environmental pollutants and lifestyle factors such as a lack of exercise, obesity and, in particular, smoking make it difficult to maintain all the nutrients that protect the heart and arteries. There is therefore a real need to take a base level of supplementation and in some cases more. In addition, you will find recommendations for a variety of treatments and remedies.

The following lists cover those nutrients I consider to be necessary as a base line as well as those that can be taken by those who want to increase their 'insurance package' or need more owing to risks or established cardiovascular disease.

Dr Sharma's Maintenance Programme

Consider this a base line package if you want to focus on protecting and improving the health of your heart and arteries. At first glance, this extensive list seems daunting, but remember, many of these nutrients can be found in the same tablet or capsule as multivitamin/mineral complexes.

MINERALS
- *Magnesium* – 500 mg once or twice daily
- *Selenium* –100 mcg nightly
  Or preferably:
- *A multimineral including the magnesium and selenium* – nearly all minerals have some part to play in the cardiovascular system.

VITAMINS
- *B-complex* – one that specifically includes vitamin B6 50 mg, folic acid 400iu and vitamin B12
- *Vitamin E* – 400iu daily[27]
- *Vitamin D* – 1,000iu daily

ESSENTIAL FATTY ACIDS
- *Omega 6* – 800 mg, taken once or twice daily
- *Omega 3* – 200 mg, taken once or twice daily
- Products with a combination ratio of omega 6 to omega 3 at 4:1

AMINO ACIDS
- *Amino acid combination* – a whey extract or a vegetable-based whole amino acid complex at the daily dose recommended on the packaging

OTHER NUTRIENTS
- *Coenzyme Q10* – 30 mg once or twice daily. (A single multivitamin may contain this.)

Dr Sharma's Advanced Programmeme
This programme is for people with symptoms of arterial damage or who have lifestyle or family risk factors. Consider the addition of these supplements after discussion with your healthcare provider.

VITAMINS
- *Vitamin B3* – if borderline hypertensive, 2,000 mg daily. (It might be useful if statins are not used in those with high cholesterol.)
- *Vitamin B12* – have blood tests and suitable intramuscular injections if needed

AMINO ACIDS
- *L-carnosine* – 200 mg daily
- *Aminoguanadine* – consider this if you are borderline diabetic or you have peripheral vascular disease. Discuss your needs with a practitioner who can prescribe this amino acid for you.

FATTY ACIDS
- *Phosphatidylcholine (PPC)* – up to 20 g of PPC (35 g of lecethin) where cholesterol is an issue and where atherosclerosis or arterial plaques are known to have formed

OTHER NUTRIENTS
- *Resveratrol* – 60 mg daily

WAYS TO REDUCE YOUR RISK

- *Magnesium* decreases the risk and incidence of stroke in men and women over the age of 60.[28]
- Meditation decreases heart attack and stroke by 47 per cent.[29]
- *Donating blood every six months*: decreases heart attack and strokes by 57 per cent,[30] decreases cardiac atherosclerotic lesions[31] and decreases blood glucose, triglycerides and fibrinogen. It increases HDL-cholesterol.[32] Donating just one unit of blood only every three years may decrease CV risk by 30 per cent.[33]

Dr Sharma's Repair Programme

This programme is for people with established heart or arterial conditions.

- *Testosterone* – 5–10 mg for a woman and 50–100 mg for a man, taken daily. This needs to be prescribed following tests and monitored by a doctor.

AMINO ACIDS

You can use certain amino acids to ease specific conditions, but see a doctor or a nutritionally trained practitioner to prescribe them:

- *L-acetyl cysteine*
- *L-methionine*
- *L-taurine*
- *L-argenine*
- *L-carnitine*
- *L-glutamine*

HERBAL REMEDIES

Discuss the following two herbal remedies with a senior practitioner or doctor:

- *Hawthorn (Crataegus)* – dosage as prescribed by a practitioner
- *Gingko biloba* – for use in atherosclerosis

OTHER NATURAL OR NON-INVASIVE TREATMENTS

Discuss the following options with a senior practitioner or doctor:

Chelation therapy

This involves the administration of certain compounds, known as chelating agents, to remove heavy metals from the body. Most cardiologists refute its benefits, but there have been many studies using the chelating agents ethylenediaminetetraacetic acid (EDTA) or dimercaptosuccinic acid (DMSA) with positive outcomes in treating atherosclerosis and blocked arteries. Encouragingly, a study completed in March 2013 known as The TACT (Trial To Assess Chelation Therapy) concluded that there was moderately reduced risk of adverse cardiovascular outcomes with chelation and further research is recommended (Gervasio et al, JAMA 2013;309 (12):1241-1250). Although chelation therapy can be taken orally, it is best administered in conjunction with intravenous treatment under specialist supervision.[35]

Enhanced external counter pulsation (EECP)

This widely available treatment, which is provided by specialists, uses three pairs of pneumatic cuffs wrapped around the calves, lower thighs and buttocks. These inflate and deflate in time with the heartbeat. The movement is monitored by electrocardiogram (ECG) signals. Painless and non-invasive, the cuffs rapidly inflate during the heart's resting phase (diastole) when the chambers normally fill with blood. This pushes blood up through the veins toward the lungs providing the heart with more oxygenated blood more quickly. At the pumping phase (systole), the cuffs deflate so that the blood leaves the heart without restriction. The effect is that the machine increases the heart output, but it also pushes blood through

SURGERY AND OTHER INVASIVE PROCEDURES

- About 1.6 million Americans undergo heart bypass surgery, angioplasty or stent procedures annually – even though evidence suggests that these procedures *do not* prolong life or prevent future heart attacks in the majority of patients.
- Roughly one in 25 patients having bypass, and about one in 65 undergoing angioplasty dies from the procedure.
- There is no data to show that the vast majority of patients receive any benefit from coronary artery bypass surgery.
- The three-year survival rate for most patients who have had bypass surgery is almost exactly the same as it is for patients with heart disease who do not have surgery.[34]

the heart arteries. It gives the added benefit that it stimulates the growth of new blood vessels in the heart. The net result is that EECP can help bypass blocked vessels. The treatment is delivered in one-hour sessions once or twice a day for up to 35 sessions, so it requires some commitment, but it can help avoid invasive procedures that may not be as successful as we would be led to believe (*see* 'Direct and Indirect Tests' box on page 143).[36]

Medicinal drugs

Over the last 60 years or so, the development of drugs geared toward cardiovascular disease has had a profound impact on the well-being and longevity of humans that have access to them. Drugs to treat high blood pressure, drugs to reduce fluid volume (diuretics), drugs used when the heart is failing, drugs that help control irregular heartbeats and drugs affecting constriction and dilation have undoubtedly benefited millions of people.

Those of us who work in Integrated Medicine and CAM, as well as individuals who read books such as this, tend to place a negative slant on the use of drugs, which can often be over the top. Drugs have their place.

There are a few fundamental points that doctors, practitioners and patients need to be aware of:

1. Is there an alternative to drug use?
2. What is the least amount that can be prescribed?
3. If a drug is taken, what can be done to negate unwelcome or harmful effects (including, but not limited to, side effects)?

Professional medical practitioners who can prescribe medication will need to deal with the first two issues, but both health professionals and patients can address the third point.

Negating the harmful effects of common drugs

One of the most important areas to consider is how certain drugs interfere with the absorption or processing of specific vitamins and minerals within the body. As a result, we can suffer a deficiency that may influence the cardiovascular system. I list here some of the deficiencies we know that drugs given to patients with cardiovascular issues can cause, as well as drugs that may in some way impinge upon some of the major nutrients involved in the health of the cardiovascular system.

It is wise when taking any of the medications in the table opposite to take supplements that will counterbalance the nutrient deficiencies, especially if you know you have a cardiovascular disease or are at a high risk of developing one.

Certain drugs have been known specifically to create cardiovascular problems, and it is worth noting the following:

- *Selective serotin release inhibitors (SSRIs)* – increase the risk of stroke[37]
- *NSAIDs* – cause heart flutters[38]
- *Aspirin and NSAIDs* – increase stroke and heart attack in those with high blood pressure and concurrent CVD[39]

I have merely scratched the surface here. I am attempting to encourage readers to search for risks and deficiencies that are not necessarily advertised or promoted by the prescribing doctor or the information sheets that come with the drugs.

I am particularly concerned that the drug companies seem to be very keen on the so-called 'magic bullet poly-pill'. The evidence for the benefits of many cardiovascular drugs is presented in statistical form, and so the suggestion is that putting them all together in one pill and providing this to all and sundry will reduce cardiovascular disease. The intention is to provide a pill including:

- aspirin;
- a statin;
- an ACE inhibitor (a blood-pressure drug);
- a beta blocker (a blood-pressure drug); and
- a diuretic (a blood-pressure drug).

This ignores the potential nutrient deficiencies these drugs can cause. The effect of statins on the pathway that makes and provides coenzyme Q10 is particularly worrying, as deficiency in this coenzyme is associated with heart failure. Statins may have benefits that are not just related to cholesterol. These might be owing to the resemblance of the molecular structure of a statin to that of vitamin D. What we do not have are long-term studies to see what happens when statins are influencing vitamin-D receptors, as this vitamin is very much associated with cardiovascular health, diabetes and the immune system's anti-cancer defence.

DRUG TYPE	MINERAL DEFICIENCY	VITAMIN DEFICIENCY	OTHER
Antibiotics	Magnesium and calcium	Vitamin B-complex	
Antidepressants: tricyclics (amatriptolene)			Coenzyme Q10
Blood-pressure medications: ACE inhibitors	Calcium, magnesium and zinc		
Blood-pressure medications: beta blockers			Coenzyme Q10
Blood-pressure medications: calcium channel blockers	Calcium	Vitamin D	
Cholesterol medications: fibrates	Most minerals	Vitamin B-complex	
Diabetes medication		B6, B12 and folic acid	Coenzyme Q10
Diuretics	Calcium, magnesium, potassium, zinc	Vitamin B-complex, vitamin C	
Non-steroidal anti-inflammatory drugs (NSAIDs – including ibuprofen)	Iron	Vitamin C	
Oral contraceptives or hormone replacement therapy	Magnesium, zinc and most minerals	Vitamin B-complex, vitamin C	
Thyroid medication	Calcium and iron		
Statins		Vitamin D	Coenzyme Q10
Valium and other benzodiazepines			Melatonin

Warfarin (coumarin) and alternatives

Doctors often prescribe this drug to thin the blood. Used also as a rat poison, warfarin is not a drug that anyone particularly likes to prescribe, but statistics clearly show (and I trust these!) that those who have irregular heartbeats or a risk of clotting (often including the group of people who have had strokes or are known to have atheroma or arteriosclerosis in the carotid arteries) benefit from taking it. However, warfarin does carry the risk of excessive bleeding and itself can cause strokes and other haemor-rhagic problems.

Doctors involved in non-drug medicine are frequently asked about alternatives. Recently, a fermented-cheese product – Natto kinase – from the Far East, has gained popularity as a treatment for heart problems. Anecdotal studies have shown that eating this cheese regularly could reduce the number of blood clots and associated problems such as stroke. We are still waiting for the conclusions of scientific studies aiming to corroborate or refute the anecdotal findings, but watch this space. Finally, other studies are looking into a new synthetic drugs such as Dabigatran and Apaxaban. Initial studies suggest that these, and others, are as effective as warfarin and may have lower risk of causing haemorrhage – one of the biggest concerns.

Exercise for the cardiovascular system

If you do only one thing to enhance your cardiac well-being, it has to be exercise. I discuss the enormous benefits in Chapter 3 and also discuss the types of exercise you can consider. Here are some facts for you:

- Exercise uses up catecholamines (the stress-causing hormones).
- Exercise releases natural chemicals and hormones that encourage repair of damaged cells.
- Exercise, through several mechanisms, optimizes the strength of the heart and the elasticity of the arteries.
- Exercise increases body temperature, causing us to sweat, which, in turn, removes many harmful chemical compounds (especially water-soluble toxins such as alcohol and its break-down products, as well as many environmental pollutants) from the body.
- Exercise uses up available sugars, particularly those easily absorbed such as the refined sugars, thereby lowering the amount of time they are in the system and capable of causing cell-wall damage through inflammation.
- Exercise increases blood flow to all organs and muscles, the skin and body tissues.

Lifestyle tips for the cardiovascular system

- Avoid drinking too much alcohol, smoking, eating excessively fatty foods and additives and preservatives – thus reducing your exposure to free-radicals.

- For the sake of your heart and arteries (as well as your lungs and skin), *do not smoke.* Cigarettes contain thousands of compounds that act as free radicals. The heat of cigarettes triggers inflammation, and inflammatory compounds produced by the body travel around, potentially triggering damage anywhere in the body. Because they travel around in the blood, they especially affect the arteries.
- Live in the country! Or spend as much time, as often as you can, away from polluted areas. Unfortunately, polluted air increases premature deaths from CVD.[40]
- Keep weight optimal for your height. The more weight you carry, the harder it is for the blood to be pushed through the fat, so the arteries have to strengthen. They do so by enlarging the arterial wall, and this leads to high blood pressure and arterial damage.

The greater your weight, the more chance you have of becoming diabetic. If you are diabetic, more sugars stay at high levels in the bloodstream, leading to inflammatory damage.

Start your day with a large mug of green tea for its protective phenolic compounds and end your day with a couple of squares of 70 per cent cocoa solids chocolate for the same reasons.

Investigations and tests for arterial health

The arteries and the bones are the only structures in the body to have recognized and established tests that indicate chronological age. Calculations can be made on the age of other parts of the body such as the nervous system and muscles, and some gizmos and computer systems claim to be able to give you a 'true age', but I am a little suspicious of such gadgets. What is important to remember is that the ageing of parts of the body is not necessarily irreversible, and changes to lifestyle and diet, as well as to treatments through nutrients, supplements and natural medication can be of great help.

The main theme of this book is to encourage people to find out about their 'oldest part', and so investigations into the health of the arteries and the heart are imperative. I think it is very important to use clinical investigations to establish the health and, where possible, age of different organs. When looking at the cardiovascular system, there are specific indications or risk factors that should encourage an individual to do minimal or advanced testing, depending on the number of risks facing them.

WHY BOTHER WITH TESTING?

According to the Framingham Heart Study, which began in 1948 and continues to monitor the health of thousands of individuals:

- 60 per cent of deaths in men aged 45-75 occur with no prior evidence of CAD.
- 32 per cent of deaths among men aged 20–64 are attributed to CAD, with 25 per cent of those showing no symptoms of heart disease prior to the event.
- 64 per cent of women that die suddenly of heart or artery disease had no previous symptoms.
- 50 per cent of CAD cases are missed by routine 'lipid profile' blood tests.
- 80 per cent of those that have a heart attack have similar cholesterol levels to those who do not.
- 25 per cent of premature heart attacks (below 65 years of age) have elevated LDL-cholesterol alone.

DIRECT AND INDIRECT TESTS

- Measurements of components in the blood are indirect tests that can highlight the potential of a problem: for example, high LDL-cholesterol or hs-CRP is not in itself dangerous, but is an indication of the potential for damage to occur.
- Direct measurements of the heart and arteries, on the other hand, give us a view of how things are structurally or functionally at that precise moment.
- Arteriography is underused and may be better than the current gold standard stress ECG.
- Some of these direct, more accurate tests can be invasive or dangerous in themselves. A radiologically opaque 'dye' may need to be put into the body, or they may require radiation treatment. The dye allows X-rays to capture images of the arteries more accurately, but putting anything into the body runs the risk (albeit very low) of an allergic or toxic reaction, as well as risking introducing infection at the needle puncture site. Less than 1 in 500 of these invasive tests causes a problem, and most of those are minor, but fatalities can occur.
- Magnetic resonance imaging (MRI) is not radiation, although it may utilize invasive procedures. It does not view the heart and arteries quite as accurately (although MRI experts may disagree), and it is, at the moment, a little more expensive than the other tests mentioned.

First-line investigations

We need to differentiate between non-invasive, less expensive and accurate testing and the potentially risky, more expensive invasive investigations.

I feel that everybody over the age of 40 should consider having investigations done. Spotting a problem early can make a profound difference and, as I have said, cardiovascular disease is reversible – therefore, the earlier it is caught, the better the potential outcome.

If test results are returned as normal and there is no obvious risk to the individual, then repeating tests every three to five years can give an indication of the speed of deterioration. If a problem is found, more frequent investigations and early follow-up treatment may help prevent or reverse disease and enhance longevity.

SOME BASIC MEASUREMENTS

1. *Height and weight* are used to calculate body mass index (BMI).
   A person's weight in kilograms is divided by their height in metres squared. It is a simple calculation often used to predict the risk

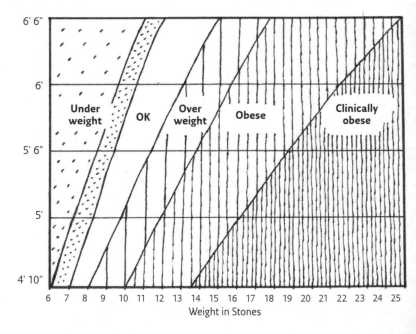

Figure 8: **Body Mass Index**

of cardiovascular disease. However, it is not always the most accurate measure as it does not differentiate between lean body mass (including muscles) and body fat, meaning that people with a particularly muscular body will have relatively high readings (because muscle is heavier than fat).

2. *The waist-to-hip ratio* is a measure of deposition of abdominal fat (central obesity) and used as an important indicator for the so-called metabolic syndrome, a common condition that is associated with insulin resistance (diabetes), high blood fats, hypertension and an increased risk for cardiovascular disease. A waist-to-hip ratio of 0.95–0.90 or less is considered healthy for men and a ratio of 0.85–0.80 or less is considered a sign of good health for women. A reading of 1 or higher signals an increased risk and indicates that some action should be taken.

3. *Blood pressure* is the pressure of the blood against the walls of the arteries. It is always given as two numbers. The higher (systolic) number represents the pressure while the heart contracts to pump blood to the body. The lower (diastolic) number represents the pressure when the heart relaxes between the beats. Blood pressure around 120 over 80 mmHg (millimetres of mercury) is considered optimal for adults.

4. *Heart rate* is the number of heart beats per minute (bpm) when we are at rest. In a healthy individual, it is usually between 60 and 80 beats per minute. The resting heart rate can to an extent indicate your basic fitness level. The better trained your body, the less effort and fewer beats per minute it takes your heart to pump blood to your body at rest. It rises with age or with certain medical conditions.

5. *Peak expiratory flow or peak flow volume* is dependent on an individual's size and age and is one of the important measurements of lung function. It measures how much air a person can exhale during a forced breath and is used to diagnose obstructive conditions such as asthma or chronic obstructive pulmonary disease (COPD).

6. *Chest* expansion is another measurement to assess lung function. The chest expansion measures the difference between inhalation and exhalation around the chest in centimetres.

7. *VO2 Max or other fitness evaluation test.* VO2 Max is a measure of how fit you are and is considered the best indicator of cardio-

respiratory endurance. Fitness can be measured by the volume of oxygen you can consume while exercising at your maximum capacity. VO2 Max is the maximum amount of oxygen in millilitres you can use in one minute per kilogram of body weight. Those who are fit have higher VO2 Max values and can exercise more intensely than those who are not as well conditioned. Calculation of your figure is described in Chapter 3.

The following tables list VO2/kg in ml/min/kg for a range of ages and levels of fitness:[41]	Men				
	20-29	30-39	40-49	50-59	60-69
Low	<38	<34	<30	<25	<21
Somewhat Low	39-43	35-39	31-35	26-31	22-26
Average	44-51	40-47	36-43	32-39	27-35
High	52-56	48-51	44-47	40-43	36-39
Very High	>57	>52	>48	>44	>40

8. *Percentage body fat* is ideally between 15–20 per cent for men and 20–25 per cent for women.

9. *Percentage body water content.* Aim at 60–70 per cent water content on the basic testing equipment.

10. *Vision by eye chart* highlights possible visual difficulties that might represent damage to the retina owing to blood vessel problems.

FIRST-LINE BLOOD AND URINE TESTS
Lipid profile
Your doctor can arrange this minimal cardiovascular profile known as a *lipid profile*. This measures cholesterol levels in your blood and differentiates between HDL and LDL, free fats known as triglycerides – and not much else. Unfortunately, only around 55 per cent of patients carrying cardiovascular risk would be identified through these tests. This percentage increases to around 84 per cent if you routinely undergo the more specific investigations listed in the 'preferable' section.[42]

URINE ANALYSIS

Red blood cells	*negative*	Positive results in any of these can
White blood cells	*negative*	be an indication for certain diseases:
Protein	*negative*	for example urinary tract infections
Bilirubin	*negative*	(nitrates positive +/- blood cells),
Urobilinogen	*negative*	diabetes (glucose positive +/-
Glucose	*negative*	ketones) or certain kidney diseases
Ketones	*negative*	(protein positive +/- blood cells),
Nitrates	*negative*	and so on.
Specific gravity	1.0	normal result
	Urine pH	

Blood glucose test
It is important to ensure that the arteries are protected as well to test for their general health. A blood glucose test can indicate whether or not you have prediabetic status, which can, in turn, lead to damaged arteries.

Urine analysis
This test rules out diabetes and early kidney changes, which can be a first sign of arterial disease (*see* box, above).

OTHER FIRST-LINE TESTS
Arteriograph
This simple-to-use, non-invasive piece of equipment is highly underrated and underutilized and, in my view, considerably more reliable that the commonly used ECG (see following pages). The simplest way to measure arterial stiffness, the marchine is often used by research labs as it gives exactly the right data for pharmaceutical companies as they develop hypertensive (high blood pressure) medication. One of the largest and longest-running studies worldwide, The Framingham Study, has used the arteriograph in its assessment of heart and arterial disease over the last three decades.

The arteriograph can identify:
• the stiffness of arteries;
• the possibility of blockage in large and small arteries;
• the overall efficiency and flexibility of the arteries;
• the fitness of the heart;

ARTERIOGRAPH RESULTS

Results from the arteriograph:
- correlate closely to the most accurate, conventional, invasive test on heart arteries, known as the angiogram;
- closely correlate to the coronary calcium score;
- give 72 per cent correlation to carotid arteriosclerosis. They distinguish between early- and late-stage changes and are thereby able to give an 'age' of the arteries.[43]

- the central blood pressure – a more accurate measurement of risk than the pressure in your arm.

In 2007, there were only about 300 arteriograph machines in use and available to the public throughout Europe; during 2013 in the UK, there were seven in use in research laboratories, but only two available for public use. One, I am pleased to announce, is in my clinic.

The medical community acknowledge arterial stiffness as a sensitive predictor of cardiovascular disease. The arteriograph measures the speed with which the pulse wave flows along an artery and, using simple calculations, gives information on the flexibility of arteries and the probability of the build-up of atheroma (the clogging of arteries) and an accurate assessment of blood pressure in the central main artery of the body, the aorta. It also gives an indication of cardiac fitness.

The arteriograph test itself requires you to lie down and rest for about seven minutes. A nurse places a blood-pressure cuff around your arm and attaches it to a special computer. The nurse measures the length of your aorta (the main artery leaving the heart) using a tape measure from the little notch at the top of your chest (the sternal notch) down to the bone in your pelvis at the bottom of your abdomen (the pubic bone). The whole test takes three to four minutes and within 15 minutes you have a clear picture of the health of your arteries.

Peripheral resistance monitoring
Peripheral resistance is a term used to describe the flexibility and patency (openness) of the very small arterial blood vessels (known as arterioles) and the microscopic blood vessels (known as capillaries) through which oxygen, other gases and nutrients are exchanged with the body tissues. It is all very

well having flexible, bouncy large arteries, but if the small blood vessels are still or blocked, blood (and so nutrients) cannot get to your organs. Unfortunately, diabetes, atheroma and hypertension (high blood pressure) all impact upon the health of the smaller arteries to a greater extent than the health of the larger ones. Of course, an organ or a tissue in the body may have many different blood vessels leading to it, so the occlusions of some may have little impact on that particular organ or tissue. However, areas such as the eyes, brain and kidneys seem to be overly sensitive to the loss of the patency of small blood vessels. Monitoring and keeping an eye on peripheral resistance is exceptionally important.

The test involves various pieces of equipment ranging from small clip-on devices that attach to a finger to more complex pieces of equipment with many leads and straps. The finger clips seem just as accurate at measuring peripheral resistance.

The stress or exercise electrocardiogram (ECG)
The stress ECG is currently the conventional 'gold standard', non-invasive test for arterial health. Unfortunately, like its cousin, the resting ECG, the stress ECG can give fairly inaccurate results and is likely to show that there is something wrong only once disease is well established. For these reasons, I think the arteriogram is a much better testing device – although it is much less widely available.

The stress ECG compares the electrical activity of the heart at rest to the electrical activity of the heart during different forms of exercise to a maximum heart rate of around 80–100 per cent of its resting level. Heart muscle that is either damaged or not receiving enough oxygen as a result of blockages in the coronary arteries will transmit electricity differently to healthy tissue.

However, this test has some drawbacks:
- Although it may be a useful test if you have coronary artery disease (CAD), the stress ECG appears to be accurate only when monitoring the male physiology; its results are not as accurate in women.
- The stress ECG may not show changes until there is obstruction of 70 per cent or more of one of the main coronary arteries. In other words, you may be aged 25, with 69 per cent blockage (markedly abnormal), but the ECG will not show that anything is wrong.
- Even with 70 per cent occlusion, the test will identify abnormality in only about 50 per cent of cases.

- An abnormal stress ECG, potentially highlighting a coronary artery blockage, is not good at predicting a heart attack. Many people who have unexpected heart attacks have had a normal stress ECG results.
- A normal ECG does not rule out CAD. The Coronary Artery Surgery Study (1975–1979) found that in patients struggling with symptoms such as angina (chest pains from a lack of oxygen to the heart) who had blocked arteries shown by special heart X-rays known as angiography, 29 per cent demonstrated a normal resting ECG.[44]

Second-line investigations

This level of testing is for those who want to know more about their current and potential risk status for cardiovascular disease (CVD). I would advise it for people with borderline family history or those who are just outside the optimum levels of fitness or body weight or who are a little wayward with regard to lifestyle.

Lipoprotein A blood test
If a blood test shows high levels of this genetically determined protein, you have an important risk factor for CVD, leading to the need for significant lifestyle changes. Taking garlic capsules may help prevent it contributing to arterial blockages, while supplements of vitamin B3 could lower levels altogether.

Lipoprotein PLA 2 blood test
This is a more sensitive and prognostic indicator than lipoprotein A and tends to be more expensive.

Apolipoprotein B;A1 ratio test
'B' needs to be low. It is genetically predetermined, but, again, lifestyle changes can stop the genes 'expressing' (becoming active).

Homocysteine blood test
Manufactured in the body, this protein is essential to our normal cellular function. However, too much homocysteine can damage the arteries. Homocysteine is found in the pathway that makes glutathione – one of the most important antioxidants manufactured in the body and a crucial component in our detoxification system. A good intake of vitamin B6, B12 and folic acid, as well as pyridoxine 5 phosphate and betaine help to regulate homocysteine levels in the body.

Hs-CRP
This is a measurement of the inflammatory response in the body. Too much inflammation causes inner artery endothelial damage.

Vitamin D blood test
This vitamin protects the health of the arteries. However, more than 50 per cent of the populations in the developed world are deficient, which makes it a useful marker when establishing optimum health for the heart and arteries.

Testosterone test
Low levels of testosterone in men are associated with increased CVD risk.[45] I discuss this more fully in Chapter 8.

8-OHdG test
This is a marker of oxidative stress, which, in turn, is a reflection of free-radical activity. (This test is not in common use.)

Thyroid function test
Low thyroxin levels are associated with a weak heart and the potential for arterial damage. High thyroxin levels apply pressure to the heart, increase blood pressure and can damage arteries.

Helicobacter pylori (HP) test
HP infection is known to contribute to heart and arterial disease. You should definitely consider this test if you suffer from indigestion or reflux or you have a history of stomach inflammation (known as gastritis) or a peptic ulcer. There are several ways to test for HP infection: a blood antibody test, a stool antigen test, a urine test or the carbon urea breath test (which involves drinking ^{14}C- or ^{13}C-labelled urea, which the bacterium metabolizes and produces labelled carbon dioxide that can be detected in the breath). However, none of the test methods are completely failsafe.

Nutritional evaluation
Ideally, this would be a first-line test. If we maintain our nutritional status, we have a much reduced risk of inflicting damage to the heart and arteries. The minerals magnesium, zinc, selenium and chromium and the vitamins B6, B12, C, E and K, as well as folic acid and beta-carotene, are all vital to cardiovascular health. The amino acids taurine, argenine and carmatine are all protective, as are the essential fatty acids in correct balance, but particu-

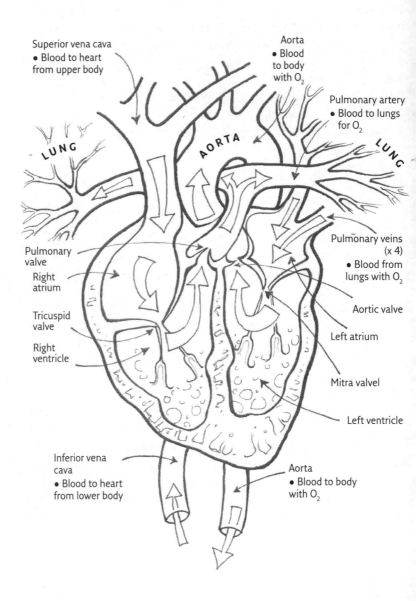

Superior vena cava
• Blood to heart from upper body

Aorta
• Blood to body with O₂

Pulmonary artery
• Blood to lungs for O₂

LUNG

AORTA

LUNG

Pulmonary valve

Right atrium

Tricuspid valve

Right ventricle

Pulmonary veins (x 4)
• Blood from lungs with O₂

Aortic valve

Left atrium

Mitra valvel

Left ventricle

Inferior vena cava
• Blood to heart from lower body

Aorta
• Blood to body with O₂

Figure 9: **The heart and its valves**

larly omega-3 and -6. One of the most important nutrients is coenzyme Q10: it is vital for mitochondrial function to provide energy to the heart muscle.

Metal toxicity
Our exposure to metals, including mercury, lead, arsenic and aluminium (see Chapter 4), increases the potential for free radicals in the body. Furthermore, heavy metals can become trapped in the sticky cholesterol plaques that adhere to the inner lining of the arteries.

Food allergy
Food allergy is considered to be a potential cause of inflammation and arterial thickening, both of which are issues for cardiovascular health and possibly hypertension.[46]

Genomics
One of the genes measured is *APO E*. We have genes coding for subsections of this gene – *APO E2, APO E3* and *APO E4*. If we have *APO E4*, we have a higher risk of arterial disease and need to pay more attention to our lifestyle and diet: for example, a low fat diet makes a bigger difference in *APO E4* carriers than it does in those with *APO E2* and *E3*; alcohol has no beneficial effect in *APO E4* carriers, whereas a couple of units daily will benefit others; only strenuous exercise makes a difference in *APO E4* carriers, whereas other variants benefit greatly from moderate exercise. Furthermore, cardiogenomics can now tell us how we will react to arterial and heart drugs such as ACE inhibitors, beta blockers and statins, and can also tell us whether or not some natural products such as ginseng, gingko and garlic may or may not benefit us.

OTHER SECOND-LINE TESTS
Carotid artery ultrasound
The carotid arteries are found on either side of the neck and are among the first branches off the aorta, the main artery leaving the heart. These two arteries subdivide and are the main feeders of blood to the head and brain. It is easy to view the patency of these arteries using ultrasound. Measurement of their blood flow has been shown to be a good reflection of arterial health throughout the body.

Carotid Doppler ultrasound receiver
Sound waves travel differently through soft, as opposed to hard, tissue. When an ultrasound is held over the arteries, sound waves bounce back to the transceiver and, with further calculations within the computerized system, advise of the speed of the blood flow (the Doppler effect) through the arteries themselves. This gives an indication of arterial health. A non-invasive, simple test, you would need to lie flat with your head turned first to one side and then to the other for no more than a few minutes, while the expert technician moves the transmitter and receiver over your arteries.

Echocardiography
The ECHO cardiogram is frequently referred to as a cardiac ECHO or simply ECHO. A computerized technique, it uses sound waves to build up a picture of the heart. It is mainly used to assess the structure of the heart and can give information about leaky or damaged valves.

This test is rather specialized and not commonly used at a basic level of screening unless the doctor has some suspicions of a faulty valve within the heart. ECHO will spot damage only once it has occurred. Unfortunately, a mechanical problem such as a faulty valve generally requires a mechanical answer – surgery.

Advanced investigations
If you fall into one of the risk categories below, you should ask for advanced investigation into the health of your cardiovascular system.

- You have hereditary or genetic risks. You are at a greater risk of arterial disease if you have close family members who have had a history of heart or arterial disease, or stroke; a father, mother or sibling who has had problems with their heart or arteries below the age of 65; family members with high blood fats (triglycerides); high cholesterol; and any history of diabetes.
- You have high blood pressure (hypertension).
- You have other specific diseases that affect the heart and arteries, such as thyroid disorders and diabetes.
- You suffer from obesity or you are overweight.
- You do not exercise enough (see Chapter 3).
- You drink too much alcohol (three or more units a day for men and two for women).

- You use recreational drugs, including (in particular) being a smoker, or some prescription medication.
- You eat fewer than nine or ten portions of fruit or vegetable per day.

ADVANCED TESTS
CT calcium score
Using a special X-ray system known as computed tomography (CT) scanning, this test looks for the deposition of calcium in the artery or arterial walls. The test can check for the early stages of disease, but should not be used too often as, depending upon the precise equipment, it could deliver the equivalent of 750 chest X-rays' worth of radiation. Newer machines will deliver lower doses of radiation, so ask before you take the test.

Coronary angiography or CT, MRI or virtual angiography
A doctor is likely to refer a person with a severe risk of, or who has signs or symptoms of coronary or arterial disease, to a cardiologist. This specialist heart surgeon will have a wealth of sophisticated equipment available for measuring cardiovascular health. Most pieces of machinery involve radiation or the invasive administration of X-ray opaque material. It is worth discussing with a complementary medical practitioner how best to protect yourself from the risks of these kinds of test: for example, by taking anti-oxidants, which counteract the influence of the free radicals that radiation produces.

Chapter 7

The Nervous System

I think if philosophers were asked where the soul lies, some would argue not within the physical body. The more poetic among them might say that the soul lies within the heart; but the scientists would be hard pushed to go beyond the nervous system. Few would argue that the conscious self, as opposed to the 'soul', is at the very least a perception created by the brain or at most the summation of brain activity in its entirety. So, however we look at ourselves, as the nervous system deteriorates, so does the 'self' or the 'soul'.

In less ethereal terms, if our nervous system deteriorates, we recognize changes in our senses and our ability to recall, learn and communicate. As a consequence, we lose our ability to expand our minds, interact with others effectively and, quite simply, enjoy life's many pleasures.

Our sense of being and our senses – as defined by science – combine to create our perception of all that we are, have been and anticipate becoming. In order to maintain who we are, we might consider that all other parts of the human body are sections of a life-support system for the brain and nervous system. Hospital life-support systems keep organs alive to support the nervous system – but there is no artificial nervous system.

The senses

This chapter describes how we can protect the nervous system from age-related degeneration. However, first I think it is important to understand how the nervous system governs our lives and to review the relevance of each sense in turn.

Vision
Over time, the eye lens is exposed to many environmental factors (sunlight, wind, and so on) and pollutants, and it inevitably sustains some damage.

The muscles that constrict and dilate the pupil (the sphincter papillae muscles), thereby governing how much light enters the eye, and the muscle that controls the curvature of the lens (the ciliary muscle), thereby allowing for long and short sight, lose blood supply and also stiffen and weaken.

Blood vessels – small as they are in the eye – become blocked, leading to diminished oxygen and nutritional supply to the retina (the back of the eye containing the rods and cones that are the light receptors), which, in turn, leads to retinal degeneration. Other conditions such as diabetes and high blood pressure can also cause the retina to degenerate. Macular degeneration – of which there are two types, 'wet' (leakage of blood) and 'dry' (lack of blood) – is predominantly related to age and is the direct result of the degeneration of of nerve tissues that supple the eye.

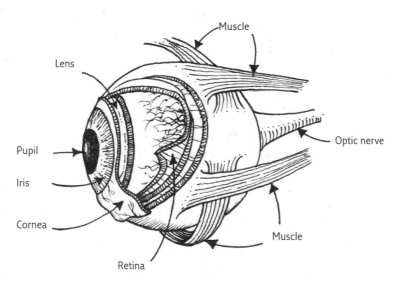

Figure 10: **Lens muscles in the eye**

NUTRIENTS AND THE EYES

- Cataracts were reduced in those eating eggs, those taking higher doses of vitamin C and those using n-acetyl carnosine.[1]
- Macular degeneration damage progressed more slowly in those taking vitamin D.[2]
- High glycaemic index foods (such as, refined sugars and processed foods) damage eyesight and may contribute to macular degeneration.[3]
- Goji berries were being explored at Kansas State University in 2010 as a possible supplement that may slow down macular degeneration.

Hearing

The interpretation of sound is dependent upon many factors and an explanation could fill a book in itself. However, having a brief understanding can help us to see how the dos and don'ts of healthy ageing can affect this important sense.

As sound waves travel down the ear canal and pass through the ear drum, they vibrate small bones (ossicles) in the middle ear. These bones are connected through joints and held in place by small ligaments.

The ossicles transmit sound vibrations to the inner ear, which connects with the auditory nerves leading to the parts of the brain that interpret sound. Furthermore, the inner ear, connecting with a part of the brain called the cerebellum found at the top of the spinal column, is associated with our ability to balance. Ageing processes affecting these nerves can interfere with stability, leading to a drop in our enjoyment of movement and exercise – a sure way to speed up the ageing process.

Deafness or hearing loss may vary from mild loss of particular pitch or notes to a complete inability to hear sound. At whatever level, hearing loss leads to social difficulties. Establishing the cause of deafness is paramount – check any worsening in your ability to hear with your medical practitioner who might refer you to an ear specialist. Incidentally, evidence suggests that the drug Viagra may encourage loss of hearing.[4] *Note that acute or sudden deafness must be treated as an emergency and should be reviewed by a specialist.*

Deafness can be divided into two groups: conductive and neurological (perceptive).

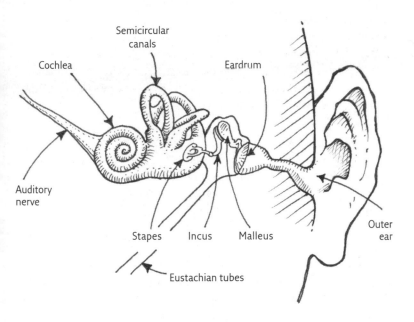

Figure 11: **Ear ossicles and the hearing nerves**

TREATMENT OF HEARING LOSS

- Obstructive causes should be removed if possible. Obstruction may occur because of fluid in the middle ear (infected or not).
- Conductive deafness through damage or arthritic conditions in the ear ossicles may respond to naturopathic treatment, but this needs to be specific.
- Do not hesitate to use hearing-aid appliances. If naturopathic treatments do not help and no surgical procedure will benefit, then the use of hearing aids can make a profound difference.
- If specific problems such as cholesteatoma, labyrinthitis or glue ear are the cause of deafness, follow through with conventional advice in conjunction with natural options for the few causes that can be influenced, such as arthritic ear bones and neurological diseases.

Conductive deafness

Sound is transmitted from the external ear canal through the eardrum and the ear ossicles into the vestibular canal, which houses the ends of the auditory nerve fibres. This part of the ear can be considered the conductive part. Trauma, obstruction, infection and bone diseases such as arthritis of the ossicles can all be a cause of hearing loss.

Neurological (perceptive) deafness

Deafness that occurs because of damage to the neurological system may be a result of trauma or infection in the vestibular canal, neurological disease (including tumours such as cholesteatoma) or trauma or infection along the auditory nerve to the part of the brain that registers sound.

Smell

The human nose has hundreds of thousands of olfactory nerves. These nerves are sensitive to gaseous molecules and penetrating through a thin bone, the cribiform plate, that join together and travel to the part of the brain that deals with smell. As humans have evolved, even though our other senses have become sharper, our ability to discern smell has diminished in comparison to many other animals. Nonetheless, smell still advises us of danger (the scent of toxic or noxious gases), gives us pleasure, and plays an important role in sexual arousal. Deterioration of the nerves associated with smell is therefore likely to lead to a reduced sense of well-being.

Taste

There are approximately 9,000 taste buds on our tongue, differentiating sweet, salt, bitter and sour. A lot of what we consider to be taste is, in fact, smell. Our taste buds constantly have to deal with tough, poorly chewed foods as well as toxic compounds such as alcohol and heat from hot drinks and soups. Our taste buds, disappointingly, deteriorate in their sensitivity as we age. Women's taste buds deteriorate from about the age of 40, and men's from around the age of 50.

Touch and sensation

Touch and sensation include itching, pain, hot and cold and pressure (which governs balance), as well as our ability to discern texture, which is so vital in our lives with regard to everyday pleasure, arousal and sexuality.

Sixth sense

Apart from our five basic senses, we also have a so-called 'sixth sense', do we not? For this we rely upon intuition, which many scientists would consider a combination of memory and cognition and our ability to 'make sense' of all sensory experience. Deterioration in our ability to comprehend and learn through experiences would make our life meaningless. This 'sense of being' is governed by the nervous system.

Where deterioration of the nervous system occurs

Deterioration of the nervous system occurs in three main ways:

1. Global degeneration

This is where the whole nervous system, including the brain, spinal column and peripheral nerves, loses its functionality. Maintaining our nervous system function as best as we can for as long as we can defers memory loss and, it is to be hoped, prevents dementia or Alzheimer's disease from setting in.

2. Specific degeneration

If certain parts of the brain start to deteriorate, specific nervous-system disorders may ensure. Parkinson's disease, macular degeneration and stroke, which are all predominantly age related, fall into this category.

3. Event-related deterioration

Physical trauma or infection, which can be acute (sudden) or develop chronically (long term) can lead to a loss of nervous-system function. Strokes (cerebral infarction or bleeds) overlapping with specific degeneration are the most common problem within this group, but so are trauma-related peripheral neuropathies (loss of sensation, tingling or numbness in the digits or limbs as a result of an accident, for example), infection and nutritional deficiencies such as lack of vitamin B12 and folic acid.

The structure of the nervous system

It is useful to understand a little about the structure of the nervous system to understand its ageing process.

Nerves are divided into those belonging to the central nervous system (CNS) – the brain and spinal column – and those in the rest of the body, known as the peripheral nerves. The CNS is bathed in cerebrospinal fluid (CSF). The nerves at different levels of the spine command different organs, tissues and muscles depending on where they leave the spinal column.

The peripheral nervous system (PNS) is subdivided into motor nerves (which control movement) and sensory nerves (which control our experience of sensation).

The motor nerves are divided into upper and lower motor neurones (the medical term for a nerve). The upper mostly belong to the CNS and the lower are mainly peripheral or outside the spinal column. Nerves in the human can be very short (microscopic) or up to 1 metre (3 feet) in length, but most short nerves create length by meeting at junctions known as synapses. Nerves controlling muscles end in neuromuscular junctions, while sensory nerves end in receptors.

A nerve is made up of a cell body (or control cell) with an axon covered in an insulating and conductive sheath known as the myelin sheath. The cell body connects to other nerves through tentacles known as dendrites.

External stimuli or our internal thought processes trigger the production of chemical messengers or neurohormones in the body, which, in turn, trigger electrical impulses that run down the axons to the synapses, then on to receptors on the next nerve or the tissue being affected.

Not all motor nerves are under our control. The autonomic (non-controlled) nervous system (ANS) governs the beating of our heart, our non-conscious respiration, our involuntary bladder and anal valves, and so on. The ANS is subdivided into sympathetic and parasympathetic systems, which act in opposition to each other: for example, the parasympathetic nervous system slows down the heart, whereas the sympathetic nervous system speeds it up. Adrenaline and noradrenaline are the most common hormones or neurotransmitters to affect the sympathetic and parasympathetic systems in different ways.

There are hundreds of events, diseases and conditions that can affect the nervous system, and the older we are, the more likely we are to suffer with any number of them. However, when we look at the ageing process, there are actually only a handful of age-related diseases that are likely to affect our nervous system.

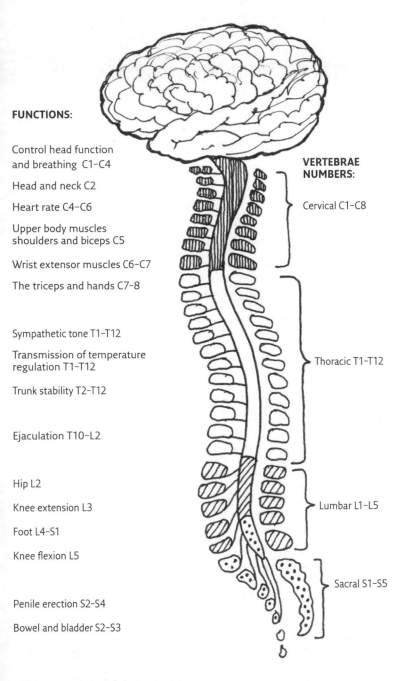

FUNCTIONS:

Control head function
and breathing C1–C4

Head and neck C2

Heart rate C4–C6

Upper body muscles
shoulders and biceps C5

Wrist extensor muscles C6–C7

The triceps and hands C7–8

Sympathetic tone T1–T12

Transmission of temperature
regulation T1–T12

Trunk stability T2–T12

Ejaculation T10–L2

Hip L2

Knee extension L3

Foot L4–S1

Knee flexion L5

Penile erection S2–S4

Bowel and bladder S2–S3

**VERTEBRAE
NUMBERS:**

Cervical C1–C8

Thoracic T1–T12

Lumbar L1–L5

Sacral S1–S5

Figure 12: **The spinal column**

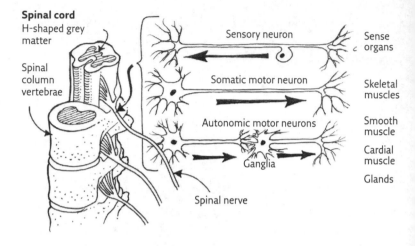

Figure 14: **Neuromuscular connections: motor neurons**

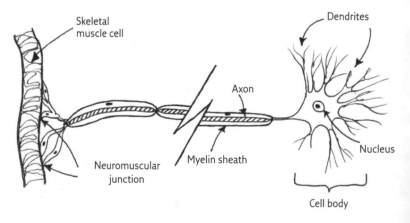

Figure 15: **Neuromuscular connections: dendrites**

Dementia

The term dementia means different things to the general public and often within the medical profession itself. Dementia describes a set of symptoms, all or any of which can be mild or severe and do not necessarily have to be related to age. There are many causes of dementia, and there are many subdivisions. Let me simplify this.

Symptoms

The primary symptoms of dementia are:

- *Memory loss* – Initially in dementia, this tends to be about things that have happened recently and is known as short-term memory loss. The difference between memory lapses that we all struggle with and memory loss is that if we have a memory lapse, when reminded of what we have forgotten, most of us say, "Oh yes, of course." People with dementia, on the other hand, do not recall the event, even when reminded of it. As dementia worsens, mid-term and eventually long-term memories disappear as well.
- *Mood changes* – Feelings of unhappiness, sadness or anger in response to an event or occurrence in our lives is a perfectly normal reaction with which most – if not all – of us are familiar. In general, we feel in control of our emotions, able (eventually, even if not immediately) to take action to change our mood. In dementia, mood changes are not related to specific events, nor are they controllable. Even drug treatments, which might be used for someone with depression, tend not to be effective if dementia exists – they may even make matters worse. In dementia, there is no obvious cause for a mood shift, except that it may be associated with memory loss or any of the other symptoms listed here.
- *Confusion* – Initially the confusion associated with dementia is frustrating and then, as it continues or worsens, it becomes frightening. Even simple tasks such as reading a book that a person with dementia may have performed throughout his or her life may cause confusion. During the late stages of the condition, sufferers may lose the ability to cook, clean or look after their own personal hygiene.
- *Poor communication* – People suffering from dementia tend to 'lose' words or may have difficulty in forming the correct speech patterns, far beyond the temporary forgetfulness of everyday stressful existence that we all experience from time to time. In dementia, poor communication can also be a failure to understand what is being said.

Types of dementia

There are various types of dementia classified, depending upon the cause or description.

Senile dementia

A term nowadays rarely heard or used in medical circles, senile dementia has been incorrectly replaced in the vernacular as Alzheimer's, which many people think covers all forms of age-related dementia. Senile dementia actually refers to the development of dementia symptoms as we age. It is, I believe, an inevitability of growing old, owing to the effects of our environment on our nervous tissue and DNA. It is not so much that we have genes that guarantee us eventual brain dysfunction, but rather that some genes are more likely than others to encourage processes in the body that lead to nerve damage. These genes are turned on or off by good or bad environmental triggers. In other words, while we may all carry genes that could trigger demential, lifestyle choices can increase or decrease the likelihood of them switching on.

Two or three decades ago, doctors also used another term, pre-senile dementia, to categorize dementia symptoms that occurred before old age. Again, it is a term that you will rarely hear any more. That is because we now have a much better understanding of the underlying causes of dementia, which means that we can describe dementia more accurately.

Alzheimer's disease (AD)

Back in 1901, Dr Alois Alzheimer spotted what he described as patches or plaques and tangles within the brain of individuals showing the sympoms of dementia. The subsequently named Alzheimer's disease is, in fact, the result of specific proteins depositing in the space outside the nerve cells and axons in the brain. The most common proteins involved are known as amyloid (beta amyloid) and Tau proteins (*see* p172 Tangles). These proteins cause plaques and tangles that bind to and obstruct the brain's blood vessels, cutting off the brain's oxygen and nutrition supply, thus limiting the amount of rebuilding and repair that can occur within the brain. The result is slow degeneration of brain matter.

Vascular dementia

The symptoms of vascular dementia appear indistinguishable from those of senile dementia and Alzheimer's disease, but they develop because of a lack of blood flow to the brain, leading to a loss of brain tissue. There is, of course,

DEMENTIA STATISTICS

- Alzheimer's disease (AD) affects approximately 24–33 million people worldwide.
- There are currently 750,000 people with AD in the UK, and it is estimated the figure will rise to over a million by 2021.
- Two-thirds of people with AD are women.
- Only 40 per cent of people with AD are correctly diagnosed with this condition.[5] However, it has been suggested in the past that we may be over-diagnosing dementia.[6] This study produced in the middle of the 1990s has yet to be disproved and the medical fraternity is well aware of the need to define dementia, perhaps with measured biomarkers, to ensure correct treatment options are available.[7]
- In the US, 5.3 million people have AD, of which 5.1 million are aged over 65.
- Less than 1 per cent of AD is caused by specific genetic variations (involving chromosome 21).
- US figures suggest that by 2050 the number of people with dementia is expected to reach between 11 and 16 million.
- In people over 65 years of age in the US, 8 per cent show some characteristics of dementia. This rises to 45 per cent of those aged 80.[8]

an overlap between VD and AD, because the amyloid plaques in AD cause a certain amount of VD as a symptom of AD. Nevertheless, VD is a form of dementia in its own right. (Chapter 6 describes what causes damage to the arteries and therefore all the things that predispose an individual to VD.)

Dementia associated with Lewy bodies
Named after the scientist who discovered them, Lewy bodies are complexes found *inside* the nerve cell. This debris interferes with cellular function, eventually rendering the nerve useless, which leads to dementia.

Dementia as a result of other disease
To list all the diseases that could cause dementia would take too much space, but there are two significant examples: HIV/AIDS and Creutzfeldt-Jakob disease (CJD), also unkindly called 'mad cow disease'. Other conditions such as motor neurone disease, multiple sclerosis, Parkinson's disease and

Huntington's chorea can all trigger dementia, depending upon which part of the brain is affected: for example, one particular type of dementia affecting the front and side of the brain is known as fronto-temporal dementia.

Parkinson's disease

James Parkinson, a British 18th-century physician, described a clinical state characterized by the following:
- an expressionless face;
- infrequency of blinking;
- a paucity and slowness of voluntary movement;
- rigidity of muscles with a rhythmic three- to four-per-second tremor which becomes more pronounced at rest;
- a stooped posture and a wide-legged walking stance (caused by a loss of the normal postural reflexes);
- a shuffling walk;
- impeded initiation and cessation of movements (crossing a road may, in extreme cases, be difficult because timing is important and being able to stop is difficult);
- memory loss and an inability to concentrate.

Causes

Parkinson's disease may occur in middle or later life as a result of the degeneration of cells in the brain that produce a chemical called dopamine. Dopamine has a pronounced effect on the control of muscles and posture.

There are various reasons why the dopamine-producing cells may degenerate, among which are encephalitis or poisoning from certain drugs, or toxicity as a result of exposure to aluminium,[9] manganese, copper and pesticides.[10] [11]

PARKINSON'S AND PESTICIDES

- There is a direct link between pesticides and Parkinson's.[12]
- Keep your copper levels at an optimum by taking an absorbable copper supplement at a level of 1 mg per 30 cm (1 ft) of height.
- There is a 10-fold increased risk of developing Parkinson's for those exposed to garden pesticides.[13]

Because most chemicals that are harmful to the body are destroyed in the liver, Parkinson's disease is associated with poor liver function, as well as with deficiencies in certain minerals – particularly magnesium and calcium – and in antioxidants,[14] vitamin D,[15] and the amino acids phenylalanine and tyrosine, a lack of which can inhibit dopamine production. In other words, long-term poor diet may trigger the condition.

Stroke

A stroke, also sometimes known as a cerebrovascular accident (CVA), is the term given to a neurological dysfunction that shows itself most frequently as the paralysis of one side of the body with or without an effect on the other side.

This weakness may develop within minutes and is usually associated with an arterial problem in the brain that results in the brain being starved of oxygen. However, a stroke may develop over a much longer period of time, even months. When this happens, it is likely that it is some other disease in the body that is causing the stroke – most commonly a tumour.

Causes

Approximately 95 per cent of strokes occur because a blood vessel in the brain is blocked by a clot, is closing up because of atheroma or is going into spasm through some neurological or chemical influence. Atheroma may cause fragility in the blood vessel, which then bursts or leaks causing a haemorrhage. To stem the bleeding, a clot forms at the rupture site and obstructs blood flow. Thus, most strokes are cerebrovascular accidents. A stroke is further classified by whether the event is complete or still evolving, and also by the type and severity of the neurological problem.

Any condition that can lead to vascular damage increases the risk of a stroke. High blood pressure may burst the small vessels in the brain, although the mechanism to protect brain blood pressure is one of the most evolved in the human being. Atheroma and the eventual clogging up of the arteries, with the increased tendency for a clot to form in such blood vessels, is much more likely to cause a stroke, and small emboli (clots from other parts of the body) may fire off atheroma plaques in other vessels or come from diseased heart valves to occlude the arteries. Preventing any of these factors is the primary means of preventing or fighting a stroke. Even if a stroke has taken place, active therapy against these conditions may prevent a worsening of the effects of stroke or a recurrence.

STROKE FACTS AND FIGURES

- Stroke is the third most common cause of death in the Western world, behind heart disease and cancer.
- It is the most common cause of severe chronic disability and happens to two out of 1,000 people each year in the UK.
- Three-quarters of this number are over the age of 65.
- The event is twice as common in black people as it is in the white population.
- 1 in 500 adults at the age of 65 or more will have a stroke.

Hypertension increases the risk of a stroke by six times, which brings the risk to 1 in 83 people. However, although many people are frightened that their high blood pressure will cause a stroke, the chances are still low (only 82:1), even without treatment for hypertension.

Prevention is the key word in stroke, because full recovery from neurological deficit is rare. Nevertheless, many people get 90 per cent of function back, although this tends to be in the first three months post-incident. Most individuals who have anything other than a major stroke will have some degree of recovery.

Immediate first-aid and orthodox emergency medicine reduce the risk of death. Cardiopulmonary resuscitation may be necessary because a stroke can affect breathing and cardiac response.

Transient ischaemic attack (TIA)

A transient ischaemic attack is a temporary neurological deficit, usually comprising a dimming of vision, a lack of power or movement on one side of the body, numbness, dizziness and difficulty in speaking that usually lasts 10 minutes or under, but may last as long as 24 hours. These attacks are usually related to a temporary blockage in a blood vessel in the brain caused either by spasm of an already atherosclerotic vessel or by an embolism (travelling blood clot or other matter). The longer the attack, the more probable the effect was caused by an embolism. Recovery is usually complete, but TIAs usually recur and may be a warning of an impending stroke.

Tremor and trembling

A tremor is a regular, rhythmic oscillation of a part of the body caused by alternate contractions of muscles either side of a joint. Trembling is simply an exacerbation of a tremor affecting a larger part of the body such as an arm or a leg.

Anything that affects the nerves or the neuromuscular junction can potentially cause a tremor. The most common causes are fever, the toxic effect from alcohol withdrawal (*delirium tremens*) or overindulgence in caffeine or other stimulatory drugs such as amphetamines or cocaine. An excess of thyroxine or adrenaline (as would occure in extreme nervousness) may cause tremors and may indicate underlying conditions such as hyperthyroidism or adrenal tumours. Other symptoms such as sweating and weight loss are usually associated with tremor.

Neurological diseases, including Parkinson's disease (which can cause a tremor when resting) or stroke (which may affect the coordination centres), can be differentiated from neurodegenerative tremor that is associated with age – often by the fact that this does not disappear on intentional movement such as picking up a pen.

A twitch is the involuntary contraction of a single muscle group and is usually an indication of an entrapped nerve or peripheral neurological damage. A twitch is known medically as a fasciculation and may be an indication of more serious neurological conditions such as motor neurone disease.

What causes the nervous system to age?

Understanding all the different factors that damage the CNS and the PNS provides us with all we need to to know to identify which tests and therapies can help us to slow down the ageing of the nervous system in general.

Our genes and the environment govern the speed with which normal physiological ageing occurs – ageing is fundamentally the body's inability

---

BRAIN MATTER

Most tissues in the body are pink because of the blood that flows through them. The white and grey matter of the brain is predominantly fatty tissue with little blood flowing through it. Most of the brain's blood vessels are in the the meninges and dura, which cover the brain. Oxygen and nutrients diffuse into the CFS creating a rich solution in which the brain effectively 'bathes'.

to replace parts or molecules, both in the cell walls and in our DNA, that have become damaged over our lifetime. Over time we are exposed to many environmental toxins that, both directly and through gene interaction, damage the nervous system.

Causes of central nervous system (CNS) damage

Plaques

These are misshapen and useless proteins found in the ageing brain. Amyloid, one of the most studied of all plaques, forms when normal proteins, which are meant to be within the brain performing structural and functional activities, change shape. All proteins have a particular structure and, like a lock and a key, fit into receptors or bind with other proteins or compounds to produce a normal physiological effect. When a protein changes shape it is said to 'fold'. These folds are caused by electro-charges in the molecules of toxins (such as heavy metals or pollutants) or by the presence of free radicals or the influence of hormones and other chemical reactions. As these folds occur, the shape of the 'key' changes and may not fit into the lock at all or jam there once inserted. The result is that the proteins do not interact as they should or they get sticky and block normal cell function. When this happens in a nerve cell wall, in a synapse or in the production of a neurotransmitter, that nerve or group of nerves stops functioning.

Tangles

This simple term describes the alteration of specific proteins known as Tau by toxins – often metals such as mercury or aluminium[16] – that get into the nerve cells. Thin tubes (microtubules) made up of Tau proteins allow the transport of nutrients through the cell. Damage causes the Tau proteins to interlink and block the tubules' ability to provide nutrition.

Lipofuscin

This is one of the more common compounds to be laid down in the nervous system tissues and is normally found in cells as an end product of the breakdown of free radicals. The more free-radical, or oxidative, damage there is, the more lipofuscin deposits there are and the more they clog up the function of the brain, in particular.

Advanced glycation end products

Abbreviated to AGEs, advanced glycation end products are proteins formed by the heat produced during the body's metabolism of sugars. The brain's only source of energy are the sugars that our diet provides via our blood-stream. When we have too much sugar in our system, the metabolic process produces too much heat. In turn, this leads to an excess of AGE products, which then damage the brain and other nerve tissue.

Toxins

Although the brain has a membrane known as the blood-brain barrier, which aims to protect the brain from pathogens, toxins – particularly heavy metals and certain chemical pollutants such as pesticides – are able to travel across the barrier. The same toxins that damage the nervous system itself may also cause a 'leaky blood-brain' barrier. These toxins are increasingly found in brain diseases such as Alzheimer's and Parkinson's diseases, so their removal through detoxification is important.

Oxidative stress

We need high levels of antioxidants to avoid oxidative damage (*see* Chapter 6). Melatonin, one of the major hormones found in the brain and predomi-nantly involved in the regulation of sleep, has strong antioxidant activity that counteracts the free radicals causing oxidative stress.

Other diseases

There is a number of diseases that can lead to neurological damage. Conditions such as high blood pressure and diabetes lead to brain-tissue loss and damage.

Nutritional deficiency

Poor diet is a major cause of premature neurological ageing. Although the brain uses only sugar for energy (it cannot use fats or proteins), it needs many nutrients to ensure complete nerve function and particularly for the production of neurotransmitters. Essential fatty acids and proteins are par-ticularly important (for example, glutamic acid or glutamate, which is a constituent of protein foods, is needed in the correct concentration as a direct neurotransmitter), but the brain needs many vitamins and minerals, too. (Interestingly, though, too much glutamic acid can itself cause dementia issues.)

Amino-acid deficiency

Your body needs the amino acid taurine to make dopamine – a deficiency in this neurotransmitter is one cause of Parkinson's disease. We need tryptophan, another amino acid (this time essential – that is, derived from food) to make our 'happy juice' serotonin.

Decreased blood supply

As previously discussed, vascular dementia is caused by narrowing and stiffening of arteries, including the deposition of amyloid causing cerebral amyloid angiopathy.

Inflammation in general

Any damage to the cells in the nervous system leads the body to attempt to repair itself – and this requires inflammation. Unfortunately, inflammation tends to create heat, which encourages plaques, tangles and AGE products, thereby resulting in a vicious circle. Nerve-tissue infection such as meningitis (an infection in the tissue covering the brain) is generally an uncommon cause of inflammation. However, as we age, our immune system becomes weaker and this puts nerve tissue at increased risk.

Radiation

X-rays and electromagnetic frequencies (EMFs, such as from mobile phones) may cause neurological disorders. EMFs are highly controversial, with some authorities considering that this kind of radiation may cause up to 30 per cent of childhood cancers[17] and other cancers and conditions.[18] However, studies of the ageing population are inconclusive at the time of writing.

Direct injury

Authorities working with Quantitative Electroencephalography (QEEG) suggest that even minor head injuries and whiplash[19] lead to damage and scarring of parts of the brain. This, in turn, can impinge on the blood flow to the brain in general and speed up the ageing process as we get older. Investigation of such damage is an advanced test that should become more available in the future.

Causes of peripheral nervous system damage

Peripheral nerve damage is an unfortunate outcome of infection, major injury, toxicity (especially alcoholism) and metabolic conditions such as diabetes. Chemotherapeutic drugs, but also common medications for blood and heart conditions, can cause problems. Nutritional deficiency, particularly of vitamin B12, is a problem as we age – we tend to lose our ability to absorb B12 as we get older due to a loss of a particular chemical produced by part of our bowel, the jejunum, and also by a loss of our bowel flora which produce a lot of vitamin B12. Loss of collagen, which protects the peripheral nerves and makes our skin 'elastic', added to injuries collected over the years all impinge on the function of our PNS.

Whatever the underlying cause, PNS damage may simply be boiled down to:
- inflammation from disease and injury;
- inflexible arteries reducing repair capability;
- nutritional deficiency;
- toxic molecules and other components in the blood.

HOW TO SLOW DOWN OR REVERSE THE AGEING PROCESS IN THE NERVOUS SYSTEM

You can maintain the health of your nervous system and, to a degree, reverse damage to it by reviewing your options in the following categories:
- Nutrition and dietetics
- Exercise
- Lifestyle changes, including avoiding toxins
- Supplementation and medication
- Naturopathic therapies

The basic advice about diet, exercise and lifestyle are covered in Chapters 1 to 3, but the advice in this chapter is geared specifically toward the nervous system.

Nutrition

So much of what I have described so far emphasizes how important nutrition is with regard to maintaining the structure of the central and peripheral nerves and how important vitamins and minerals are in defending the nervous system against free radicals and oxidative damage; you will also have an idea of how your body needs nutrients to make neurotransmitters and keep nerves functioning.

Fruit and vegetables

A good supply of vitamins and minerals comes from nine or ten portions of fruits and vegetables a day. Please reread Chapter 2 and consider juicing to help you maintain high levels of these nutrients. Here is a quick reminder of what you need:

- Cherries and berries (particularly blueberries), which contain flavonoids, are important for the general health of the nervous system, but specifically for the age-related conditions of macular degeneration and cardiovascular-related dementia.
- Potassium-rich foods (*see* Chapter 5).
- Nuts and seeds containing good levels of essential fatty acids.
- Folic acid (predominantly derived from vegetables) and vitamin C, which have been found to be deficient in patients with dementia.[20]
- Vegetables and other sources high in vitamin A, which are beneficial for age-related conditions such as sicca (dry eye syndrome) and (senile) keratoses. The former can benefit from vitamin-A eye drops.
- Deficiencies in general have been shown to be more pronounced in those with dementia than in controls.[21] Vitamin B6 and B12 and folate are particularly relevant.[22]
- Vitamin E in its role as a 'free radical scavenger' (a powerful antioxidant) is very relevant according to many studies.
- The minerals copper, manganese and zinc have all been associated with an increased risk of dementia, and all of these are found in good fruit and vegetable diets.

Fibre

Some authorities involved in the care of the various forms of dementia comment that a high-fibre diet is of benefit. As fibre is known to bind toxins and prevent their absorption into the blood stream and as most high-fibre foods tend to carry nutrients, it would seem logical that the body needs fibre in order to combat the symptoms of dementia.

Fibre is important also because, anecdotally, we know that regular bowel movements help prevent sluggish thought processes and weaken some of the symptoms of dementia.

However, it is important to remember that fibre is difficult to chew and to digest. As we age, our teeth weaken and our stomach acid levels fall, making fibre even more likely to cause bloating, discomfort and indigestion. Keep a careful balance – eat enough fibre to stay healthy, but not so much that you end up with stomach problems. Listen to your body.

Protein

Not only do proteins form building blocks for the structure of the nervous system, but most of the neurotransmitters, the chemical messengers within the nervous system, are protein based, too. Furthermore, several amino acids (the breakdown products of proteins) are important in the normal functioning and repair of the nervous system.

Healthy organic meats and vegetables that are high in protein (*see* Chapter 2) are important – with one main exception. For sufferers of Parkinson's Disease, low-protein intake, particularly in the morning, can enhance the efficacy of the drug L-DOPA, which is prescribed to combat the symptoms of the disease.

When I was starting my training in nutritional medicine, over 25 years ago, Dr Bruce Milliman, past Clinical Director at the Bastyr University, Seattle, explained to me that even he and his family, despite being fundamentally vegetarian, aimed to have one animal protein meal a week to cover the range of essential amino acids that would otherwise require eating too many vegetables.

The following specific proteins are the most important for neurological health. However, it is important to have a good intake of a variety of these and other proteins to ensure that your diet contains all essential amino acids.

- *Lecithin.* Taken as a supplement (1 tablespoon 3 times daily), this protein is involved in the production of the neurotransmitter acetylcholine. An increase in blood levels of this may benefit memory and dementia. Fish (particularly its roe), eggs, and unprocessed nuts and grains have a good lecithin content, but the best source is the oil of the soya bean.
- *Tyrosine.* This is a precursor of L-3, 4-dihydroxyphenylalanine (commonly abbreviated to L-DOPA). This is a building-block of dopamine, the neurohormone that is deficient in Parkinson's disease and that we also need for mood regulation. It is found in soy products, avocados, sesame seeds, pumpkin seeds and almonds.
- *Phenylalanine.* Converted into DOPA, this protein is found mostly in meats and animal produce such as eggs. Vegetarians can get reasonable amounts through soya.

As we age, we produce less stomach acid. This is particularly detrimental to the breakdown of proteins and so a hydrochloric acid supplement with any protein or large meal (preferably taken in the middle of the meal) is likely to be beneficial. We need stomach acid to help the body more easily absorb nutrients from our food, particularly vitamin B12, an important vitamin in the general functioning of the nervous system.

Fats

Certain oils and fats interfere with the absorption of essential fatty acids (EFAs) and can particularly influence the fat-rich nervous system. Try to avoid corn oil and excessive amounts of trans fats (which will be labelled on products). As 70 per cent of the brain is made up of fatty acids, the fewer bad ones you put in, the better.

EFAs are vital to the function of all organs and most bodily processes. Because the nervous system is predominantly made up of EFAs and other fats, ensuring good intake is vital.

Phosphatidylserine is predominantly made in the body and is not abundant in our diets, so you should try to eat foods containing it. Mackerel and tuna are the best sources, although it is also found in dairy products, wholegrain rice and root vegetables. Liver and kidney (as well as brain, for those real carnivores among us) are also good sources.

Dr Patricia Kane, a researcher in a pioneering cell membrane and nervous tissue repair therapy, phospholipid exchange, recommends taking omega 6 (linoleic acid) and omega 3 (alpha linolenic acid) at a ratio of 4:1 for maintenance and therapeutic care of the nervous system. Balanced oils such as these are available online, but please ensure that any oil you buy is manufactured using cold-pressing techniques and is from a reputable source.

To ensure a balanced intake of oils try making the following – you should aim to have 2–3 tablespoons daily, perhaps as a salad dressing or in soup, or drunk mixed into juice:

Sunflower oil or walnut oil (3 tbs); flaxseed (linseed) oil (1 tbs)

Carbohydrates (sugars)

Avoid high levels of fructose and of corn syrup. These are generally found in processed foods, but also in a lot of fizzy drinks (sodas).

Keep refined sugars to a minimum. There is a theoretical correlation between sugars in the brain and the tangles associated with dementia.

Essential fatty acids

Phospholipids

Phosphatidylserine is best obtained from unrefined soya products and oils and phosphotidylcholine is found in wheatgerm, broccoli, Brussel sprouts, peanut butter and milk chocolate. These are useful in the treatment of Alzheimer's Disease in particular, but also of any cognitive problems or nerve damage.

Other foods

Turmeric, a spice frequently used to flavour Indian food, may help avoid the formation of amyloid plaques that are characteristic of Alzheimer's disease. Regular dietary intake of turmeric may prove to be of benefit – although because the spice is not easily absorbed (it is not very soluble), it may be useful to take supplements. Drugs under development that enhance delivery are likely to be needed to get the turmeric to the brain.[23] At this time it appears that perhaps you would need to take up to 2 grams daily to help in the treatment of Parkinson's disease.

Excess salt reduces cognition if associated with decreased exercise.[24]

Fluids

Water

Dehydration is well accepted as causing confusion and will worsen dementia. Ensure that you drink at least 1 to 1.5 litres (1¾ to 2½ pints) of fluid a day.

Alcohol

Some studies suggest that 1–2 units of alcohol daily, particularly of red wine, may enhance cognitive function (as well as reduce the risk of stroke). I take the view that a little bit of what you enjoy does you good.

Coffee

Studies generally suggest that 1 or 2 cups of medium-strength filter coffee or 2–4 cups of tea (about 150 mg of caffeine) may reduce the incidence of dementia. Much of the early research on animal brains is a little inconsistent. Currently, research suggests that high caffeine intake does not risk cognitive impairment nor the development of dementia, and possibly those who took over 277.5 mg per day had fewer brain lesions indicative of dementia than those who took in less than 115.5 mg. A couple of cups a day may benefit us from mid-life onward.[25]

Dr Sharma's Programmes

Dr Sharma's Maintenance Programme

This is a basic programme to protect and improve the nervous system. At first glance, this extensive list seems daunting, but remember, many of these nutrients can be found in the same tablet or capsule as multivitamin/mineral complexes.

MINERALS

- *Magnesium* – 500–1000 mg daily. This helps overcome anxiety, depression and very often unexplained fatigue. There is some evidence of its benefit for combating some forms of dementia.
- *Selenium* – 100–200 mcg daily if you suffer from macular degeneration and cataract. It also increases defence against viral illnesses, a problem for the elderly – especially winter-associated influenza.
- *Silicone* – 1 mg daily. Inhibits aluminium absorption, which may reduce the risk of certain types of dementia.
- *Zinc* – generally available with copper in a ratio of 15 mg:2 mg. It helps slow down macular degeneration and some forms of hearing loss.
  (Be wary of taking large doses of zinc, as too much zinc in the system may lead to folic-acid deficiency.)

VITAMINS

- *Vitamin B-complex* – containing B2, B3, B6 and B12.
- *Folic acid* or the more active form, *methyl tetra hydroxyl folate* – at least 400 mcg taken daily.
- *Vitamin D* – at least 1000 iu taken daily, but dosages up to 10,000 iu daily are likely to be of most benefit.[26]
- *Natural source Vitamin E* – minimally 200 iu.

ESSENTIAL FATTY ACIDS

- *Omega-6 and omega-3 oils* – at a ratio of 4:1. This supplement will help relieve the symptoms of tremors, all other neurological diseases and constipation, which can exacerbate the symptoms of dementia.

AMINO ACIDS

- *Whey* – if you are vegetarian or eat very little animal protein, take a whey supplement at the dosage recommended on the label. If you are vegan, take a plant-based amino acid supplement such as aloe vera-based protein powder.

OTHER NUTRIENTS

- *Melatonin* – 2–3 mg taken nightly. This is a powerful antioxidant and there is particular research backing its use in treating (therefore possibly avoiding) macular degeneration. It may also help stave off glaucoma and sleep disorders (particularly those associated with ageing) and can help slow down the effects of degenerative disease such as dementia.[27]
- *Antioxidants* – although a small study on 78 patients[28] suggested that antioxidants were not useful in dementia, the use of pharmaceutical-grade nutrients should not deter from the vast amount of evidence to support supplemental use.[29]

Dr Sharma's Advanced Programme

This programme is for those with symptoms of nervous-system damage, or lifestyle or family risk factors. Discuss taking these supplements with your healthcare provider or take them if you want to enhance the protection of your nervous system.

VITAMINS

- *Riboflavin (vitamin B2)* – 10–100 mg taken daily may slow down the development of cataracts and help in macular degeneration.
- *Vitamin B3 (niacin)* – 5 mg taken twice daily may be beneficial and is known to help in depression and anxiety.
- *NADH (made up from niacin)* – 5–10 mg taken daily may reduce tremors and ease the symptoms of Parkinson's disease.
- *Vitamin B12* – a subcutaneous or intramuscular injection of around 1000 to 3000 mcg may be of benefit in the treatment of dementia. Methyl B12 can be taken in drops you place under your tongue to be absorbed through the membranes of your mouth. Its benefit in neurological conditions is well supported.[30]

MINERALS

- *Potassium* – although it is best to increase your potassium intake by eating more fruit and vegetables, under medical supervision (by prescription), potassium supplements may help ease symptoms such as postural hypotension (feeling dizzy when standing up suddenly). A dose of around 300 mg daily can help ease the symptoms of nervous-system disorders, may improve muscle strength and may help prevent stroke.

AMINO ACIDS

- *L-tryptophan* – 1,000 mg taken twice daily (on an empty stomach, preferably with a small amount of carbohydrate) may help relieve depression and insomnia.
- *L-tyrosine* –1,000–2,000 mg taken daily. This amino acid is a precursor to dopamine – necessary for preventing Parkinson's disease. However, it may also help relieve depression.
- *Taurine* – 1.5 g taken daily may help slow down the effects of macular degeneration. Taurine is predominantly found in animal-based proteins and is therefore important to take in supplement form if you are a vegetarian.
- *Glutamic acid (glutamate or L-glutamine)* – 1–2 g taken daily may improve mental function.

ESSENTIAL FATTY ACIDS

- *Phospholipids* – phosphatidylserine and phosphatidylcholine should be used in the treatment and prevention of Alzheimer's disease, cognitive decline and nerve damage.

OTHER NUTRIENTS

- *Ginseng*, the benefits of which have been remarkably well researched, acts in several different ways in the brain and on the genes.[32]

Dr Sharma's Repair Programme

This programme is for those with established conditions. Consider adding the following to the recommendations above if you have specific neurological problems:

VITAMINS

- *Vitamin A* – eye drops can be of benefit for *sicca* (dry eye syndrome); 'senile' keratoses (age spots) may need doses as high as 100,000 iu per day for up to 20 months – by prescription only.

PHOSPHOLIPIDS

At the British Society for Ecological Medicine's Scientific Conference in November 2010, leading experts from around the world presented research and evidence on the potential use of phospholipids (special fats predominantly used in cell structure) in the repair of nervous-system damage. Treatment is both oral and intravenous, and as well as including an array of fatty acids, it utilizes minerals and vitamins with growth factors and a carbohydrate-limited diet.

Results demonstrate that this therapy, currently termed 'Phospholipid Exchange', may reverse prevalent symptoms, stabilize imbalanced chemistry in the nervous system and potentially be a treatment for currently incurable disease. More formal trials in the UK, the USA and Germany are underway and, if they support initial findings relating to the efficacy of this treatment, may offer a new therapeutic strategy for neurological and possibly other diseases, particularly those involving toxic exposure. If you are interested in finding a doctor with a specialist interest in this field, contact the British Society of Ecological Medicine.[31]

MINERALS
- *Lithium orotate* – 120 mg taken weekly. Advocated by some integrated physicians, particularly in the USA, lithium is used in drug form to deal with severe psychiatric disorders such as schizophrenia and bipolar disorder. I am not a great supporter of its general use and believe we get enough in our diet. To ensure good levels, make eggs, lemons, potato skins and seaweed frequent parts of your diet.

AMINO ACIDS
- *L-methionine* – up to 3 g taken daily. Vegetarians in particular have low levels of this amino acid. It is good for staving off the effects of Parkinson's disease.
- *Phenylalanine* – 1,000–2,000 mg taken daily if you suffer from Parkinson's disease. Half that dose may help relieve the symptoms of depression.
- *L-leucine or L-isoleucine* – up to 15 g in divided doses throughout the day if you suffer from motor neurone disease.
- *L-threonine* – 2–4 g taken daily if you suffer from motor neurone disease.

- *N-acetylcysteine (NAC)* – up to 200 mg taken three times a day if your doctor has established metal toxicity associated with dementia.
- *Acytyl L-carnitine* – 500 mg taken twice daily can help ease the symptoms of dementia and particularly early Alzheimer's disease.

OTHER NUTRIENTS

- *Coenzyme Q10* – 30 mg taken once or twice daily if you have periodontal disease (often associated with some forms of dementia).[33] Doses as high as 1,200 mg taken daily may be suitable for those suffering from Parkinson's disease.[34]
- *Hydergine* – up to 5 mg taken daily may help relieve the symptoms of dementia.[35]
- *Huperzine* – 0.4 mg taken daily improves cognitive activity and, seemingly working on a brain enzyme called acetyl cholinesterase, appears to improve the symptoms of Alzheimer's disease.
- *Vinpocetine* – limited research into this nutrient means that its efficacy is still in question; it may help stave off cognitive impairment.
- *Ghrelin* – this hormone, discussed briefly in Chapter 8, is associated with increasing appetite. Levels appear to have a direct effect on Parkinson's disease (PD) – higher levels appear to increase dopamine production. This suggests that a low calorie intake may be beneficial in combating the symptoms of PD. Keep an eye out for the development of pharmaceutical analogues (pharmaceutical 'copies' of a natural compound, in this case ghrelin) as taking them under medical supervision may help treat PD.

HERBAL REMEDIES

- *Gingko biloba* – standardized extracts are usually made up of approximately 25 per cent of the active component *Gingko heterosides*. Aim for about 40 mg taken 3 times daily if you suffer from age-related mental decline, macular degeneration or hearing loss. It may also be of benefit in treating age-related impotence.
- *Mucuna pruriens* – acts as a natural L-DOPA provider. Latest research from 2009 suggests that this herbal extract may relieve the uncontrolled movements of Parkinson's disease, even at low doses.[36]

HORMONE TREATMENTS

- *Thyroxine* – prescriptions of thyroxine (whether natural extracts or pharmaceutical grade) have to be monitored by doctors, but may be beneficial for combating age-related cognitive issues and possibly for delaying the development of neurological disease.

- *Dehydroepiandrosterone (DHEA)* – discuss taking this hormone (10–25 mg daily) with a medical practitioner.
- *Testosterone* – if tests show that you have low levels, this hormone may be considered as a treatment for memory loss and dementia, although we need more studies to be wholly confident in its efficacy.[38]

THE USE OF DRUGS

Drug treatment in Parkinson's disease has its place. Most neurologists would have us start medical intervention as late as possible as the body seems to become resistant to their effects. Keep an eye out for the availability of *Mucuna pruriens*, as mentioned already, in your area.

Beyond Parkinson's treatment I am not convinced that there is much benefit from the use of drugs in age-related neurological disease *at this time*. However, considerable research is ongoing, so keep an open ear and mind. For example, one of the world's leading researchers into ageing, Dr Aubrey de Grey, PhD, suggests that research into anti-amyloid vaccines may well influence deposits associated with Alzheimer's disease.

- *Aminoguanadine* – 75–150 mg taken daily can act as an antioxidant in living cells, neutralizing the effects of particular damaging free radicals and preventing the damage to cell walls and membranes that cause premature cell death.[39]
- *Centrophenoxine* – reduces lipofuscin levels, the latter being associated with dementia. It works by increasing levels of acetylcholine (*see* 'Acetylcholine' box below), which is a good thing as acetylcholine is good for brain function.
- *Dimercaptosuccinic acid (DMSA)* can help the body expel mercury if heavy metal tests reveal that you might have toxic levels in your brain.

ACETYLCHOLINE

Acetylcholine is good for brain function. It performs 'cholinergic' functions that are important in brain activity, such as memory and understanding. Many drugs taken as we age for conditions such as depression or high blood pressure block acetylcholine through their anticholinergic side effects. These drugs have been shown to worsen dementia.[40]

The harmful effects of drugs

What is concerning is that 76 drugs used commonly for a wide range of medical (not only neurological) disorders may actually *cause* memory loss and dementia. Around 40 drugs cause Parkinson's, 35 cause insomnia, 147 cause confusion and delirium, and over 300 can trigger depression, psychosis or even hallucinations.[41]

In Alzheimer's, the cholinesterase inhibitors (Aricept, Galantamine and others) only show limited effect in some areas of dementia and only in those with mild to moderate disease. Improvement seems to work only for 12 months or so. This group of drugs may be associated with premature death from other causes. The second type of Alzheimer's drug, known as N-methyl-D-aspartate receptor antagonist (NMDARA), blocks the production of glutamic acid (glutamate), which is a useful neurotransmitter but harmful in excess. Damaged brain tissue appears to increase glutamic acid levels.

Doctors have little option but to offer medication that counteracts symptoms of illness, but, unfortunately, many drugs actually worsen dementia.

It is extremely important that any drug you are given, at any age but particularly from mid-life onward, has little or no dementia-like side effects. I would encourage you to look very closely at the listed side effects of any drug prescribed. I will mention a few groups in particular.

Antipsychotics

Avoid antipsychotics in favour of more natural approaches and treatments for as long as possible, as these drugs often exacerbate the symptoms of dementia. A mixture of antidepressants and antipsychotics increases four-fold the speed with which dementia worsens.[42]

One out of every six patients prescribed antipsychotic drugs, many of which are known to have little long-term benefit in the elderly and are used mainly for their sedative effects, are causing significant harm in people with dementia and the general ageing population. The problem lies in the methodology of looking after our ageing population. As dementia creeps in, symptoms that make an affected individual difficult to live with increase. Frustration leads to anger and agitation, and direct or indirect symptoms of depression, neurosis and anxiety all contribute to 'cries for help' from the individual or the carers.[43]

Selective serotonin re-uptake inhibitors (SSRIs)
These are popular antidepressant drugs. Some reports suggest that these drugs increase cognitive performance in the ageing brain, but when researchers looked at the data, the evidence for this was weak.[44]

SSRIs have been linked to a number of harmful side effects:
- They have been shown to shrink an important controlling part of the brain known as the hippocampus.[45]
- Falls caused by unsteadiness are associated with SSRIs. Prozac is one of the more famous in this group.[46]

Tricyclic antidepressants
These cause damage to the brain.[47]

Statins
I discuss statins at length in Chapter 6. Some controversy has arisen with regard to the use of these drugs as a treatment for dementia. In 2003, research suggested that statins, despite potentially altering cholesterol levels and indirectly maintaining a good blood flow to and in the brain, had no role in either the prevention or the treatment of dementia.[48] In 2008, a ten-year study conducted in collaboration with the University of Michigan School of Public Health suggested that statins may halve the risk of dementia, but by

COMMON DRUGS THAT MAY CAUSE DEMENTIA SYMPTOMS

- Amitriptaline
- Atenolol and other, but not all, beta blockers
- Beclomethasone
- Captopril
- Cimetidine and Ranitidine
- Codeine
- Diazepam and other benzodiazepines
- Fentanyl
- Fluoxamine
- Morphine
- Nifedipine
- Paroxetine
- Prednisolone/prednisone and hydrocortisone
- Warfarin

2011 we were, again, informed that statins are of no benefit.[49] Furthermore, statins have been associated with memory loss – among these, lipitor, mevacor, zocor, and pravachol all had reports of memory loss, with over 900 such cases for lipitor alone since 2004.[50]

Exercise

I think I can create an argument based on solid scientific research that there is no part of the body that does not respond beneficially to exercise. The nervous system is perhaps best served, and there appears to be so much evidence based on animal experiments, population studies and measurements of various neurotransmitters that I wonder why it is not compulsory for any ageing population to exercise! Consider the following:

- Exercise has been found to increase levels of 'brain-derived neurotrophic factor'; other studies have found that exercise increases levels of serotonin, dopamine and noradrenalin (norepinephrine). These are neurohormones that are good for the brain.
- Exercise triggers the production of endorphins, the body's natural opiates (morphine-like compounds), which may have an effect in enhancing happy and positive feelings, which, in turn, benefit the brain.
- Aerobic exercise protects against dementia.[51] It is as simple as that!
- Studies have shown that exercise both prevents and slows down the development of Parkinson's disease.[52]
- Exercise keeps down blood pressure, reduces the incidence of diabetes and encourages blood flow, thereby reducing risks of vascular dementia and macular degeneration – frankly, it will benefit most neurological conditions.
- Exercise has been shown to alter levels of beneficial amino acids in the brain, thereby enhancing the function of neurotransmitters.[53]
- Exercise alters stress hormones such as adrenalin (epinephrine) and noradrenalin (norepinephrine), with numerous metabolic effects throughout the nervous system.
- Studies show that learning and memory are improved with exercise as is our mental acuity and activity.[54]

To benefit the nervous system, exercise needs to be aerobic, but specific exercises that require balance are most beneficial. Balance is controlled in part by specialized nerves called proprioceptors of which there is an abundance in the soles of the feet. The impulses that travel up to the brain are sorted out in the part of the brain at the top of the spinal column (the cerebellum) and in the brain stem at the base of the skull (the pedunculopontine nucleus). This coordinates with visual centres and to a degree with information from other senses. Studies show an increase in blood flow to the cerebellum when we do balancing exercises.[55]

A lot of Eastern exercise systems such as yoga and martial arts like tai chi focus on balance, but even the simple experience of walking on uneven terrain helps. Your recommended 30–40 minutes of brisk walking every day is best practised 'off road' – walking up and down hill and dale and across ploughed fields.

Exercise contraptions based on the old concept of a 'wobble board' can, markedly stimulate the brain to reduce the neurological consequences of ageing when practised for just a few minutes a day. You can find wobble boards in most gyms.

Lifestyle

Sleep

Owing to its slower rate of repair, the nervous system – perhaps more than other parts of the body – benefits from rest. Time spent sleeping and in relaxation or meditation is well proven to enhance nervous-system health, activity and capabilities.

To a degree, everyone has an optimum sleep pattern that may vary within a certain range. Science suggests that fewer than five hours' sleep a night is detrimental, and, outside of the teenage years, anything more that 10–11 hours is probably a pathological condition.

The suggestion that we should rise from slumber at dawn and go to sleep at dusk is probably a sound but unrealistic expectation. We are not exercising and burning up calories through the daylight hours as we used to before the Industrial Revolution, and going to sleep is not as easy as it used to be because of light and noise 'pollution' after the sun sets. Furthermore, as we age, bladder sensitivity and other disturbances at night break our sleep pattern.

We require different levels of sleep depending on our physical and mental activity over the course of any particular day, but the simple rule of thumb of going to bed when tired and awaking without being awoken is the ideal. This may be possible for many at weekends, but through most working weeks it is not so easy, and going to bed a little earlier (as it is usually the need to get up that shortens our sleep) is a sensible ploy. Sleeping six to eight hours a night with an average of seven hours seems to be the most often recommended by sleep experts, with some authorities suggesting nine hours is optimum.

The science behind sleep is vast and complex. Put very simply, sleep can be divided into two broad types: rapid eye movement (REM) and non-rapid eye movement (NREM) sleep. NREM is often further divided into stages N1, N2 and N3.

During a full night's sleep we undergo between five and seven differing cycles of approximately 90 minutes. When we first fall asleep, we have the longest periods of N3 (deep) sleep and short periods of REM (dreaming) sleep. When we are closest to waking, periods of N3 are at their shortest, and we spend most of each 90-minute cycle in N2 (light) sleep and REM (dreaming) sleep.

Some imaging studies clearly demonstrate that nerve function and, eventually, damage occurs when we do not get enough sleep. Having one hour less than we need each night quickly accumulates to neurological dysfunction. Although the brain can recover by sending us more quickly and for longer periods into N3 sleep at our next sleep opportunity, there are suggestions that prolonged lack of sleep enhances age-related neurological damage.[56] A lack of REM sleep in particular has been hypothesized for some time as being relevant to the development of Alzheimers disease.[57]

EVERYDAY TIPS

- Ensure you brush your teeth twice daily. Chronic inflammation of the mouth increases the risk of developing Alzheimer's disease.[62]
- Avoid electromagnetic frequencies (EMFs) as brain tumours known as gliomas and possibly others known as meningiomas have an association with these.[63]
- All forms of meditation and prayer have been shown to reduce depression in ageing populations.[64]
- An active social life slows cognitive decline up to the age of 80.[65]
- Nine hours every day of bright light reduces incidences of both dementia and depression.[66]
- Music reduces depression in ageing populations.[67]
- Music decreases anxiety, depression and aggressiveness, while increasing memory capability in those with Alzheimer's disease.[68]

Meditation

As we reach middle age, and even earlier, a few minutes a day in a meditative state may markedly benefit age-related nerve conditions. Many studies support the benefits of meditation in maintaining cognitive awareness and function, and preventing the onset of age-related neurological problems.

The process of meditation switches the brain into particular electrical patterns and activity that demand less from the nervous tissues, thereby reducing the amount of waste material that can cause damage. Zen meditation is known to have neuroprotective effects and reduces the cognitive decline associated with normal ageing.[58]

Theoretical biochemical reasons are plentiful to support why meditation, in association with yoga, can improve attention and cognitive deficits even in those showing dementia.[59]

Meditation is not a simple technique to learn, and for some it requires marked shifts in their perception and understanding of what true relaxation is. There are many different forms and techniques, and everyone should try to learn a technique that suits them.

Other factors

Low levels of the brain's 'happy juices' such as serotonin and noradrenalin (norepinephrine) are linked to depression and influence memory generally. Deficiency in both can speed up dementia. According to one paper, counselling can potentially defer and slow down the effects of dementia.[60]

Many studies show that keeping the brain active can prevent dementia. Learning a second language in middle age actually delays onset and may even prevent dementia. Bilingual patients had delayed onset of dementia by an average of about four years.[61]

Investigations and tests

I have described changes that can occur in the nervous system owing to the deposition of toxins, the formation of tangles and plaques, and so on. Amyloid and lipofuscin build up in the nervous tissue, and if we were able to get a clear view of this and other microscopic changes, we might be able to compare alterations to specific age groups and give an actual, as opposed to a chronological, age of the nervous system. There are no simple, non-invasive tests that can do this.

Measurement of reflexes, memory, learning and understanding (cognition) are all so variable and dependent on factors such as genes, IQ, previous education, stress and depression levels, plus many other factors, that it is not possible to create a comparative table of age-related actions. That said, in my opinion there is considerable benefit in undergoing various levels of testing as we are aware that deficiencies and toxins – both avoidable factors – can be corrected through treatment.

Establishing if past injuries such as bangs on the head, whiplash, oxygen deprivation or toxic events have impacted on brain blood flow or function can advise us on levels of treatment or lifestyle alterations that may prevent premature deterioration or even the development of diseases such as Parkinson's disease.

First-line investigations

This level of investigation should be considered by everyone interested in optimizing their health.

BLOOD AND URINE TESTS
- *A broad nutritional analysis* including tests for:
  - vitamin B-complex;
  - folic acid;
  - essential fatty acids;
  - mineral profile;
  - antioxidants.
- *Toxic metal screening* – I recommend this as a first-line assessment because of the increasing evidence that deposits of mercury and aluminium in the brain may trigger age-related conditions.

Second-line investigations

This level of testing is for those who want to know more about their current and potential risk status for nervous system diseases or age-related neuro-logical disorders. It would be wise for those with a family history of dementia or neurological disease to opt for these investigations.

BLOOD TESTS
Neurogenomics
There is limited evidence that most age-related neurological diseases are genetically passed on, but environmental influences affecting a parent may persist through the lives of their children and therefore pose a risk if they interact with genes. We may have been exposed to risks in the first 20 years simply by living in the same environment as our parents. We also tend to copy

their lifestyles and continue with risks that we may have been brought up with.

The nervous system and its health relies upon us protecting it from free-radical activity. It is able to detoxify through two processes: methylation and the use of glutathione. We can examine which genes govern these activities, and any changes we find can provide a warning that the patient may have a faulty detoxification system.

Genomic profiling for neurological problems does not search for genes that 'cause' age-related neurological disorders. There are genes that are associated with dementia and Parkinson's disease, but these make up a low percentage of those who suffer from these diseases.[69]

Haemoencephalography (HEG)
This is the study of blood flow in the brain using an optical probe that shines light through the skin and skull to assess the colour of the blood. Oxygenated blood is red, while deoxygenated is blue. Healthy brains have a specific blood flow, but brain areas that are damaged or demanding increased oxygen or nutrition will appear redder.

This simple test requires nothing more than sitting with electrodes on the scalp. The electrodes are also attached to a computer that uses electrical information from the brain to determine how perfused the brain is. Research suggests that conditions that may be picked up during analysis of the computer reading, or even predicted, include:

- ageing memory loss;
- Alzheimer's disease;
- stroke;
- toxic encephalopathy (brain damage).

Advanced investigations
These are necessary for those who show signs of any of the neurological conditions discussed in this chapter, including dementia, Parkinson's disease and tremor, and those who have had transient ischaemic attacks, strokes or other neurological diseases.

Quantitative electroencephalography (QEEG)
QEEG is an assessment to measure the electrical activity of the brain. It is becoming more widely available and there appears to be plenty of evidence that is as accurate a method of pinpointing pathology as other tests.[70]

The QEEG was found to predict dementia in Parkinson's disease three years prior to discernable characteristics of deterioration.[71]

The procedure takes about an hour. A cap containing sensors is placed over the scalp to measure electrical activity in the brain. Brainwave patterns, how different parts of the brain interact and the efficiency of the brain all form part of the analysis. The process requires the individual to sit with their eyes open and then closed while carrying out some basic tasks (often using a computer screen).

MRI and CT scanning

I do not discuss here in detail the advances that are being made in conventional scanning, such as magnetic resonance imaging (MRI) and computed tomography (CT), but work through your general practitioner and specialists is of course important.

Florbetapir (^{18}F) testing

I feel it is worth mentioning one new test involving a chemical called Florbetapir (^{18}F), as it highlights an important point about testing in general. Florbetapir (^{18}F) is a radioactive diagnostic agent that binds to amyloid plaques to evaluate their presence in Alzheimer's disease. This may differentiate this type of dementia from other forms, but as 20 per cent of people have amyloid with no dysfunction, surely we have to be a little wary of a radioactive compound being sent into the brain? Until we have specific treatments for amyloid, I think perhaps it is prudent if offered this, or frankly any other test, to ask the question: "What is the therapeutic, as opposed to the academic, worth of this test?"

Chapter 8

Hormones

Hormones are vital chemical messengers produced in very small amounts by tissues in the body known as glands. A hormone travels from one place to another and affects organs and systems via receptors on cell walls or in the cells themselves. The diagram on the following page illustrates the major glands in the body.

Neurohormones are chemicals made by one end of a nerve that influence another nerve or a receptor on the cell wall of a muscle or organ. These are called hormones, but really we should call them transmitters.

Most hormones travel from the gland, through the bloodstream or through the fluid in the nervous system, to other parts of the body.

All glands, like other parts of the body, lose functionality with age and are affected by pathological conditions. Some hormones are not influenced by nutrition, supplements, natural therapies or even drugs, but many can be – to varying degrees. This chapter focuses on those hormones that we can influence through naturopathic techniques. It's these that give us the power to be able to slow down, or possibly reverse the ageing process.

How do hormones affect ageing?

As hormones travel in the bloodstream they may affect every part of the body. Specific hormones have a profound influence on:

- the brain and nervous system;
- the cardiovascular system;
- the bones and muscles.

All stimulate the cells they affect, increasing activity and speeding up repair. As a hormone level diminishes, so does the activity of the organ or system over which that hormone has an effect.

As we reach the end of our reproductive years, the glands making our sex hormones, the ovaries in women and testicles in men, stop working as efficiently as they once did. Ovaries 'fail' on average when women reach their mid-40s, while men find their testicles can remain active until death, although the production of testosterone and sperm declines after the age of 60 or so. As the levels of sex hormones fall, so do their effects on muscles, nerves, skin and hair. As a result, falling hormone levels affect not only our ability to reproduce but also our strength, libido, moods, emotions and appearance.

The neurotransmitters, adrenalin (epinephrine), noradrenalin (norepinephrine) and others found in the nervous system or produced in the adrenal medulla (the inner part of the adrenal glands) influence nerves throughout the body. To help balance this, another part of the adrenal gland, the adrenal cortex, produces a stress-coping hormone called cortisol. Without cortisol, our bodies would operate on a prolonged state of high alert, in turn speeding up the ageing process, particularly in the cardiovascular, structural and nervous systems.

An understanding of how we can test to see if we have sufficient amounts of hormones and how we can treat deficiencies (or excesses) using natural (or drug) therapies is vital to optimizing health and slowing down the ageing process.

HOW TO SLOW DOWN THE AGEING OF THE GLANDS

The production of hormones from our endocrine system (the collective name for our hormone-producing glands) not only influences the health and activity of the target organs, but also directly affects our mood, sexuality and ability to enjoy life. Failure to keep our hormone levels in an optimal state and the receptors functional may lead to unhappy and unhealthy later years.

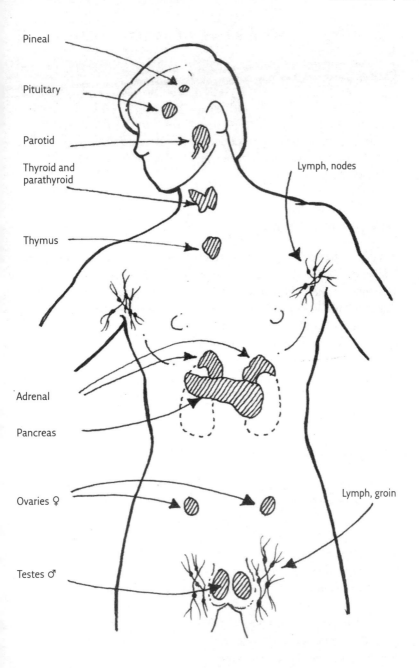

Figure 16: **Glands of the body: the endocrine system**

NOT REAL GLANDS

Some tissues in the body are referred to as glands, but they are not truly glands at all. Lymph nodes (found all over the body, not just in the neck as we often assume), for example, are meshworks of protein strands that trap white blood cells and debris, but do not make hormones. Other non-glands include Bartholin's glands (found in the vagina), salivary and parotid 'glands' (which produce saliva) and sebaceous glands in the skin that make our protective skin secretions.

The pituitary gland

Found in the brain, the pituitary gland makes several hormones that influence the functionality of other glands. The production of these hormones is not easily influenced by supplements and natural products, but maintaining general health and psychological well-being will keep the pituitary gland functioning better for longer. Stress is relevant to the pituitary and its control of other glands.[1]

A medical practitioner will use blood tests to measure levels of the pituitary hormones, but only when specific illnesses or ailments demand it. Only ACTH, HGH, TSH and oxytocin, have a direct relevance to ageing well.

Human growth hormone (HGH)

Studies in growth hormone since the 1970s clearly indicate that the process of ageing is markedly influenced by growth hormone.

Growth hormone is known to:
- influence cell growth;
- influence cellular repair;
- decrease telomerase activity (influencing cell activity and preventing cancer);
- stimulate the immune system;
- improve depression and anxiety;
- have a positive effect on memory;
- act against insomnia;
- increase libido.

Pituitary hormone	Organ or tissue influenced
Adrenocorticotrophic hormone (ACTH)	Adrenal cortex (the part of the adrenal gland associated with stress response)
Antidiuretic hormone	Kidneys and bladder
Human growth hormone (HGH)	All body tissues
Follicle-stimulating hormone (FSH)	Ovaries
Luteinizing hormone	Ovaries
Melanocyte-stimulating hormone (MSH)	Melanocytes in the skin (tanning)
Oxytocin	Brain and breast tissue
Prolactin	Breast tissue
Thyroid-stimulating hormone (TSH)	Thyroid

In a few studies, HGH has been found to improve quality of life, reduce fatigue, help maintain lean body mass, lower cholesterol levels and protect against atherosclerosis, thereby working against the onset of heart disease.[2] There is evidence that HGH may influence diabetes, rheumatism and osteoporosis, and generally benefit healthy longevity.[3]

Signs and symptoms of HGH deficiency

The word that best sums up HGH deficiency is 'sagging'. Facial changes such as droopy eyelids, sagging cheeks and a downward inflection of the mouth giving a sad grimace are all standard signs as is a general aged look. Hair loss, longitudinal lines in the nails and particularly a loss of muscle tone may all be related to HGH deficiency.

Psychologically, anxiety, depression, a lack of self-worth and the inability to find a 'happy place' may all be associated with insufficient HGH, especially if this is a marked shift from a person's normal attitude.

Testing for HGH

HGH is broken down quickly in the bloodstream and so measuring it directly is an inaccurate means of testing. A compound in the blood known as insulin-like growth factor (IGF-1), also called somatomedin C, acts in the body in conjunction with HGH, and as levels are proportionate to each other, it is better for doctors to measure IGF-1 levels instead. In essence, they gain a reflective reading of HGH. Some medical centres also offer a test known as IGF-BP-3, which is slightly more accurate. As with most hormonal tests, symptoms have to be taken into consideration when looking at the results.

Once we are over the age of 25, our HGH levels drop to a low threshold, stabilizing and showing little fluctuation. This makes testing for levels a little pointless. Most anti-ageing researchers specializing in hormones consider that HGH levels are not as relevant as the concentration of HGH in the blood. In order to maintain good health, they believe that it is better to bring up HGH concentration to that which we might expect in a 25-year-old. Measurements of IGF-1 between 120–500 umol/L are considered optimal, although one authority[4] suggests IGF-1 levels should be 300–350 umol/L for men and 220–300umol/L for women.

As HGH can drive down the stress-coping hormone cortisol, it is sensible to measure cortisol level on and off to ensure stability within expected ranges. You should not use HGH if your cortisol level is low; wait until it is brought back into the normal range before resuming treatment.

Treatment

Considering all the potential benefits, why is HGH not high on the list of treatments available to all of us and particularly as we age?

HGH is considered safe to use when it is medically necessary: for example, to treat dwarfism if this is detected early enough. However, side effects of HGH, especially if it is administered at too high a dosage, can include overgrowth of bone and tissues (acromegaly), which is best characterized by those few 'giants' that used to fascinate circus-goers in days gone by. Other than that, high levels of HGH can cause fluid retention, painful joints, enlarged breasts in males and liver damage. A few studies have suggested an increased risk of cancer in adults who have taken HGH, but a study in 2004[5] claims to have demonstrated that only a small increased risk of colon cancer and Hodgkin's disease (a cancer of the lymphatic system) exists. Even studies where HGH was used by people with cancer were not particularly conclusive in establishing there is a risk.

So, why is HGH not used widely? I do not know! Could it be that the use of HGH would reduce the incidence of diseases in our ageing population to such an extent that it would cost the pharmaceutical industry a substantial amount of profit?

Like many other hormones HGH is quickly broken down in the gut, therefore treatment involves injecting it into muscles. However, there is ongoing research into sprays and sublingual absorption (lozenges that go under the tongue). HGH *must* be prescribed by a medical practitioner – never

SIDE EFFECTS OF
HUMAN GROWTH HORMONE

According to the World Anti-Doping Agency (2007), commonly
reported side effects for HGH abuse include:
- diabetes in prone individuals;
- worsening of cardiovascular disease;
- muscle, joint and bone pain;
- hypertension and cardiac deficiency;
- abnormal growth of organs;
- accelerated osteoarthritis.

These problems seem to correlate quite closely with the conditions
HGH might treat! As is often the case, too much of a good thing can
be harmful.

risk injecting a product that you buy over the Internet. Unfortunately, while
the authorities stick to their poorly supported scepticism about HGH as an
anti-ageing treatment, it is too often available through unlicensed sources.

A medical professional should start with a low dosage and monitor your
signs and symptoms, adjusting the dosage as necessary.

Non-conventional and naturopathic options

If you are considering the use of unprescribed growth hormone, I strongly
advise you to look at the following options instead:
- Maintaining a lean weight seems to encourage cellular response to
  our naturally low levels of HGH.
- The same can be said for getting enough sleep, reducing stress and
  particularly avoiding tobacco and other drugs.
- Getting levels of the other hormones correct, particularly the sex
  hormones, the sleep hormone melatonin and the thyroid hormone,
  can all influence HGH levels.

SUPPLEMENTATION

Oral absorption of compounds known as secretagogues is theoretically,
rather than scientifically, considered to be a potential treatment for HGH
deficiency. Secretagogues stimulate the pituitary gland to produce
HGH and have no recognized risks or side effects. At this time, a product
known as symbiotropin has anecdotal evidence of efficacy. Sermorelin is

another secretagogue, which is taken as instructed on the label – usually under the tongue.

HGH production is controlled by a hormone known as growth-hormone-releasing hormone (GHRH) made in the hypothalamus, a part of the brain that controls certain functions within the pituitary gland. There is some encouraging data regarding GHRH given by injection, but these studies tend to be on younger people. If you decide to try supplementation, it is worth noting the following:

- The efficacy of HGH secretagogues seems to diminish if you take them continuously. Instead, try a pattern of four weeks on and four weeks off.
- Ensure you read the dosages and side effects on any product you choose and that you tell your doctor that you are using it.
- To encourage HGH secretagogue activity, consider supplementation with niacin (vitamin B3) – take 500 mg twice daily. (If you get hot or flush when taking niacin, buy the non-flush type.)
- Take an inexpensive whey product or other complex essential amino acid formula, because several amino acids are required for HGH production. (Be wary of expensive products claiming to be HGH-releasing factors that simply contain amino acids as there is no guarantee they will get to your brain to have an effect.)

Oxytocin

Interesting research, conducted predominantly in the USA, highlights the anti-ageing potential of the hormone oxytocin. Released from the posterior part of the pituitary gland, oxytocin was one of the first hormones to have its structure of nine amino acids discovered. Its name evolved from the Greek for 'quick birth' after scientists in the early 20th century discovered that it enhances the contraction of the uterus. Historically, Oxytocin was thought to have little influence elsewhere in the body other than encouraging the flow of breast milk. However, in the last few years, its association with several other areas of health have come to light.

Oxytocin has potential uses in:

- anorgasmia – an inability to orgasm;
- enhancing erection and ejaculation;
- increasing sociability with knock-on effects for overcoming feelings of isolation and improving our sense of connectedness;
- autism and Asperger's syndrome;

- post-traumatic stress disorder;
- the pain of fibromyalgia, and other muscular aches and pains;
- psychopathic behaviour, narcissism and manipulative behaviour;
- general well-being and stress.

Some of these problems are common age-related changes in physical and psychological character. Experiments on rats and anecdotal evidence in humans have demonstrated that oxytocin has effects on heart muscle, and both animal and human studies show that supplementation can benefit stress levels and the sexual dysfunction of delayed orgasm or an inability to climax.

Oxytocin is known as the 'love' hormone as it is produced when we cuddle. More intimate or sexual activity increases oxytocin production and attention paid to the nipples in particular can flood the system with this hormone. An orgasm peaks oxytocin levels in the blood. Importantly, oxytocin may help couples remain bonded as they age – at a time when we might begin to feel taken for granted.[6]

Treatment

To ensure good levels of this hormone in your system (levels are easy to measure), maintain intimate contact throughout your life. Oxytocin is also available in the following forms:
- *Injection* – best for labour and aches and pains.
- *Nasal sprays and sublingually* – easier to use and effective in sociability and sexual issues.
- *Slow-release ingestible capsules* – however, the hormone is swiftly broken down in the gastrointestinal tract, so its effects are diminished.

Blood test results and symptoms of deficiency will help your medical practitioner prescribe you the correct dosage of this hormone supplement. An average daily dose is 5iu, starting at perhaps half that to monitor for side effects. Doses of up to 50iu may be used to treat autism.

The risks of taking this hormone in pharmaceutical form are not well established, but ensure that your doctor monitors your levels of stress-coping adrenal cortisone (a deficiency may show up as fatigue). Becoming over-affectionate – 'clingy syndrome' – is a sign that the dosage is too high. Side effects appear to be short-lived and disappear swiftly on stopping or reducing the dosage.

Melatonin

Melatonin is best known as the jet-lag hormone. It is produced by a small piece of tissue known as the pineal gland, which delivers melatonin directly to the bloodstream, and is also made in small amounts by white blood cells, bone marrow cells and some epithelial (inner lining of tubes) cells. Melatonin production is inhibited by natural daylight. As the sun goes down, less light reaches the pineal gland from nerves at the back of the eye and so melatonin levels increase at night time.

Fifteen years ago, I wrote that we should be wary of using melatonin as a supplement because not enough was known about its safety. However, in the last decade a plethora of evidence has emerged to suggest that my caution was unfounded. In fact, if I were able to take only one product to supplement my health, it would probably be melatonin.

Study after study is showing how melatonin appears to have an influence in many different areas:

- *Alzheimer's disease* (*see* Chapter 7).
- *Parkinson's disease* and possibly other neurological degenerative diseases (*see* Chapter 7).
- *Sleep disorders* associated with a break in circadian rhythm such as jet lag, but also in those who work night shifts, 'burn the candle at both ends' or have age-related insomnia.
- *Macular degeneration.* This disease comes in two forms – dry and wet (*see* Chapter 10). Both forms seem to benefit from melatonin and it appears more effective than current injection treatments, which are the gold standard.[7]
- *Glaucoma* – a condition in which increased pressure in the eyeball damages the retina and vision.
- *Arterial hypertension* (high blood pressure; *see* Chapter 6).
- *Gastrointestinal diseases.* Studies show the benefits of melatonin in inflammatory bowel disease and spasmodic abdominal pains, as found in irritable bowel disease.
- *Depression.* Agomelatine is a melatonin analogue – that is, it has a similar chemical structure to melatonin and has recently been released as an antidepressant working on circadian patterns. The analogue has a similar strength to approximately 75 mg of melatonin. Used predominantly in patients with psychiatric disorders, this new antidepressant should encourage research into higher dosages of melatonin by itself as an antidepressant.
- *Chronic fatigue syndrome* and *fibromyalgia.*

- *Rheumatoid arthritis (see* Chapter 10*)*.
- *Cancer* – evidence of efficacy in treatment outcomes[8] and in counteracting the side effects of chemotherapy and radiation.[9]
- *Syndrome X (metabolic syndrome).,*
- *Immunity (see* Chapter 9).
- *Hormone production in pregnant women* (but actually reducing follicle-stimulating hormone and luteinizing hormone if not pregnant).[10]

How melatonin works

As you might assume, in order to have so many different benefits, melatonin has multiple modes of action. Primarily, it works as *a powerful antioxidant*. Its antioxidant activity is probably the reason for its benefits in macular degeneration, where it is considered a 'rescue factor' – one that actually repairs as much as prevents deterioration.

Melatonin is the most potent antioxidant in the nervous system and, as a result, has a direct influence on our susceptibility to neurological disease. This hormone increases levels of leptin, the appetite suppressant that the body produces to tell us that we have eaten enough. It is through this connection that melatonin probably influences metabolic syndrome and diabetes.

Furthermore, melatonin influences mitochondria. The actual production of energy involves molecules known as NAD/NADH, and melatonin appears to act at this particular point. And, finally, melatonin also appears to influence our very DNA. It modulates the cleaving off of telomeres responsible for the natural death of cells and the prevention of immortal cells that are generally poor in function or potentially cancerous.

Melatonin and ageing

By the time we reach 80 years of age, the body produces only 25 per cent of the amount of melatonin that we had in our youth.

The US National Library of Medicine cites more than 65 medical research papers relating longevity to the use of melatonin supplementation in both animals and humans. The same database provides more than 14,000 papers on melatonin's antioxidant activities and other processes!

Testing for melatonin

The body produces between 30 and 100 mcg of melatonin per day. Saliva samples and urinalysis enable doctors to gauge levels of melatonin's breakdown product 6-sulphatoxy-melatonin. The urine test is probably the most accurate.

Melatonin deficiency is hard to define except by tests, as the signs and symptoms are similar to those of anyone who is not getting enough sleep – for example, poor quality of sleep, lack of dreams, feeling tired on waking, anxiety, depression, tendency to become emotional and irritability. Physical symptoms such as high blood pressure, muscular tension and others associated with a bad night's sleep are often present, but not specific.

Melatonin levels should be tested in anyone who has any of the conditions mentioned above, particularly those with heart conditions such arrhythmia or a past history of stroke or heart attack.

Lifestyle and nutrition

Melatonin is produced in darkness. Try to make your sleeping quarters as dark as you can and, conversely, in order to encourage the circadian aspect of melatonin production, try to get into direct sunlight as much as possible during the day and especially as early in the morning as you can. Many of the wavelengths of light that are relevant to health – including relevant to the stimulation of melatonin production – are cut out by window panes and spectacles. You need to get outside, but remember not to look directly at the sun and avoid sunburn.

Melatonin production is known to be decreased by caffeine, alcohol and tobacco, as well as by electrical devices close to your head and high electrical currents.

Melatonin treatment

If you plan to take melatonin, discuss your dosage with a physician. In the UK it is a prescription-only medication, but that is not the case worldwide. Throughout this book I have not, generally, recommended dosages for medication that are best prescribed by a doctor. However, as this hormone is widely available off the shelf, I feel it is best to direct those who unwisely choose to self-medicate.

Below the age of 40	1.5 mg nightly before bedtime
Over the age of 40	3 mg nightly before bedtime

Take the tablets around 30–60 minutes before going to bed for your melatonin levels to peak three to four hours later.

One authority believes that the use of selenium and zinc at the same time helps with melatonin uptake and activity.[11]

PARTNER WITH RESVERATROL

Research suggests that melatonin may interact with resveratrol, a compound found in the skin of red grapes, that is in itself a potent antioxidant that delays age-related cellular deterioration.[12] Melatonin seems to activate the beneficial compounds within resveratrol, so using the two together seems sensible.

There are no known contraindications to taking melatonin, although studies have not been performed on those under the age of 18, nor on pregnant women and breastfeeding mothers. If you take too much, reversible depression, tiredness and a loss of libido may occur. You are likely to be overdosing on melatonin if you are waking early, feeling headachy in the morning and noticing strong heartbeats with or without sweating. Intense dreaming and excessive sleep are an indication of overdose.

Supplementation may increase human growth hormone production, so seek medical advice before you take melatonin if you are already taking HGH secretagogues or injectable HGH.

Melatonin increases the conversion of thyroxine T4 to T3, so those on thyroid supplementation might need to take less. Please ensure your doctor tests your thyroid levels – both T4 and T3) – as well as TSH (*see* thyroid, below).

THE THYROID GLAND

The thyroid gland is an H-shaped structure about the size of a palm, situated along and under the Adam's apple. Thyroid cells synthesize thyroid hormones, the most prominent being thyroxine (T4) and tri-iodothyronine (T3). These both include iodine and the amino acid tyrosine. (The thyroid gland also contains a small amount of tissue known as the parathyroid. This produces a hormone called calcitonin, which controls calcium levels in the body.)

The thyroid hormones are responsible for regulating the metabolism of cells throughout the body. The amounts of thyroid hormone in the body are controlled by a chemical released from the pituitary gland known as thyroid-stimulating hormone (TSH). This itself is controlled by another hormone called TSH-releasing hormone (TRH), which comes from a part of the brain known as the hypothalamus. An increase in the level of thyroid hormones depresses the production of TRH, which has a knock-on effect for the production of TSH. In turn, levels of T3 and T4 fall. This cycle attempts to maintain a constant level of circulating hormone within a suitable range. This is an example of a biofeedback mechanism. As we age, this control mechanism becomes less efficient.

T3 is about four times more potent than T4. It is made inside cells by the removal of one of the iodine molecules. The effects of thyroxine are therefore much greater inside cells. Cell-wall damage by free radicals and other environmental chemicals may interfere with receptors to such a degree that thyroxine may not be able to enter cells, thereby reducing efficacy even in the presence of normal levels.

Hypothyroidism (low thyroxine levels)

The thyroid hormones and their axis of control affect nearly all the cells in the body and deficiency is well referenced as being associated with ageing. A lack of thyroid hormones not only influences cell function, but increases the amount of damaging free radicals, while reducing antioxidants. A decrease slows down detoxification, muscular function and cell metabolism. The symptoms of hypothyroidism may occur in any part of the body and should be considered if two or three of the symptoms in the table above persist.

Quite frankly, we all might feel many of these symptoms at any time, so diagnosis is rather dependent on testing.

Hypothyroidism may be divided into primary (failure of production within the thyroid itself) or secondary (caused by other influences on the thyroid). If left untreated early in life, this will lead to a marked mental inability known as cretinism. It is not a directly age-related condition (for more information, see my book *The Family Encyclopedia of Health*) and there are many causes:

- *Iodine deficiency.* This occurs in specific parts of the world where there is insufficient iodine in the food chain. Seafood in particular is high in iodine, and people living in mountainous areas where fish is not part of the regular diet are more prone to iodine deficiency.
- *Goitrogens.* These are food substances (including soya bean, peanuts, millet, turnips, cabbage and mustard) that prevent the utilization of iodine by damageing the thyroid. Cooking usually deactivates goitrogens.
- *Cortisol.* This stress hormone is known to block the production of T3.
- *Non-recognition.* In rare cases, thyroid levels may be normal (or even raised), but symptoms of hypothyroidism continue. This may be because the cells of the body do not recognize the thyroid hormones.

Heavy metal, chemical or elemental (arsenic, cadmium) toxicity may be a root cause of this condition.[13]

- *Destruction of normal thyroid glandular tissue by tumours, operations or radioiodine.* The latter two are more frequent because these are common treatments for hyperthyroidism.
- *Autoimmune thyroiditis.* Also called Hashimoto's disease, this most commonly affects middle-aged women and is because of antibodies being formed against different constituents of the thyroid gland. Put simply, the body attacks its own thyroid.
- *Drug-induced hypothyroidism* may be caused by certain prescribed drugs including those used for heart arrhythmias, some tranquilizers, antiepileptic drugs and others.
- *Reduced TRH or TSH associated with disease or tumour* in the pituitary gland or the hypothalamus.

Ageing is associated with a reduced production of THS, T3 and T4 as well as their cell receptors. A lack of thyroid hormone activity affects all of the following age-related issues:

- apoptosis, normal cell death
- nutrient absorption

HALOGENS IN THE HOME

- *Iodine* is a halogen and is in the same category in the chemical periodic table as fluoride, bromide and chlorine. Any compounds including these elements may therefore influence the effects of thyroxine.
- *Bromine* is found in polybrominated biphenyls (PBBs), which are contained in flame retardants, manufactured materials and many plastics in our homes.
- *Polychlorinated biphenyls* (PCBs) are PPBs' chlorinated cousins and are found in new sofas, curtains, carpets, and so on.

Buy new home furniture in the spring and spend as much time as possible with your windows open to blow away the toxic substances. Try to avoid letting babies crawl on new carpet and avoid exposing newborns to new furniture and fittings. Perhaps look out for clean and hygienic second-hand furniture for babies and hold on to 'hand-me-down' baby clothes.

Symptoms of hypothyroidism		
Depression	Anxiety	Insomnia
Poor concentration	Loss of memory	Numbness or tingling
Carpal tunnel syndrome	Dizzy spells	Weight gain
Sensitivity to the cold	Poor vision	Fatigue
Abnormal circadian rhythms	Water retention	Hoarse voice
Slow heart beat	Slow speech	Decreased immune function
Irritability	Palpitations	Brittle hair and/or nails
Decreased appetite	Constipation	Infertility/miscarriage
Irregular periods	Absent periods	Hair loss (notably eyebrows)
Muscle cramps	Dry skin	

- the ability to repair
- immune system activity
- psychological well-being, especially depression, as well as overall quality of life
- memory
- heart and arterial health by failing to prevent atheroma and high blood pressure
- age-related illnesses, such as cancer, diabetes, arthritis and osteoporosis

Testing for thyroid hormones

Blood tests are now readily available to establish thyroid-hormone levels in the blood. However, what is considered a 'normal' level varies from lab to lab, let alone from country to country. Ranges are based on population studies and not on individuals, and too many doctors now are reliant on the test results alone rather than also listening to the patient.

This situation has been made worse by guidelines from the Royal College of Physicians (RCP), England, in February 2009. The guidelines state that the only validated method of testing for thyroid function is blood and need only include serum TSH (thyroid-stimulating hormone) and a measure of free thyroxin (T4). This has led to physicians and experienced practitioners being criticized and, in some cases, taken to task for considering the relevance of other thyroid hormones such as T3 (which I have already explained is much more potent); the guidelines ignore the health of cell membranes and the functionality of thyroxin receptors and furthermore diminish the potential benefits of measuring thyroid hormones in urine. Some authorities in Europe consider that urinary T3 and T4 thyroxin measurement is a better reflection of thyroid-hormone status.

Individuals with a TSH at the top end of the normal scale and with T4 at the lower end of the reference range would not be considered, by conventional attitudes, for thyroxin replacement or as having thyroid health issues. A patient with a few or a multitude of the aforementioned symptoms who falls into normal ranges therefore may not be treated as a hypothyroid case. Physicians in the UK and the USA have found themselves up against their governing body – on occasions on the losing side – for prescribing thyroxin to hypothyroid symptomatic patients with 'normal' results.

In summary, though, I recommend the tests below.

BLOOD TESTS
- *TSH*
- *Free T3*
- *Free T4*
- *Total T4* – this includes the T4 bound to proteins, which is how it is transported around the body.

URINE TESTS
- Free T3
- Free T4

OTHER IMPORTANT TESTS
Autoimmunity
Despite the RCP's determination in 2009, many endocrinologists accept that one of the main causes for hypothyroidism is autoimmunity. This is where the individual's body's immune system attacks its own thyroid. When this happens, two specific antibodies are formed and these should be measured in anyone with symptoms or in routine screening, because raised levels of these antibodies can be predictive of eventual hypothyroidism. I therefore recommend the measurement of:
- anti-thyroperoxidase;
- anti-thyroglobulin.

Genomic testing

A test for the polymorphism of a gene DI02 indicates the ability of the body to recognize and convert T4 to the more active T3. In cases where T4 levels are normal, but T3 is low, or when T4 replacement seems not to be helping, this test guides doctors to the use of T3 supplementation instead or as well. Other polymorphisms may indicate which of us is likely to struggle with thyroid problems throughout life and particularly as we age, allowing consideration of supplementation sooner rather than later.

Urine testing for iodine

Some authorities, particularly in the USA, consider iodine deficiency to be an area that is markedly underdiagnosed. This is highly controversial at the moment, but a debate that appears moderately well reported can be found at the Iodine Group.[14] Several eminent physicians, Abraham, Fletchas, Hakala and Brownstein, are very pro-iodine supplementation generally. I watch with interest and consider urinary iodine testing in many cases of suspected hypothyroidism and in all my age-related screening.

Basal body temperature (BBT)

Measuring basal body temperature (BBT) is a useful way to evaluate thyroid status. BBT gives some indication of the body's cells' metabolic rate. This, in combination with the blood tests and symptoms of hypo- or hyperthyroidism, provides a much better guideline.

To measure BBT, place a thermometer beside your bed before sleeping and then, first thing on waking, before you get out of bed, put the thermometer under your tongue. Stay in bed like that for at least five minutes. Repeat the test on ten consecutive days, then add together all ten readings

---

TESTING AND TREATMENT TIPS

- Get checked for nutritional deficiencies, specifically tyrosine (the amino acid), iodine, zinc, copper, iron and selenium, all of which are necessary for good thyroid function.
- Ask your doctor to check for mercury, lead and other chemical contamination, using blood or urine samples, and to treat you accordingly.
- Try acupuncture to try and stimulate the thyroid.

and divide by ten to give you an average BBT. Normal body temperature is between 36.4°C (97.6°F) and 36.7°C (98.2°F).

A lower than normal BBT combined with thyroxine levels in the lower half of the normal range may indicate a hypothyroid state. Numbers at the other end of the scale may indicate hyperthyroidism.

Treatment for hypothyroidism

Thyroxine replacement therapy replenishes the blood levels, but does not attempt to isolate or treat the cause of hypothyroidism. Holistic practitioners may try to restimulate the thyroid once they have removed any possible underlying causes of hypothyroidism, but as restimulation is frequently unsuccessful, they may have to resort to thyroxine replacement.

Many patients are reluctant to consider having to use medication for the rest of their lives, but it is important to remember that in the case of hypothyroidism it is simply a replacement for what the body produces naturally. Natural thyroid, made from desiccated cow (bovine) or pig (porcine) thyroid, is available. This provides T3 and T4 as well as proteins, vitamins and minerals potentially geared toward thyroid health. However, the artificial pharmaceutical form, which comes as T4 (except in rare cases where an endocrinologist prescribes T3) is purer and a physician knows exactly how much is being given.

A doctor will prescribe all orthodox treatment and monitor your progress. However, some patients feel better on 'natural' sources – perhaps because of the T3 content. In any case, ensure that you have your blood levels and BBT tested every four weeks until your thyroid function is normal.

SUPPLEMENTS

Supplementation with the following specific nutrients, in the presence of normal levels of other vitamins and minerals, has been shown to benefit both thyroid function and receptor recognition.

- *Iodine* – as Lugols Iodine (3 drops) or Iodoral (a mix of potassium iodide 7.55 mg and elemental iodine 5 mg), taken two or three times per week. Some authorities consider it necessary to take iodine daily, but I strongly recommend getting tested for iodine levels first. If not tested, I recommend only low doses as shown here.
- *Selenium* – 100 mg taken daily
- *Zinc* – 15 mg with *copper* 2 mg taken nightly
- *Tyrosine* – 500 mg taken twice daily

THE OVARIES

Oestrogens

There are three types of oestrogen in the human body:

- Oestrone (estrone) – E1
- Oestradiol (estradiol) – E2
- Oestriol (estriol) – E3

The steroidogenic pathway diagram on the following page shows that E2 and E3 are derived from E1 (although E2 can be made from testosterone).

Although men do make some oestrogen (in the adrenal glands and fat tissue), women make much more because oestrogens are produced predominantly in the ovaries. These tiny glands harbour millions of cells that have the potential to become eggs. Only about 300–400 of these cells will reach maturity and be part of the fertility cycle that may lead to pregnancy. As the ovaries age, they stop producing oestrogens, the remaining cells stop maturing and the menopause arrives.

Through the reproductive years, women have E2 in abundance. During and post-menopause, it is E1 that takes centre stage because it tends to be made from hormones stored in body fat. Under normal circumstances, E3 is the weakest, or least prevalent, of these main oestrogens – however, during pregnancy the body makes it in large quantities. E3 seems to be a protective hormone, and is the oestrogen most effective in avoiding vaginal dryness. This makes it the most suitable topical treatment for exactly that problem. E1 is much weaker in effect than E2. However, if E1 becomes more prominent owing to lower levels of E2, it may actually promote breast and uterine cancers.

Progesterone

Made predominantly in the ovaries, progesterone is a precursor to the stress-coping hormone cortisol. In women, it triggers the inner lining of the uterus (endometrium) to prepare for the arrival of a fertilized egg. Progesterone amounts remain high if implantation occurs and, along with high oestrogen levels, maintain a healthy pregnancy.

Figure 17: **The steroidogenic pathway**

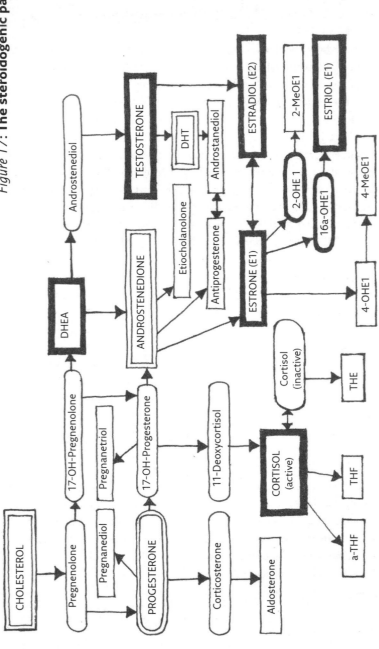

Testing for oestrogen and progesterone

Oestrogen and progesterone can be measured in blood, saliva or urine samples.

BLOOD TESTS

Most doctors use blood tests to measure levels of oestrogen and progesterone in the system, but controversy exists as to the usefulness of such tests except when a doctor already suspects that the patient is ill. Most conventional doctors do not use urine and saliva tests.

SALIVA TESTS

Considerable research suggests that saliva tests may provide more useful information than blood and spot urine test samples because oestrogen and progesterone concentrate over a period of time in the saliva, giving, arguably, a more accurate picture of an individual's overall levels.[15] Saliva tests measure bioactive hormone – that is, the amount of hormone that is effective in the body (much hormone in the blood binds to proteins and is not active).

Analysis of saliva samples that are taken over the course of one day will show variations in hormone levels and changes relating to the circadian (daily) rhythm.

URINE TESTS

Single, on-the-spot urine samples can be useful, but 24-hour urine sample collection is the most accurate of all the tests as it gives a longer-term view – that is, it is not variable owing to hour-by-hour fluctuations found in saliva and certainly blood. It is well established in medical literature as a reliable method of assessing physiological hormone levels, but is underutilized.

Menopause

For women, the physiological cessation of menstruation, the menopause usually occurs between the ages of 45 and 52 (often, for those wishing to predict, within two years either side of the age at which the woman's mother went through it). Colloquially known as 'the change' and medically termed 'the climacteric', the menopause is arbitrarily considered to have happened once a woman has had no periods for 12 months.

There are three stages of menopause:

- *Premenopause* – where periods are still regular and present, but any of the symptoms mentioned below may begin to occur.
- *Peri-menopause* – commonly lasting two to five years, this stage is characterized by irregular periods, lighter or heavier bleeds, hot flashes (blushing) and flushes (sensations of heat), night sweats, vaginal dryness, fatigue, weight gain and insomnia, as well as mood swings, forgetfulness and loss of libido.
- *Post-menopause* – no more periods. Periods recommencing after 12 months are unusual, and although they are rarely anything to worry about, you should consult your doctor. Once you are through 'the change', the physical symptoms (except fatigue) disappear, but the psychological symptoms may persist.

The menopause begins when a woman's body experiences a drop in its levels of oestrogen and when progesterone production ceases altogether. The peri-menopause symptoms particularly affect the arteries and nervous system, via the hormone receptors, but the symptoms are primarily caused by adjusting to a loss of these hormones rather than the low levels themselves.

Treating the symptoms of menopause

The 'treatment' of peri-menopausal symptoms and the psychological and physical effects of menopause vary according to each individual woman's experience. Furthermore, many women do not have access to natural or pharmaceutical therapies and have to rely upon advice offered by older women and their own personal experimentation to cope with the symptoms. I divide treatment into three categories: lifestyle (including diet and exercise), natural supplementation and hormone replacement therapy (HRT).

LIFESTYLE

If you experience flushes, steer away from carbohydrate foods, particularly refined sugars or white grains. These exacerbate symptoms because they are rapidly converted into sugars that cause a quick insulin release, which, in turn, causes your blood sugar levels to drop. The results can be sweating and flushes. For similar reasons, avoid alcohol, caffeine, spices and smoking.

Meditation or relaxation techniques help ease both the physical and the psychological symptoms.[16] Specific therapies such as acupuncture, shiatsu and osteopathy may also help – but we need more research to be sure.[17]

NATURAL SUPPLEMENTATION

Changing hormone levels increase free radical and oxidative stress.[18] This means that antioxidant supplements may ease the symptoms of menopause. Use of some or all of the following supplements:

- *Gamma linoleic acid* (usually from evening primrose oil) – up to 1,000 mg taken three times daily
- *Calcium and magnesium* – taken at a ratio of 500 mg:1,000 mg twice daily
- *Vitamin B6* – 100 mg taken once or twice daily
- *Vitamin E* – 400iu taken twice daily
- *Inositol* – 1,000 mg taken two to three times daily
- *Zinc and copper* – at a ratio of 15 mg:2 mg taken nightly, immediately before bedtime

I am not generally in favour of self-prescribing herbal medication, but you can discuss with a trained practitioner the use of *Agnus castus* and black cohosh (*Cimicifuga racemosa*), and phytoestrogens such as genistein and daidzein, the isoflavins typically found in plants known as 'natural oestrogens'. There is a high content of these in soya bean foods and extracts,

MENOPAUSE SIGNS AND SYMPTOMS

- *Psychological symptoms* – mood swings, short temper, depression, anxiety, usually lowered but occasionally raised libido and insomnia.
- *Physical symptoms* – hot flushes, sweats (especially at night), water retention, fat deposit increase, headaches, aches and pains, malaise and lethargy, and cystitis-like symptoms.
- *Physical signs* – loss of breast tissue, vaginal dryness, osteoporosis (bone thinning) and skin changes such as water retention, fat deposit increase, change in skin texture, wrinkling and dark 'staining'.

Seven out of ten women will have some or all of these symptoms for a short period – say up to 12 months – but one in two will have some or all of these symptoms for up to five years. The symptoms make the menopause sound like a disease process affecting only women (a concept that the pharmaceutical industry is only too ready to exploit), which of course it is not. Many men who do not have such a dramatic drop in hormone levels will also have many of these symptoms.

and this may account – at least in part – for societies that have a high intake showing low rates of breast and ovarian cancer. *Dong quai* (*Angelica sinensis*) and Siberian ginseng (*Eleutherococcus senticosus*) are often found in Eastern herbal treatment programmes.

HORMONE REPLACEMENT THERAPY (HRT)

When lifestyle changes and natural therapies do not ease the symptoms of menopause, I advise you to consider HRT. First, though, it is important to clarify the differences between natural, synthetic and bioidentical HRT.

Natural HRT is based on natural hormones, which occur in plants or may be extracted from other animals, but are not necessarily bioidentical (exactly the same as) the hormones that the human body produces for itself.

Synthetic HRT uses hormones that the pharmaceutical industry manufactures to replicate the hormones our bodies produce. Like natural hormones, these are not identical to our own, but they may have similar effects. Artificial progesterones are known collectively as progestins; artificial oestrogens do not have a collective name and are named individually instead. As a rule of thumb, natural hormones act ten times less potently than our own hormones, while manufactured hormones act ten times more aggressively.

Bioidentical HRT (bHRT) uses hormones that are identical in chemical structure to those that are found in the human body and are named in the same way.

Hormones influence the body by attaching to hormone receptors, which are integral parts of cell membranes or are found within cells. Natural and synthetic hormones do not fit perfectly into receptors, whereas the hormones used in bHRT have exactly the same shape as our own hormones, so they do. Natural and synthetic hormones, once locked into the receptor, may not be recognized by the natural enzymes designed to remove hormones from the cell wall, thereby creating either a block of that receptor or persistent, longer-lasting effects. Consider the analogy of a lock and key. The lock can be forced open or 'jimmied' with a piece of wire or a key with predominantly similar shape; however, persistent use of such a key is liable to damage the lock, break off in it or get stuck.

The benefits of natural and bioidentical progesterone are as follows:
- Essential for inner lining of uterus in pregnancy
- Protect against breast cysts
- Natural diuretic

- Stimulate bone formation
- Lower cholesterol
- Prevent arterial disease
- Reduce cancer risk
- Improve sleep as well as libido
- Enhance thyroid hormone activity
- Influence healthy blood clotting
- Normalize blood-sugar levels
- Help control zinc and copper levels
- Help relieve depression and anxiety

The risks of pharmaceutical hormones (progestins) are as follows:
- Dizziness
- headaches
- vaginal dryness
- acne
- breast pain or tenderness
- mood swings
- depression
- decreased energy
- abdominal bloating
- decreased libido
- fluid retention
- weight gain

The benefits of natural and bio-identical oestrogens are as follows:
- Improved blood sugar control
- Positive influence on protective HDL cholesterol
- Decrease in blood pressure
- Influence flushes/flashes
- Reduce risk of arterial disease

The risks of manufactured oestrogens are as follows:
- May adversely alter cholesterol and other fats in the blood
- Increased weight
- Increased fluid retention
- Enhanced breast tenderness and engorgement
- Increased blood pressure
- Increased sugar cravings

- Enhanced depression
- Hair loss
- Irregular vaginal bleeding or spotting
- Muscle aches and cramps
- Increase in coughs and colds
- Numerous other minor side effects

Bioidentical HRT consists of medication prescribed by doctors trained in the use of conventional and bHRT treatments. I am yet to meet a doctor trained in prescribing bHRT who uses synthetic hormones in preference.

Doctors will prescribe a dosage based upon each individual woman's needs and complaints, and depending upon whether the hormones are taken via a lozenge that sits under the tongue, or are injected through the skin.

TESTOSTERONE

Most often thought of as a male-only hormone, testosterone has an essential role in secondary sexual characteristics, influencing such bodily features as increased muscle mass and the growth of facial hair. It inhibits fat distribution to the hips and thighs and has a powerful effect on libido (sex drive) and aggression. The female body also produces testosterone, but at levels approximately 20 to 25 times lower than those in men. Although women also have fewer testosterone receptors on their cell membranes, libido nevertheless is benefitted by even low levels of this hormone.

In men, testosterone is mostly made in cells known as Leydig cells in the testes. A little is also made in the adrenals. In women, around half of the testosterone is made in fat and skin cells, with the other half made in the ovaries and adrenals.

In men, testosterone levels generally decrease from a peak around the age of 20 to about half-peak levels once the man reaches 70. Overall, the amount the male body produces during old age is enough to maintain height and, to a degree, muscular structure, as long as men continue to exercise throughout their lives. By the time a woman reaches the age of 40, she is producing about half her peak levels of testosterone, but this does not have a profound effect on her height or muscles because female form is predominantly governed by oestrogens and progesterones. Women therefore lose the psychological and health benefits of testosterone some 30 years sooner than men.

Recognizing Testosterone Deficiency

Recognizing testosterone deficiency depends upon a combination of signs and symptoms. Both men and women experience fatigue, memory and concentration loss and a loss of muscle tone. Because testosterone levels are higher in men than in women, these symptoms are more pronounced for men than they are for women. The effects of testosterone deficiency are set out on the following pages.

IS MY TESTOSTERONE LOW?

The following questionnaire is adapted from recommendations in Morley et al's *Metabolism* 2000:49 pp1239–1242.

1. Is your sex drive tailing off?
2. Do you lack energy?
3. Is your strength and/or stamina failing?
4. Have you lost height?
5. Do you feel you are enjoying life less?
6. Are you often unhappy or irritable?
7. (Male) Are erections less strong?
8. Have you lost sporting prowess?
9. Do you fall asleep after meals?
10. Is your mental work or performance deteriorating?

TESTOSTERONE SUPPLEMENTATION – THE RISKS

No hormone supplementation is likely to give benefit without having some risks. For example, testosterone supplementation may adversely increase the size of the prostate. Men who have issues with their urinary flow (one of the symptoms of prostatism) must especially pay attention to the worsening of their symptoms if they are taking testosterone supplements.

There is some evidence of increased prostate infection and that prostate cancer will become more aggressive under the influence of testosterone supplementation. Whether or not testosterone actually causes prostate cancer remains a subject of much debate, although the current consensus is that there is no direct evidence of causality.

Women, having less testosterone throughout their lives than men, may find that supplementation causes increased facial hair, and hair around the nipples, genitals and in the arm pits. Supplementation is contraindicated if it begins to cause hair loss on the scalp. Because the female body converts testosterone into oestrogens, those with oestrogen-sensitive breast cancer

HEALTH BENEFITS OF TESTOSTERONE

System/Organ	Men	Women
Arteries	Potent effect on maintaining arterial dilation (keeping the arteries open) and reducing the age-related thickening of the arterial muscle wall	Similar but weaker effect to that in men
Heart	Increases heart contraction and strength and increases blood flow to the heart	Similar but weaker effect to that in men
Blood pressure	Reduces blood pressure	Poor evidence of any benefit with regard to blood pressure
Psychological effects	Increases libido, benefits mood generally and benefits memory; reduces anxiety	Similar effects as for men
Sexual benefits	Increases libido and sexuality; enhances the health of the genitals and the prostate, but may increase prostate size	Increases libido; benefits the health of the female genitals
Hair growth	Some effect on hair growth in those with a specific genetic pattern; male pattern baldness is more associated with an excess of a protein prostaglandin D2 (PDG2)	Some effect on genetically influenced individuals
Bone density	Increases bone density	Increases bone density
Blood constituency	Reduces blood tendency to clot	No strong evidence of benefit
Body mass	Decreases obesity and fat storage, while increasing muscular strength and lean mass	Weak effect on body fat, but with equivalent effect on female muscles as that of men
Sugar control	Reduces risk of diabetes	No influence on sugar control
Brain activity	Increases certain connections between neurones in the brain and benefits the nervous system through increased blood supply	No marked evidence of influence

and those with a family history of breast cancer should not take testosterone supplements at all.

In men, the conversion of testosterone to oeostrogen may cause side effects that include increased breast tissue (gynocomastia) and lowered sex drive. Supplementation may increase aggression, trigger or worsen acne and interfere with sleep.

Testing for testosterone

Testosterone is derived from cholesterol and the pathway includes the production of progesterone and DHEA. The body can convert testosterone to oestradiol, a potent oestrogen, and also to androstanediol that has effects similar to DHEA.

Measures of testosterone alone may not give the whole picture. Testosterone contradicts certain metabolic processes encouraged by oestrogens and progesterone, so knowing the level of testosterone alone might not give the whole picture. High levels of oestrogen and progesterone may counteract what appear to be normal levels of testosterone.

As a result, it is best to have a comprehensive hormone profile. Ideally, blood tests should measure free testosterone, particularly in men, because it is free testosterone that is active although the majority of this hormone travels around the body bound to Sex Hormone Binding Globulin and another liver made protein, albumin. SHBG slows down the breakdown of testosterone and also interferes with its conversion to another active metabolite known as dihydrotestosterone. A measure of the ratio Total testosterone:SHBG is a useful guide.

For those considering accurate supplementation by prescription, it is better to test for androstanediol glucuronide, a major metabolite reflecting androgen activity.[19]

Urine and saliva tests are useful to confirm testosterone deficiency in men, but are less telling in women as the amounts of testosterone in the urine and saliva are already small, and they do not necessarily relate to how much testosterone there is in the bloodstream and its efficacy.

In the presence of low normal or deficient testosterone results, but no obvious symptoms of lowered testosterone levels, you might be able to discern if testosterone therapy would be of benefit or harm if you undergo the following tests:

- Doplar ultrasound of carotid arteries – showing increased thickness of the muscle walls or early development of atherosclerosis
- Dual-energy X-ray Absorptiometry (DEXA-scanning) – showing

Symptoms of testosterone deficiency	
Men	**Women**
Receding hair at the sides of the forehead	Small wrinkles around the eyes and mouth
Loss of thickness of beard and moustache	Softening muscles
Tendency to dry eyes	Dry vagina associated with painful intercourse
Decrease in pubic and armpit hair	Thinning body hair (testosterone appears not to influence female pubic hair)
Increase in breast tissue	Decreased interest in physical activity
Increased abdominal fat	Decreased clitoral and nipple sensitivity and reduction in orgasm
Erectile difficulties (although psychology and arterial disease must be considered)	Increase pacificity and submissiveness
Testicular size reduction	Cellulite and varicose vein development
	Reduction in height (also a symptom of decreased oestrogen and progesterone levels)
	Tendency to slump

decreased bone density for the age of the individual.
- Research Genetic Cancer Centre Testing – showing the presence of prostate cancer cells in men and breast cancer cells in women – a contraindication to the use of testosterone supplements

Lifestyle effect on testosterone
Optimal, as opposed to excessive muscle-building (resistance) exercise, increases testosterone levels in both sexes. Excessive exercise uses up testosterone and leads to an overall decrease in levels. This is temporary unless the excessive exercise is from endurance sports.

Emotional stress uses up testosterone, whereas spending time happy, listening to uplifting music and encourageing sexual contact and sexy thoughts all increase testosterone levels and activity.

Being overweight reduces testosterone as fat makes the enzyme that converts testosterone to oestrogen – aromatase.

Sleep increases testosterone production and a deficiency is associated with sleep apnoea – a brief cessation in breathing during sleep that is often associated with snoring.

Diet

Protein and cholesterol foods may raise testosterone levels, whereas sugar and refined carbohydrates decrease them. Fibre binds with testosterone and removes it from the body. Testosterone, being a steroid hormone, is recycled through the liver, and the breakdown products as well as certain amounts of testosterone leave the liver through the bile into the gut. Fibre has its benefits in other areas, but like with most things, everything in moderation. A diet too high in fibre may lead to reduced testosterone levels.

Supplementation

The following have evidence of increasing testosterone levels:

- Vitamin D
- Magnesium
- Zinc

Reasons to use testosterone supplementation

Always consult your doctor before considering testosterone supplementation. Take it only if you have had tests that indicate your levels are low and supplementation is not contraindicated in any way. It is also appropriate to *consider* treatment for those with levels in the lower half of the normal range who show symptoms of testosterone deficiency.

Transdermal testosterone gel, preferably in a form know as liposomal, is the best way to raise testosterone levels. Oral treatments are common, but digestive juices break them down in the stomach and the testosterone also has to pass through the liver, which further breaks it down – all before it reaches the bloodstream.

Women should consider taking around 3 mg daily.

Men should take 50 mg daily.

These dosages can be increased to three times the levels, depending on symptoms and test results. Make sure your testosterone levels are frequently monitored because taking more than you need is unlikely to be of benefit.

Men seem to react more quickly than women to testosterone supplementation, seeing benefits sometimes within a few days. However, as a general rule, men should expect to see increased energy levels (a first indication that supplementation is working) within three weeks, and improvement in erectile function within ten weeks.

Women should see emotional and benefits in libido levels at around four weeks, but physical improvements such as increased muscle strength and bone density can take up to nine months.[2]

The adrenal glands

The adrenal glands, made up of the adrenal medulla and adrenal cortex, sit on top of the kidneys. The adrenal medulla manufactures catecholamines (such as adrenaline; *see* below), while the adrenal cortex manufactures testosterone and aldosterone. Levels of these hormones rise and fall in response to physical and psychological stress on the body. Aldosterone influences most systems in the body, including the kidneys, governing the absorption of minerals and thereby balancing the levels of electrolytes (sodium, potassium, calcium, magnesium, and so on) in the blood.

In conventional medicine, the adrenal glands are either:

- not working – leading to a lack of stress hormones and cortisol, causing Addison's disease;
- are diseased and producing too much cortisol – leading to Cushing's syndrome; or
- producing too much adrenalin (epinephrine) from tumours such as pheochromocytoma or cancer.

In the absence of these conditions, the adrenals are considered to be working within normal ranges. There is no grey area, no high or low normal function – just black and white. There is no adrenal fatigue, imbalance or dysfunction.

Many practitioners consider conventional medicine to be missing evidence of insufficiency by looking only at marked deficiency. Here are some of the symptoms of adrenal dysfunction as noted by Dr J L Wilson:[21]

- Tired all the time – TATT
- Tired beyond that which you deserve
- Awaking tired
- Not coping emotionally or physically
- Needing, or only coping with, stimulants such as caffeine or sugar
- Slow recovery from minor illnesses
- Losing joy and motivation; nothing is fun
- Low libido

Adrenalin and noradrenalin (epinephrine and norepinephrine)

Our entire evolution could be attributed to our ability to produce our stress recognition hormones, adrenalin and noradrenalin (called epinephrine and norephinephrine in the USA and other parts of the world). Collectively these are known as catecholamines. As people evolved, the gene mutations that favoured rapid production of catecholamines were more likely to keep their owners alive. This is the process of natural selection: if early humans heard a rustle in the bushes, those with genes that enabled a fast production of catecholamines (to quickly override calming neurohormones) were more likely to escape danger in time. Fear triggers fight and flight reactions, calmness does not.

Catecholamines activate a speeding-up process in the body – quickening metabolism, raising heart rate, increasing blood pressure and increasing respiratory rate. The results are that more oxygen enters the blood and blood vessels to the muscles open up so that oxygen and other nutrients (particularly sugar) are available for survival response.

In times of danger, catecholamines, built up from amino acids, are essential. Overproduction leads to a powering-up of the organs and body survival systems, while oxygen and nutrients are diverted from organs such as the bowel, liver, kidneys, and so on. We go pale when facing a fearful situation because blood is pulled away from the skin.

In the long term, prolonged stress response leads to excessive deprivation of oxygen and nutrients creating damage of tissues, with illness and premature ageing the outcome.

In the West, we fortunately no longer have to face predators, famine, droughts and warring tribes, but we do have to overcome the toxic environments that we ourselves have created, as well as deal with the stress of modern life and reduced time for exercise and leisure. We also have poorer nutrition. All of these modern stresses lead to catecholamine release.

Testing

The body rapidly both produces and breaks down catecholamines, which makes it difficult to measure levels of these hormones in the blood. A preference is to measure the breakdown products that occur in the urine. This includes assessing the levels of the compounds that help us deal with stress – cortisol in particular – or our calming neurohormones such as serotonin. If looked for, the metabolites of noradrenalin and adrenalin, vanillylmandelic acid (VMA) and homovanillic acid (HVA) are found in relatively small amounts in samples from non-stressed people.

Measurement through heart-rate variability tells us about the sympathetic and parasympathetic levels (*see* Chapter 7) and that gives a much better understanding of our overall stress levels. Haemencepalography and quantitative electroencephalography (QEEG) testing are more advanced and expensive methods of looking at stress effects but much more useful than the measurement of catecholamines.

Treatments and therapies

Techniques such as meditation, relaxation therapy and regular prayer, as well as good levels of physical exercise, all keep catecholamine response in check. Read the sections in this book on exercise, lifestyle and diet as a first step to making sure your body is responding to stress appropriately.

SUPPLEMENTS

Catecholamines are vital to our survival, and because these are predominantly built up from amino acids, they require a range of vitamins and minerals, particularly vitamin B-complex, vitamin C and magnesium. Supplements that will help balance catecholamine production are:

- *Specific amino acids* such as 5 hydroxytriptophan, acting as a precursor to serotonin. Also, consider L-theanine tyrosine and glutamate.
- *Gamma-aminobutyric acid (GABA)* decreases anxiety. Take 500 mg two or three times daily.

Cortisol

Produced in the adrenal cortex, and in the brain and gut in small amounts, the 'stress-coping' hormone cortisol belongs in a group of hormones known as glucocorticoids.

The effects of cortisol are seen throughout the body. Cortisol is essential for the production of gastric acid, kidney function, acid-alkaline balance, good levels of sodium and potassium (which we need for proper muscle function) and copper, as well as many other metabolic functions.

Cortisol is made from cholesterol via a pathway that includes progesterone. Levels follow a circadian rhythm, reaching a high point as the sun rises and a low point about 12 hours later. This links in with helping the body cope with stress during the daytime, while acknowledging that we do not need as much cortisol during sleep.

Melatonin, one of the hormones that trigger the onset of sleep and influences cortisol and vice versa, so that low levels of melatonin can lead to overactivity of cortisol at night, which can disturb sleep.

Cortisol and ageing

With regard to ageing, cortisol has a number of influences:
- Increased release in response to adrenalin levels (stress).
- It opposes the actions of insulin getting sugar into cells, although it

does work in a similar way to insulin by increasing glycogen (rapid access energy stores) synthesis in the liver.

- It suppresses the activity of the immune system, specifically T-cell activity involved in infection and fighting cancer.
- Reducing inflammation, which is useful in acute situations, but may inhibit repair and protective processes in the body in the long term.
- It reduces bone formation and reduces calcium absorption in the gut.
- It is involved in the formation of memories, but in excess damages the ability to learn and recall.
- It can increase blood pressure.
- It helps detoxification through the liver.
- It can increase or reduce appetite.
- At the correct level it enhances mood and motivation to do things, whereas an excess reduces these.
- It helps control pain.

As we age, the adrenal glands secrete less cortisol, and lower levels are compounded by the fact that the damaged cell membranes of older cells make it hard for cortisol to be absorbed. In this way, levels of cortisol circulating in the blood, in fact, rise. Increased evening and nighttime levels may have an adverse effect on sleep.

SYMPTOMS OF CORTISOL DEFICIENCY

- Poor coping when stressed
- Depression, often with mood swings
- Poor recall and confusion when under stress
- Paranoia and neurosis, often with irritability
- Quick to lose temper and have inappropriate emotional responses
- Fatigue
- Lightheadedness or even dizziness if rising rapidly from sitting or lying
- Muscle and joint aches
- Tendency to acute infections
- Hair loss
- Bloating, loose stools and abdominal pains
- Skin has a tendency to tan easily and skin creases become brown

Measuring cortisol levels

Integrated physicians and those trained in more natural approaches recognize that cortisol deficiency can lead to many physical and psychological complaints.

Blood tests are generally of use only when Cushing's or Addison's diseases are suspected and these are not really age-related issues. Analysis of urine samples taken over 24 hours is popular with some integrated practitioners as it gives more accurate reading than the 'flash' view of a blood test. However, it does not tell us much about variations in cortisol levels throughout the day.

My preferred method for assessing cortisol levels is saliva testing. However, this has poor support from most mainstream endocrinologists who tend to be faced with patients with disease rather than those who are 'tired all the time' or those who have various stress-related symptoms. It is best to take four or more saliva samples over the course of the day and plot the cortisol readings against the levels expected for the age of the individual. Ask your doctor to perform these tests at the same time as taking and testing dehydroepiandrosterone (DHEA) and melatonin samples. Cholesterol is the precursor to many different steroid-like hormones. The pathway that takes cholesterol to cortisol is different from that which leads to DHEA. A depression in DHEA levels can indicate favouritism for the pathway leading to cortisol, so that a low DHEA level with low normal cortisol can be indicative of the body having long-term stress, but still managing to cope.

Treatment for cortisol deficiency

Treatment for cortisol deficiency aims to increase levels of this hormone through the use of synthetic substitutes – prednisone, prednisolone, hydrocortisone or other stronger forms. Only a doctor should prescribe these and only when specific medical conditions require it.

A pregnenolone tablet, or progesterone taken under the skin or tongue, can enhance cortisol activity without the need for direct artificial supplementation. The body converts these compounds to cortisol when it needs to. Provided your doctor monitors your cortisol levels and administers the medication, these treatments are less likely to incur the potential risks and side effects of steroid administration.

Eating certain foods such as flaxseed and soya and reducing salt intake can also influence cortisol levels. Reducing obesity, exercising more and spending more time practising relaxation or meditation therapies will also have an effect.

Aldosterone

Altered levels of this hormone can occur if you are taking blood-pressure-lowering medication. These medicines may also cause electrolyte imbalance – the correction of which requires aldosterone. Although falling aldosterone levels are rare, they can be associated with hypertension. Ask your doctor to test your levels using a urine sample.

Dehydroepiandrosterone (DHEA)

DHEA is a complex structure derived from cholesterol. The body converts it into our sex hormones (testosterone and oestrogens), but it also has direct activity in the body. The steroidogenic pathway diagram shows how DHEA becomes testosterone and oestrogens. On the way it is converted to androstenedione and androstenediol. These and DHEA appear to have similar activities, although DHEA-S (attached to a sulphur molecule) appears to be the most potent.

DHEA acts particularly on the immune system through specific receptors and the endothelium, the inner lining of blood vessels.

Some studies show that DHEA has a protective effect in arterial disease and reduces the incidence and risks of heart attacks and strokes. There also appears to be evidence of DHEA supporting the following functions:

- *Improved appearance of skin* – DHEA increases skin thickness and moisture and may decrease 'age spots'.
- *Improved ability to achieve erection* – but not as much in those with diabetes or nerve disorders.
- *Improved bone mineral density.*[22]

The Natural Medicines Comprehensive Data Base (2011) concluded that DHEA was ineffective in Alzheimer's disease and cognitive patterns in ageing populations.[23] There appears to be little to support its use for overcoming menopausal symptoms or the symptoms of Parkinson's disease. However, a lack of evidence does not necessarily mean that DHEA is ineffective – it may be that we do not yet have enough studies to support its use in the treatment of these conditions. Remember, it behoves the finances of the pharmaceutical industry to disprove natural products that can influence health as we age, so studies on these are not performed on any great scale. A lack of evidence is not necessarily a lack of efficacy.

Lifestyle and DHEA

Exercise and psychological stress increase levels of DHEA in the body. Obviously, the first is a good thing, while the second is merely a reflection of the need of DHEA by the body when under stressful conditions. It may simply be that DHEA rises when the body demands more of its stress-coping hormone, cortisol, because they both share 17-OH-pregnenolone as a precursor.

Proteins and fats seem to increase the body's production of DHEA, but we might expect that as both are often associated with increased cholesterol intake through the diet. Interestingly, sugars and fibre reduce DHEA production.

Smoking reduces DHEA production, as does the process of ageing. By the time we reach 70 years of age, we produce only around 20 per cent of what we were making when we were 25.

Testing for DHEA

Whatever test you have, ensure that it measures your levels of dehydroepiandrosterone sulphate (DHEA-S). A blood test is one option. Although DHEA-S is broken down quite rapidly in the blood, low levels on repeated occasions would suggest a deficiency. Alternatively, DHEA's major metabolites are known as 17-ketosteroids and these can be measured in a 24-hour urine collection. My preference at the moment is to measure DHEA levels in the saliva as this is a simple method. Doctors can compare results with cortisol levels in the same sample to provide a clearer picture of how the body is coping with stress.

Do I need to take supplemental DHEA?

Yes! I think DHEA has an underestimated value in maintaining health as we age. The presence of receptors on the endothelium and certain white blood cells, as well as evidence that DHEA may influence mineral density in bones, suggests that supplementation is most likely to be a good thing, protecting against arterial disease, stroke, infections and osteoporosis.

DHEA's position in the steroidogenic pathway shows that it increases levels of our sex hormones, which infers another probable benefit of keeping DHEA levels up.

Only a health practitioner should prescribe you with DHEA. Start with a low dose – 10 mg taken daily, increasing up to 25 mg daily, but no higher unless otherwise recommended. Some individuals struggle with mild headaches when they take DHEA – monitor your reactions carefully.

Women may find that DHEA converts more readily to testosterone and its derivatives, which can lead to increased body hair (hirsutism), increased aggression and increased muscle tone. If you experience any of these side effects when you begin taking DHEA, stop taking it immediately and discuss taking a lower dosage with your practitioner.

Insulin

This most important hormone does not have its own section in many books on ageing. We know of its relevance to sugar control, metabolic syndrome (poor sugar control, weight gain, rising blood pressure, decreased HDL and raised free fats in the blood), diabetes and hypoglycaemia (low blood sugar), but its influence on healthy ageing is poorly reported.

Glucose is the breakdown product of most carbohydrates and is formed rapidly from refined (white) foods, sugar, bread, pasta, and so on, and more slowly from complex carbohydrates. Insulin not only controls the amount of sugar that is absorbed into cells from the bloodstream, but also has an influence on amino acids (the building blocks of proteins) and minerals such as potassium and magnesium, which have a particular influence on the strength and function of muscles.

Nearly all cells have insulin receptors that are dependent upon an amino acid known as tyrosine. Insulin levels in the blood increase when insulin is released from special cells in the pancreas known as islet cells of Langerhans in response to rising sugar levels from our diet. The surge in insulin triggers the receptors to allow more glucose into our cells.

THE EFFECT OF INSULIN ON SUGAR/GLUCOSE

- Insulin encourages sugar to enter muscles for activity.
- It influences the storage in the liver of glucose as glycogen, which the body can access very quickly.
- It encourages the conversion of sugar by fat cells into fat storage.
- Overall, insulin reduces the level of sugars in the bloodstream, which is important as the brain does not function well if sugar levels are too high or too low. Insulin in high levels when we eat lots of sugar also inhibits the breakdown of fat from fat stores, thereby preventing weight loss.

Insulin receptors are particularly high in number in the cell walls of muscles and fat cells. Interestingly, the brain and central nervous system and the liver do not require insulin, as they have other efficient methods of taking up glucose. Insulin influences liver cells to convert glucose into a store of energy known as glycogen.

Diabetes

Type I diabetes, or insulin-dependent diabetes mellitus (IDDM), is deficiency of insulin owing to destruction of the islet cells and is most frequently caused by autoimmunity – the body's immune system attacking itself – but also by viral infection, alcohol or drug poisoning and other diseases.

Type II, or non-insulin-dependent diabetes mellitus (NIDDM), can be considered as insulin 'resistance' – there is plenty of insulin around, but the cells do not recognize it.

What causes insulin resistance remains complex and controversial. There may be a genetic predisposition to the insulin receptors failing to recognize the hormone. However, insulin resistance appears usually to be associated with obesity and dietary factors – predominantly consuming too much sugar. But which comes first? Animal studies show that a short spell on a high-fat diet leads to resistance, although the good news is that an intake of the healthy omega-3 fatty acids can reduce that effect. Raised levels in the blood of free fatty acids (triglycerides), made in the liver from sugars, is also associated with diminished insulin sensitivity. Too much fruit sugar (fructose) appears to contribute to insulin resistance, and there may also be an association with a hormone known as leptin, an appetite suppressant.

A few studies show that high levels of cortisol, our stress-coping hormone, can contribute to the miscommunication between insulin and cell membranes.

A lack of exercise and a vitamin-D deficiency (we manufacture vitamin D when we are in the sunshine) are also associated with insulin resistance.

Where the fat lies

The human body has both visceral fact and subcutaneous fat. Visceral fat surrounds our internal organs, particularly in the abdomen. In excess this causes an 'apple-shape' figure, and people who are this shape appear to have a far greater risk of insulin resistance and diabetes than those with a 'pear-shape' figure. Subcutaneous fat is the fat that underlies our skin and seems to contribute only slightly with regard to sugar-balance issues.

Insulin and ageing

Sumo wrestlers, despite having large amounts of body fat, rarely report any Type II diabetes. They presumably have a considerable amount of visceral fat and yet do not develop insulin resistance. Why? When we eat sugars, glycogen is formed in the liver, and stored there and in the skeletal muscles. It is only when these storage areas are full that the insulin receptors seem to default and insulin resistance is triggered. Sumo wrestlers avoid diabetes because of the amount of exercise they do – burning off the sugars, reducing the amount that the body has to store.

Body heat can crystallize or harden sugar and even deposit it around the body, including in the arteries, blocking off the blood flow and the flow of lymph. This leaves cells without necessary oxygen, and with poor levels of glucose and other nutrients, and a build-up of damaging waste products.

This poor control of sugar and fat levels might arguably be considered a disease rather than an ageing process. However, as we age, we tend to move and exercise less, so fat builds up. Therefore, you can argue that insulin resistance is an ageing process, and if not controlled, the next step on from type II diabetes increases the risk of arterial disease, which, in turn, influences most organs and potentially shortens life.

Testing for insulin levels

Conventional medicine measures glucose in the urine and the blood-stream. A specific test for a type of haemoglobin (called HbAc 1), which is influenced by high sugar levels, also gives an indication of a loss of sugar control. However, all these tests are aimed at early detection once a diabetic condition is imminent.

I think we should give more focus to preempting or predicting diabetes.

Insulin resistance encourages the body to make more insulin to try to override the blockage, and so it seems logical to measure serum (blood) insulin levels; but fat cells absorb insulin, so testing blood levels is not as useful as they may appear normal even if the actual amount of insulin being produced is high.

There are, however, other tests that can be used to predict probable development of insulin control issues or diabetes.

Inflammation generally shows up before diabetes does, and certain markers tend to move out of the reference ranges if diabetes is developing. These are:

• Hs-CRP
• Interleukins 6 and 8

- Tumour necrosis factor alpha
- Plasminogen activator inhibitor type 1 (PAI-1)

Fat cells produce and secrete one particular compound, *adiponectin,* that regulates lipid and glucose metabolism. It influences the body's response to insulin and has anti-inflammatory effects on the cells that line blood-vessel walls. High levels of adiponectin reduce risk of heart attack and diabetes. Falling adiponectin levels are the hallmark of the first stage of progression to diabetes. A measurement of a low adiponectin level is a possible test to predict the onset of diabetes.

Many labs measure leptin levels, but I am not sure if it is a particularly useful test – in the majority of cases, leptin levels do not rise before obesity is apparent anyway. Raised leptin levels decrease appetite by acting on the appetite receptors in the hypothalamus in the brain to promote feelings of satiety. However, leptin is proinflammatory, increases blood vessel growth to cancers and decreases fertility. Measurement can therefore be used to gauge if the weight carried as fat is actually likely to be dangerous.

Another hormone called ghrelin rises when our blood sugar levels are low, such as when we fast. It increases appetite and is anti-inflammatory; it also increases gut motility and improves memory. It may increase dopamine production to have a direct effect on Parkinson's disease (PD). This suggests that low calorie intake may be beneficial in PD. Again, I am not sure of the benefit in measuring this although treatment with this may become a part of our future medical armoury.

Testing for C peptide measures the conversion of insulin from a precursor known as pro-insulin.

Dr Sharma's Programmes

Should we take supplements to encourage glands to produce hormones? Overall, I think there *is* a benefit, and this decision is made easier as many of the necessary nutrients that optimize hormone production are also supportive of the cardiovascular and nervous systems.

The bigger question is: should we take hormone supplements as we age? Again, I think the answer is yes, but only after careful medical assessment of need and measurement through accurate testing.

Dr Sharma's Maintenance Programme

This is a basic programme to protect and improve the hormonal system. At first glance, this extensive list seems daunting, but remember, you can find many of these nutrients in the same tablet or capsule as multivitamin/ mineral complexes.

MINERALS
- *Calcium and magnesium* – at a ratio of 500 mg:1000 mg taken twice daily
- *Zinc/Copper* – 15 mg/2 mg taken immediately before bedtime

VITAMINS
- *Vitamin B6* – take 100 mg once or twice daily
- *Vitamin E* – take 400iu once daily
- *Inositol* – take 1,000 mg once or twice times daily

ESSENTIAL FATTY ACIDS
- *Gamma linoleic acid* – the usual source is evening primrose oil; 1,000 mg three times daily (up to 1,000 mg taken three times daily on professional advice for treatment of symptoms or conditions)

AMINO ACIDS
- *Whey* – take an inexpensive whey product or, if vegetarian, a suitable complete essential amino acid supplement

OTHER NUTRIENTS OR REPLACEMENT THERAPIES
- *Melatonin* – take 2–3 mg nightly
- *Resveratrol* – take 20 mg once or twice daily

Dr Sharma's Advanced Programme

This programme is for those with symptoms, lifestyle or family risk factors. Consider the addition of these supplements after discussion with your healthcare provider or if you want to enhance the protection of your hormonal system. Use all of the supplements in the maintenance programme above, plus:

VITAMINS
- *Niacin* – vitamin B3 – 500 mg taken twice daily (try to get the non-flush type) if taking HGH

Dr Sharma's Repair Programme

This programme is for those with established conditions.

FOR HYPOTHYROID CASES
- *Desiccated thyroid* such as armour thyroid if poor response to conventional thyroxine.
- *Iodine* – as Lugols Iodine 3 drops or Iodoral (a mix of potassium iodide 7.5 mg and elemental iodine 5 mg) taken two or three times weekly
- *Selenium* – take 100 mg daily
- *Zinc and copper* – taken in a ratio of 15 mg:2 mg nightly
- *Tyrosine* – take 500 mg twice daily

FOR FEMALE HORMONE ISSUES
Discuss the following with a herbalist or doctor with training in the field (I do not support self-prescribing).
- *Agnus castus*
- Black cohosh (*Cimicifuga racemosa*)
- Phytoestrogens such as genistein and daidzein
- Dong quai (*Angelica sinensis*)
- Siberian ginseng (*Eleutherococcus senticosus*)

The following are medications that a physician must prescribe:
- *Oxytocin* – consider 5iu taken daily
- Pharmaceutical grade thyroxine
- Pharmaceutical hormones if bioidentical or more natural options fail to produce an improvement

Who should have tests?

Hormone testing can optimize psychological, physical or sexual performance in many people. However, I particularly recommend testing for the following people:

- Men or women who are experiencing low libido, mood issues, energy deficiency, TATT, and so on
- Those with symptoms of thyroid problems
- Those with diabetes or syndrome X (otherwise known as metabolic syndrome)
- People who are overweight, under-exercising or who have a family history of diabetes

First-line investigations

Everyone interested in optimizing their health should consider these investigations.

BLOOD AND URINE TESTS
- TSH
- Free T3
- Free T4
- Total T4
- Anti-thyroperoxidase
- Anti-thyroglobulin

(The above can usually be found together in full thyroid profiles.)

- *Insulin-like growth factor (IGF-1)*
- *Testosterone and sex-hormone binding globulin* – in men
- *Oestrogen and progesterone* – in women with persistent tiredness or peri-menopausal symptoms
- *Adiponectin*

URINE ANALYSIS
- *Free T3*
- *Free T4*

Second-line investigations

This level of testing is for those who want to know more about their current and potential risk status for deficiencies or who have symptoms. It is recommended for those with borderline family history or who are just below the optimum levels of fitness, body weight, or who overindulge.

BLOOD TESTS
- *Cortisol* – if using HGH or secretagogues
- *Melatonin* – particularly if you are using HGH or secretagogues

If diabetes is a concern:
- hs-CRP
- Interleukins 6 and 8
- Tumour Necrosis Factor alpha
- Plasminogen Activator Inhibitor Type 1 (PAI-1)

If hypothyroid:
- *Full nutritional analysis for minerals* – particularly iodine, zinc, copper iron and selenium, amino acids generally, but ensure the test includes tyrosine and tryptophan, and B-complex vitamins.

SALIVA TESTS
If you are concerned about so-called adrenal fatigue:
- Cortisol
- DHEA
- Melatonin

URINARY ANALYSIS
- *Metal toxicity testing* – consider this if any of your hormone levels are low. Toxic metals are particularly damaging to the production of thyroid hormones.[24]
- *Urinary iodine testing* – consider this if you have low levels of thyroxine or you suspect that you have hypothyroid symptoms.

NUTRITIONAL EVALUATION
- *Food-allergy test* – consider getting an accurate food-allergy test.

Advanced investigations
Consider the following tests if you are interested in optimizing your health as well as undergoing the essential investigations.

BLOOD
- *Oxytocin* – to ensure optimum levels.
- *Leptin and ghrelin* – although your results will not alter your treatment advice, knowing your blood levels of leptin and ghrelin will help your doctor generally to monitor your hormone health.

Chapter 9

The Immune System

Although cardiovascular disease is the leading cause of death in the over-65s, poor function of the immune system, leading to infections including chest infection and pneumonia, is the third highest cause of death (behind cancer) in 55- to 65-year-olds and the fourth highest after the age of 65. Furthermore, immune dysfunction is related to cancer and is the highest cause of death of people aged 45 to 64. Forty per cent of those who develop cancer over the age of 55 will die because of that disease.

We have flurries of press coverage regarding immune system dysfunction, particularly at the times of year when our elderly population is encouraged to have inoculations against pneumonia and influenza. Unfortunately, up to 75 per cent of the elderly do not actually respond to vaccination – that is, their immune systems do not create a defence response against the invading pathogens. What is more, actual safety, let alone efficacy or effectiveness, is poorly evidenced in those over the age of 65.[1]

I do not wish to explore the potential of vaccine dangers to any great extent here, but I feel I do have a duty to raise awareness about the use of mercury and aluminium along with formaldehyde as preservatives in vaccines. The potential dangers of certain compounds, known as adjuvants, that stimulate the immune response to the vaccine have not been well researched. Overall, I think that the decision to vaccinate people as they age (and our children) should occur on a person-by-person basis.[2]

The structure of the immune system

Most immunologists battle to keep up with the advances in our understanding of the immune system, but a brief overview is all that you really need to understand how best you can maintain immune function into old age for as long as possible.

For the sake of clarity, we can divide the immune system into two parts:
1. Innate immunity, also known as ancestral immunity
2. Adaptive or clonotypical immunity

Innate immunity

This kind of immunity is to do with a first-line and non-specific defence against invading organisms and altered cells such as cancerous cells that may prove harmful.

The first part of the innate immune system requires intact barriers such as the skin and the inner membrane linings (known as epithelial layers) of the gut, lungs and upper respiratory airways (nose, sinus, throat), and the inner lining of the bladder. The integrity of these barriers stops foreign organisms and toxins getting in. The membranes produce defence compounds that infuse the sebum (the slightly greasy compound in our skin), the sweat and the mucus made by the epithelial lining. These defence compounds are known as immunoglobulins and are made by specialized cells – mostly white blood cells – that sit in or close to these barrier membranes. Secretory IgA (sIgA) is made predominantly in the 10 metres (33 feet) or so of the adult small intestine. Its production is triggered in the newborn by the first breast milk, colostrum. Throughout our lives sIgA is a vital part of our innate, first-line defence mechanism.

Further components of our innate immune system are the non-specific white blood cells known as 'phagocytes', which move through the bloodstream and body tissues enveloping invading organisms or absorbing damaged and toxic cells. Other white blood cells produce chemicals that trigger inflammation, which attracts more blood-carrying defence cells, scar-tissue-forming cells, oxygen and nutrients to aid healing in the affected area. Inflammation is a vital part of our defence and repair process – until it becomes excessive or turns up in the wrong place. A lot of these mechanisms defend us by recognizing and killing off cancer cells.

Adaptive immunity

The production of particular types of white blood cells (some of which produce the defence compounds immunoglobulins), adaptive immunity tackles specific infections and toxic material. Adaptive immunity is also the linchpin of our allergy response.

Two types of white blood cell (WBC), known as T-cells and B-cells, are active in adaptive immunity. We do not go on producing WBCs for ever. As we age, naïve leucocytes, which become T- and B-cells and are very active in our youth, reduce in number and slow down their production so that overall we have fewer WBCs circulating in our system.

B-cells

B-cells make immunoglobulins known as antibodies. These are key-like compounds that recognize specific molecular shapes found on bacteria, viruses, other invading organisms and toxins. Such bugs have particular molecular shapes on their cell walls, which we call antigens. Antibodies lock into the antigen and cause the destruction of the cell wall or attract other WBCs such as some of the T-cells to envelop it.

T-cells

T-cells are so called because they are made in the thymus gland. They are recognized by a particular cell surface configuration called the T-cell receptor.

T-cells have many different functions, including:
- helping other parts of the immune system (helper T-cells);
- attacking cancer cells directly (cytotoxic natural killer T-cells);
- regulating a balance so that a defensive response to the body's hostile 'invaders' is not too aggressive;
- memory-cell activity (see below).

Memory cells

As we go through life, we encounter increasing numbers of foreign organisms. Rather than maintaining large armies of T- and B-cells, we form memory cells. These cells 'remember' individual antigens so that when we are next exposed to them, the memory cells sends out chemical messengers to naïve leucocytes triggering them to start up antibody production.

Why does ageing impair the immune system?

Senescence is the term given to aged and dysfunctional cells. Immunosenescence describes the gradual deterioration of the immune cells. This decline renders our ageing bodies less capable of fighting infection and less likely to recognize and deal with damaged, cancerous or other, non-functioning cells. Immunosenescence also prevents us responding to vaccination. It interferes with both innate and adaptive immunity.

Cellular ageing and decline

The epithelial wall of the bowel (innate immune system) fights to keep out 100 trillion bowel bacteria. Similarly, the skin defends us against infection and chemical toxins, which land on us in their thousands each day. As we age, our gum health declines, too, further adding to the burden on our immune system. As these barriers start to fail, our acquired, secondary immune system becomes overloaded. The WBCs that envelop germs or altered (cancerous) cells also lose some of their control molecules, and the correct production of defence and inflammatory control (cytokines protein messengers) diminishes, too.

The immune system throughout our life builds up memory cells and deals with scores of infections all day, every day. We produce increasing numbers of memory cells as our exposure to organisms and toxins builds up throughout our lives. Our reserve of naïve leucocytes over time converts to memory cells, so that eventually we do not have enough left to mount an adequate T-cell or B-cell response to a new infection. An analogy is 'too many generals, not enough soldiers'.

Eventually there comes a point where immune 'housekeeping' registers a lack of response and assumes the WBC present are ineffective and breaks them down. This includes a loss of memory cells, which leaves us open to infections that we had, to date, managed to deal with. This is why as we age, having had a 'lifelong' immunity to, say, chickenpox, we develop shingles; of more concern, our 'lifelong' defence against the viruses that cause influenza (flu) disappears, making flu so much more dangerous an infection as we get older.

Intracellular viruses

Another vital aspect of ageing is our exposure to viruses that are not generally dangerous, but that ingratiate themselves into cells. This means that they are hidden from our immune system. Not being particularly aggressive, they lie there dormant and are kept at a low replication rate by the intracellular defences. As we age, these viruses flare up owing to the loss of intracellular defences and overwhelm our immune system, including our anti-cancer defences. The main antagonists include:

- herpes virus;
- cytomegalo virus (CMV);
- Epstein-Barr virus (EBV, the cause of glandular fever);
- mycobacteria.

As we age, the immune system focuses too much attention on these persistent intracellular organisms and is less able to attack new ones. Its ability to recognize new infections also diminishes because persistent infection alters complex mechanisms.

HOW TO SLOW DOWN OR REVERSE THE AGEING OF THE IMMUNE SYSTEM

The processes described above prevent the immune system from functioning optimally as we age. However, the immune system can be influenced quite effectively through healthy living and supplementation. The importance of adhering to a healthy lifestyle affects all organs and systems, but the immune system can fluctuate particularly rapidly in the presence of poor habits and deficiencies.

Our genotype (genetic makeup) influences the immune system as much as it does the cardiovascular, neurological or other systems. Profiling our genetic makeup can teach us about the influence of our nutrition and toxic intake on the control of inflammation, our ability to fight viral and bacterial infections, and the control of allergy, asthma and dermatitis (eczema). Knowing our genetic profile gives us the power to design the level of control we need to exert over our environment and intake.

Nutrition

The amounts of minerals, antioxidants and essential fatty acids that we consume governs, at a genetic and cellular level, inflammation, in particular. This is one of the most important aspects of our immune and defence system.

Generally, aim for a high intake of a variety of different-coloured vegetables (red, dark green, orange, and so on). Members of the *allium* food group (onions, garlic, and so on) have an effect on controlling tumour necrosis factor-alpha (TNF-alpha) – one of the most important inflammatory compounds made by the body – to ensure that the activity of the immune system's white blood cells is neither too weak nor too strong and produce correct immunoglobulin production.

We must produce another protein, Interleukin-6 (IL6), at optimum levels to ensure correct rate and strength of inflammation and white cell response.

IL6 is positively moderated by an intake of:
- fish oils;
- a variety of fruit and vegetables;
- vitamins A and C;
- zinc.

IL6 is adversely affected by an intake of:
- carbohydrates, especially refined sugars.

Exercise

I highly recommend exercise to help boost your immune system. The specific benefits are as follows:
- Regular exercise is known to enhance the production of T-cells.
- Exercise reduces excessive inflammatory compounds such as cytokines.
- Exercise increases phagocytic activity (white cells surrounding foreign material).
- Exercise encourages normal natural killer cell activity.
- Exercise increases telomere length in white blood cells (*see* Chapter 1).
- Exercise delays the onset of immunosenescence.[3]

Lifestyle

The less we compromise our immune system through our lifetime, the more likely it is to stay well-functioning into old age. To maintain a healthy immune system, we need to try to avoid exposure to:
- *Toxins* – see Chapter 4.
- *Allergens* – avoid allergens wherever possible by understanding those airborne compounds and foods to which you know you are sensitive. Consider the use of water and air filters around the house and use dust-mite protection over pillows and mattresses.
- *Stress* – meditation has been shown to influence the immune system in a variety of ways. A most important study concluded that secretory IgA increases with meditation, improving the barrier effect of the body's membranes.[4]

Dr Sharma's Programmes

We need to keep our immunity functioning at an optimum level to maintain healthy longevity. It is all very well looking after organs and other systems, but if immunity fails, the health of any other part of the body is redundant.

All the different parts of the immune system – the skin and epithelial membrane linings of the body, the secretions, the immunoglobulins produced by the white blood cells (B-type), the acquired immunity including the specific anti-cancer cells such as natural killer cells – are dependent upon a wide range of minerals, vitamins and other nutrients. It is so important to keep the immune system functioning – especially as we age – owing to its natural tendency to falter then, and we therefore need to ensure good supplemental intake.

Dr Sharma's Maintenance Programme

This is a basic programme to protect and improve the hormonal system.

MINERALS
- *A broad-spectrum multimineral taken along with a multivitamin supplement (as below)* – I recommend this is taken once or twice daily as most minerals will have some part to play in immune function.

VITAMINS
- *A broad-spectrum multivitamin with minerals (as above)* – choose one that is high in antioxidants, particularly vitamins A and C.

ESSENTIAL FATTY ACIDS
- *Omega-6 and omega-3* – taking these at a ratio of 4:1 seems to be the best mix for controlling inflammatory response, although if inflammation is present, a practitioner may raise the omega-3 levels with fish oils such as krill oil.

AMINO ACIDS
- *Branched-chain amino acids* – many amino acids are the building blocks of proteins and so have a vital role in the normal function of the immune system. A group known as the branched-chain amino acids (BCAAs) are essential for lymphocytes (white blood cells), and a lack of BCAAs impairs immune function – particularly the

immune system's fight against invading organisms.[8] Branched-chain amino acids given intravenously show improved immunity in patients with infection and increased immunity in post-surgical patients.

• *Whey protein* – this is an abundant source of BCAAs, particularly due to the levels of leucine, isoleucine and valine, which can be taken individually in poor healing.

Dr Sharma's Advanced Programme

This is for those with immune system dysfunction, a susceptibility to infection or those over the age of 65. Consider the addition of these supplements after discussion with your healthcare provider, or if you want to enhance the protection of your nervous system.

In the advanced programme, consider taking all the nutrients from the maintenance programme twice daily. Furthermore, consider taking the following nutrients, too, as they all have specific evidence of efficacy – some at gene level – as well as having a direct effect on white blood cells:

NUTRIENTS INFLUENCING TNF-ALPHA

• *N-acetyl cysteine*
• *Green tea* – as drink or capsules
• *Probiotics* – maintains bowel flora levels benefits (not only TNF-alpha, but also supports sIgA and bowel epithelial integrity)
• *L-carnitine*
• *Glutamine/glutamate*
• *Purified thymus extracts* – recommended by certain authorities

NUTRIENTS INFLUENCING IL6 INFLAMMATORY ACTIVITY

• *Ginseng*
• *Oligomeric proanthocyanidins (OPCs)* – powerful antioxidants found in pine bark extract and grape seed extract
• *DHEA*
• *Coenzyme Q10*

Conventional medicines and therapies

Conventional medicines tend not to be developed to enhance organ or system function, but are generally geared toward attacking organisms. Antibiotics, antivirals and antifungals are the obvious examples. Other drugs based on steroid-like action reduce inflammation in an attempt to alleviate symptoms of disease rather than moderate inflammatory activity. Some drugs can and *do* increase white-cell activity, but these tend to produce side effects and are generally prescribed only by specialists.

Drugs that are prescribed for other age-related diseases and conditions such as chemotherapy for cancer or statins for high cholesterol have a direct immunosuppressive role that is rarely taken into account when dealing with an isolated disease process.

Vaccinations may not be all they are cracked up to be as we age, although statistics seems to suggest a reduction in the number of deaths from influenza and pneumonia among those vaccinated against these conditions in the over-65s population.

Overall, I do not think that any drug programme can boost the immune system generally as we age, unless we are actually ill, in which case it may be necessary to treat each case on a specific basis.

However, if you are taking medication for another condition and that in itself is hampering the function of the immune system, the supplements mentioned above will help put your immunity back on track.

One big concern is the presence of intracellular viruses such as herpes, CMV and EBV. No drugs presently available have a marked effect in combating the viruses that lie dormant within cells. Conventional medicine does not yet have in place treatment for what more recent studies consider to be a major issue in healthy ageing.

BENEFITS OF MEDITATION

The first-line or innate immune system responds to meditation practices that foster compassion. Meditation as part of a holistic Tibetan regimen may influence the outcome of multiple sclerosis (MS), which may be triggered or worsened by an over-aggressive inflammatory response of the nervous system.[5]

Furthermore, many papers cite the benefits of meditation on white-cell response by altering immune function through the process of psychoneuroimmunology.[6]

Meditation even increases the beneficial response to vaccination.[7]

Keep an eye out for the development of nanotechnology (microscopic drugs that work at an intracellular level) and meanwhile maintain good levels of zinc, magnesium and potassium, all of which are important for intracellular detoxification.

Investigations and tests

However well you may feel and however up to date you are, there is great benefit in knowing whether or not your immune system has a genetic predisposition to weaken owing to poor detoxification, a need for high doses of nutrients or if you have weak anti-cancer or strong allergic tendencies.

First-line investigations

The majority of us who do not have a history of recurrent illnesses or a history of having had to take many antibiotics might, arguably, have no need of first-line investigations. I believe, however, that a base-level understanding of personal genetic makeup can focus attention on necessary lifestyle adjustments to stimulate the immune system and prevent premature deterioration. I therefore recommend the following as first-line investigations:

Immunogenomic profiling
The amount of research presently taking place in the field of immunogenic profiling means that we will soon see huge advances in our understanding of how genes control our inflammatory and immune responses. You will need to discuss matters with your healthcare provider to discern which tests to use, but please also see Useful Websites.

Second-line investigations
This level of testing is for those who clearly have a condition related to immune deficiency, a family history of cancer below the age of 65, or who are entering middle age without optimum levels of fitness and body weight or who live life to excess.

NUTRITIONAL ANALYSIS
I recommend testing specifically for:
- vitamins A and C;
- vitamin B-complex;
- white blood cell zinc, copper and magnesium;
- essential fatty acids;

- glutathione;
- iron/ferritin.

OTHER USEFUL SECOND-LINE TESTS

There are a variety of other useful tests:

- *Amino-acid assessment* – ensure that you have been following your normal diet for at least two weeks to see if you are absorbing enough branched-chain amino acids.
- *DHEA levels* – *see* Chapter 8.
- *Viral immune activity status* – consider this testing for herpes, CMV, EBV and chlamydia.
- *Comprehensive digestive stool analysis with parasitosis* – this assesses whether you have a good, beneficial bacterial balance and checks that you are not carrying parasites.
- *Full tumour immunity profiles or tests* – these are offered by specialist laboratories looking at immunosenescence and anti-cancer immunity. They look at T-cells, memory cells and natural killer cell function, as well as inflammatory levels and important minerals such as zinc and immune compounds such as glutathione.

Cancer

Cancer rates are climbing. I discuss UK and European figures here, but the USA and other parts of the world that keep records have similar statistics. Later on, I discuss US statistics in specific cancers that can be related back to rates around the world. Latest figures suggest that the UK incidence for cancer is more than 465,000 new cases each year. More than 175,000 British people will die from a cancer or from problems related to the disease (Cancer Research UK, Nov, 2011). Statistics vary, but between 1 in 3 and 1 in 6 people will develop cancer at some point in their lives.

Statistical analysis of countries keeping records in Europe estimated that there were nearly 3.2 million cancer cases diagnosed in 2011, excluding non-melanoma skin cancers, and 1.7 million deaths from cancer.

The most common form of cancers are:

- breast cancer (429,900 cases – 13.5 per cent of all cancer cases);
- colorectal cancers (412,900 cases – 12.9 per cent of all cancer cases);
- lung cancer (386,300 cases – 12.1 per cent of all cancer cases).

STATINS AND CANCER

While some studies suggest a protective effect of statins against cancer,[9] animal studies and some evidence in human statistical observation suggest that statins might be associated with cancer.[10]

Lung cancer had the highest death rates for cancer (334,800), followed by colorectal (207,400 deaths), breast (131,900) and stomach (118,200) cancers. However, probably in part owing to the banning of smoking in public places in many European countries, there has been a levelling off of the rates of all cancers since 2005.

The total number of new cases of cancer in Europe appears to have increased by 300,000 since 2004. The ageing of the European population will cause these numbers to continue to increase.[11] European estimates suggest that an increase to 374 cases will be diagnosed per 100,000 of the population per year from the rate in 1975 of 295.[12]

Preventative measures, earlier detection and better treatment options – both orthodox and complementary – increase longevity and decrease suffering. Nevertheless, overall statistics suggest that, except in a few types of cancer, mortality rates have not improved despite these 'advances'. What we are aware of, though, is that the earlier the detection of a developing tumour, the better the outcome. A preventative lifestyle and preventative therapies reduce cancer risk considerably.

Lifestyle behaviour patterns such as smoking or exposing the skin to UV rays are well-known causes of cancer, but there is not enough emphasis on other factors such as the following:

- *Obesity* – being overweight is associated with increased risk of cancers occurring in the oesophagus, breast, endometrium (the lining of the uterus), colon, rectum, kidney, pancreas, thyroid, gallbladder and possibly other parts of the body.[13]
- *Insufficient exercise* – exercising reduces cancer rates.[14]
- *Environmental toxins* – heavy metals and pesticides have an impact.[15]
- *Stress* – immune function is impaired by chronic stress: a life-effecting stressful event increases the chances of developing breast cancer over the following five years.[16]
- *Nutritional deficiencies* – evidence indicates that vitamin and mineral deficiencies can lead to DNA damage and therefore cancer.[17]

Although we are becoming more aware of how to check for cancer, and how to behave to avoid developing cancer, self-help cancer prevention is often hard, and the big food companies do not make it any easier.

Specific cancers

This is not a book about specific cancer treatment. However, now that we are living longer, we have to face the growing incidence of age-related cancer.

PROSTATE CANCER

Prostate cancer is the second leading cause of cancer deaths in American men (behind lung cancer). The American Cancer Society estimates that through 2012, doctors will diagnose about 240,000 new cases of prostate cancer, which is just under 12 per cent of all cancers and will result in around 20,000 deaths.

The disease is rare before the age of 40, although generally two out of three people receive their diagnosis before the age of 65.

Most men diagnosed with prostate cancer do not die from that disease. Even without naturopathic intervention, which seems to have benefit even with minor supplementation, 98 per cent of men with prostate cancer will be alive ten years after diagnosis, and 92 per cent 15 years later. However, the figures worsen if prostate cancer has spread to the bones, organs or tissues away from the prostate (the five-year survival rate drops to 29 per cent). Nevertheless, even if the cancerous cells have spread regionally (to local lymph nodes), five-year survival is still close to 100 per cent with current conventional treatment.[18] In the UK, 37 per cent of men were diagnosed with prostate cancer in 2008, with just over 10,000 dying from the disease in 2009.

MINERAL AND VITAMIN EFFECTS AND PROSTATE CANCER

Vitamin-D deficiency and a low calcium intake is associated with prostate cancer.[21]

Some studies show that high levels of zinc may aggravate prostate cancer. This happens if one of the trace element protein carriers in the body, metallothionein, is at a low level as zinc bound to metallothionein regulates a vital gene (p53 gene) that suppresses cancer cell development. *If you have prostate cancer or a family history of this condition, do not take zinc without testing for this protein and measuring p53 gene activity.*

Comparing the USA's estimates for 2012 with the figures for the UK population in 2008/9, I can illustrate how regionally, despite similar interventional, conventional treatment programmes, there seems to be considerable variation in likely outcomes. This could be because the US performs treatment earlier and more aggressively, or perhaps because there are more specific protective factors or causative processes in some parts of the world. We seem to have a genuine need to diagnose early and treat the body as a whole by removing cause and boosting the immune system.

The *British Journal of Urology*[19] showed a substantial reduction in the incidence of prostate cancer in a group of just under 1,000 men treated with daily supplementation of 200 mcg of selenium over an average of five years. Statistics similar to this have been pieced together by Professor Pfeifer, former Director for Clinical Research at the Aeskulap Klinik in Switzerland. He has formulated a natural complementary therapy for prostate cancer known as *The Pfeifer Protocol*.[20]

Prostate cancer may not present with symptoms until the condition is advanced. Symptoms include blood in the urine and, very rarely, pain on urination. If you have a slowed urine stream or it is reduced in strength, or you suffer from hesitancy and urgency, you are more likely to have an enlarged prostate (prostatism), but do discuss these symptoms with your doctor.

BREAST CANCER

Breast cancer is usually discovered as a lump either by self-examination or through a routine exam. Tethering or puckering of the skin, often around the nipple and areola, is a warning sign, as is any unexpected discharge from the nipple. The statistics for breast cancer vary considerably worldwide. North America, Western Europe (including the UK), Australia and New Zealand reported more than 90 new breast cancers occurring per 100,000 women in 2011.[22]

In Eastern Europe, there were about 74 new cases per 100,000; if Russia is included, the rate drops to 57 cases per 100,000. In Africa, generally 40 new cases occur per 100,000 people, but there are geographical variances for that figure. The numbers are the same in the Middle East, but drop to a the rate of 22 per 100,000 in Indo-China.

It seems that the longer you live, the more likely cancer is to develop. Of course, there are many variables and theories behind the statistics, but it is interesting to note that incidence is higher in:
- countries with a higher sugar intake;

- countries with higher levels of obesity;
- populations that drink pasteurized, homogenized dairy products;
- countries where trace nutrients in food are lacking owing to over-farming of the arable land.

The number of women in the UK who are currently developing breast cancer is 1 in 8.[23] This is the same figure as in the USA (American Cancer Society, 2012). The chance of dying from breast cancer is about one in 36. Figures for the USA and the UK are half as good as parts of Europe and other parts of the world.

As both cancer treatment and the human makeup are much the same worldwide, there must be other factors (such as sugar intake, obesity, and so on) that can reduce breast-cancer rates in a population. The use of oral contraceptive pills (OCPs) appears to slightly increase the risk of breast cancer, especially among younger women, although the risk level normalizes after ten years of discontinuing use.

Focusing on a healthy lifestyle seems to be an important aspect of avoiding or defeating breast cancer. This book is not about dealing with specific cancers, but, from a protective point of view, pay special attention to the following:

- Be aware of what you eat and how it was produced.
- Avoid exposure to chemical pollutants.
- Drink bottled or filtered water – even the filtration processes of our tap water cannot remove all the OCP or artificial hormones that get into our water system from the urine of those who take them.
- Test for any chemicals found in the system, including heavy metals, and remove through far infrared therapy and other detoxification processes.

BOWEL CANCER

The term bowel cancer, sometimes referred to as colorectal cancer, covers cancer of both the colon and the rectum. The incidence is strongly related to age, with 70 per cent of such cancers diagnosed in people aged 65 or over. There is a sharp increase in diagnosis from around the age of 50 and strong evidence to suggest that a bowel cancer can take up to 15 years of development before it will show signs that bring an individual to a doctor.

Bowel cancer is detected either during routine screening or at a visit to the doctor – usually following the development of any of the following symptoms:

- rectal bleeding;
- change in bowel habits lasting longer than four to six weeks;
- abdominal pains;
- iron deficiency anaemia (as a result of bleeding);
- bowel obstruction;
- unexplained weight loss and fatigue.

Bowel cancer is associated with:
- poor fibre intake;
- diets high in red meat and animal fat;
- low intake of fruits and vegetables;
- poor calcium and magnesium levels;
- a genetic tendency, particularly in families that have large bowel polyps;
- those with inflammatory bowel conditions in their medical history;
- alcohol intake;
- smoking;
- obesity;
- lack of exercise.

Certain dietetic and lifestyle factors are associated with a decreased risk of developing bowel cancer. High folic-acid intake (from legumes – peas and beans and dark green vegetables, including broccoli, okra, spinach, seeds and sprouts) and live yoghurt, assumed to be beneficial because of high levels of probiotics, also reduce the risk.[24]

Aspirin continues to elicit great debate as to whether or not it is instrumental in the treatment of or resistance to bowel cancers. A low dose of aspirin (75 mg) is beneficial to the heart and arteries but ineffective in cancer protection, whereas the higher dose for cancer is ineffective in the heart and raises a risk of internal bleeding. As things stand, those with a hereditary colorectal cancer risk reduce their chances of developing the disease by taking 600 mg of aspirin per day.[25]

Overall, studies suggest that aspirin may be beneficial even for those who do not have a family risk, but taking it always needs to be balanced with the risks of bleeding and aspirin allergy (which can induce asthma, stomach ulcers or other bowel inflammatory conditions).

It is also worth noting that aspirin is an artificially made derivative of salicylic acid, which is found in the majority of fruits and vegetables and also in many herbs and spices. Scientists have yet to establish fully whether – at least in part – the salicylate (another name for salicylic acid) is the protective factor in aspirin. Certainly, statistics showing that those who eat more fruit and vegetables are less likely to develop bowel cancer. Eating good amounts of fruit and vegetable may well be providing an aspirin-like defence, negating the need for additional aspirin. Interestingly, there is no evidence that high fruit and vegetable intake increases the risk of bleeding disorders or intestinal inflammation, thereby suggesting that it is the artificial form of salicylic acid that is harmful.

The lifetime risk of developing bowel cancer in the UK is estimated to be one in 15 for men and one in 19 for women.[26] USA figures are similar. Parts of Eastern Europe have nearly 80 per cent higher rates in men, but not in women, whereas the Greek population has less than half the rate of the UK. Clearly, lifestyle and diet have a huge role to play in the development of bowel cancer.

Faecal occult blood (FOB) in a stool sample is the main way in which we test for bowel cancer. The test is only around 85 per cent accurate and is not specific for cancer – it is merely an indication of bleeding in the bowel. The result is that one in six cases of bowel cancer will be missed. Testing for specific proteins present when inflammation in the bowel is active is much more accurate (around 95 per cent), missing only one in five cases – still too many, but better nonetheless.

I think it would be better for doctors to check the stool for either calprotectin or lactoferrin. We should conduct such a test in the general population every year after the age of 50, and after the age of 40 in those with a family history of bowel cancer. As we learn more about how the environment (and specifically what we ingest or inhale) interacts with our genes, we are becoming more aware that genetic or inherited tendencies do not necessarily have to lead to an increased likelihood of developing cancer. Nutrigenomics testing (*see* page 259) can detect gene interactions and advise us how we might best prevent disease setting in.

Other scientifically validated pioneering techniques such as tests looking at the effects of natural extracts and the gene activity of cancer cells themselves are available, but they are not yet widely utilized, pending longer-term outcome studies. (In other words, the science behind the test is solid, but whether it makes a difference to the outcome of developing or living longer with a cancer is yet to be established.)

Screening for cancer

Currently, orthodox medicine is geared toward 'early' detection, and most of us (specifically, those without genetic predisposition to cancer) are not generally introduced to tests that might diagnose either a tendency to cancer or tests that isolate cancer cells in the bloodstream at a stage before we might be able to detect a tumour.

RECOMMENDED BROAD INVESTIGATIONS

Tumour immunity profile

Your body's defence against cancer is largely down to the white blood cells, known as natural killer cells, and other T-cells in your immune system. The tumour immunity profile is a blood test to indicate how well your body's specific anti-cancer immunity is functioning, as well as establishing the levels of essential vitamins and minerals circulating in your blood.[27]

DNA adducts

This blood test looks at DNA in white blood cells and isolates chemicals and metal toxins that might be attached (DNA adducts), as these might cause a cell to become cancerous. Isolating such toxins allows the possibility of removing the possible causative agent, and of gauging the necessity and levels of detoxification required. Finding a laboratory that does this specialized level of testing is tricky, so generally try to find physicians working in the field of integrated medicine and cancer (see also Useful Resources).

Nutrigenomics

The study of how different foods may interact with specific genes to increase the risk of common chronic diseases, including some cancers, nutrigenomics provides molecular insight into how pollutants and environmental chemicals (such as additives and preservatives) in the diet influence health by diverting the normal activity (expression) of genes. Through an understanding of the structure of an individual's genetic makeup (genome), nutrigenomics explains how the influence of diet on health depends on an individual's genetic makeup.

This new field of investigation has developed since 2003 when the Human Genome Project led to the identification of all the genes in the human makeup. Scientists now recognize that toxins and nutritional deficiencies may trigger incorrect cell multiplication – the underlying cause of cancer development. Certain genetic types are more susceptible to this kind of cell mutation than others.[28]

Perhaps 'ecological genomics' would be a more appropriate name as the studies look at a variety of gene markers that tell us about risks of environmental and lifestyle triggers for cancer. This test does not show whether an individual will or will not get cancer, but it will show how lifestyle changes could minimize the risks of developing the disease by avoiding certain toxins and overcoming nutritional deficiencies.

Without getting too complicated, but to give you an idea of how useful the information may be if you are genetically predisposed to weakened cancer defences, tests look at specific genes such as those involved with the production of interleukin 1-beta and TNF-alpha. The genes governing these can be influenced by taking nettle leaf extract, stomach acid (hydrochloric acid) capsules, and fish oil and N-acetyl cysteine supplements, as well as drinking green tea and taking probiotics. Reaching an optimum weight influences TNF-alpha – TNF-alpha measurements can help predict who is at a greater risk of developing cancer if they are overweight. Establishing potential causes and risk factors requires:

- a full consultation and medical history and review of lifestyle;
- the removal of potential environmental causes of tumour through detoxification and improvement of the immune system through nutrition and natural supplementation adjustment;
- a look at individual failings in dealing with stress and psychological factors.

All of these, once identified, may help treatment choice.[29]

Tumour cell detection

This test, which is still under review, isolates cancer cells from a blood sample and measures more than 20 cancer-cell 'markers' (compounds) in dilutions of as little as one cell per litre (1¾ pints) of blood. (Athough cancer cells are known to invade the bloodstream, once they are over 3 mm in size, most standard, orthodox blood tests measure markers that may show positive in only 60 per cent of cancers, and even then only when there is a substantial tumour in the system.) The laboratories go to great lengths to point out that this level of study is in research, but, nevertheless, the great potential remains for this to be the most accurate and advanced test for the recognition of very early stage tumour.

For those who may have a high risk (*see* page 259), this test may identify a problem well before symptoms arise.

First-line investigations

The best way to assess cancer risk and potentially catch the presence of a tumour is to put all of the above profiles together.

ORTHODOX SCREENING FOR CANCER

I know of no government-led screening anywhere in the world that focuses on predicting the individual risk of getting cancer – rather, orthodox screening is aimed at early detection.

Countries with socialized health systems, such as the National Health Service (NHS) in the UK, screen for the following:

- Bowel cancer
- Prostate cancer in men
- Cervical cancer in women
- Breast cancer in women

There is continued debate about what the results of these investigations actually tell us, but overall I am supportive of tests. Private screening companies can look for a tumour anywhere in the body. Full body scans are available using magnetic resonance imaging (MRI) or computerized tomography (CT or CAT) scans. CT scanning delivers radiation through X-ray – in itself this may, according to some, increase the risk of cancer.

These scans are likely to pick up a solid tumour, but generally not before it is at least 0.5 cm (¼ in) in size. Tumours above 0.3 mm are likely already to be shedding cancer cells into the bloodstream, so arguably, even this form of early detection may be too late.

BOWEL CANCER SCREENING

Stool sample tests measure various compounds. The most common and inexpensive is the use of a chemical guaiac that detects the heam molecule in blood. A second test identifies antibodies to haemoglobin, and thirdly, there are now much more expensive DNA tests which are actually isolated from cancer and pre-cancerous lesions. These tests rank about 85%–90% sensitive – missing about 1 in 10 cancers. The benefit of isolating a cancer early or even in its pre-canccrous state leads to a 15%–33% decrease in mortality over 13 years.[30]

Identification of inflammation in the gut is less cancer specific, but possibly has a 95 per cent accuracy using different markers such as calprotectin and lactoferrin. The use of tests like colonoscopy and the less expensive sigmoidoscopy (quicker process of scoping the bowel, but it does not travel so far around the large bowel) are invasive, but, surprisingly, there are no randomized controlled studies showing that these tests are of benefit.[31]

Virtual colonoscopy (VC) using CT scanning is less invasive – at least initially. Most lesions identified by VC generally lead to an optical scope colonoscopy. The reading is dependent on the skill of the radiographer reading the report, and there are far fewer of these skilled individuals than there are experienced OSC experts, but that is changing. One perceived benefit is that 16 per cent of those using VC had lesions discovered outside of the colon, making the VC a broader investigation.[32]

BREAST CANCER SCREENING
Mammography
In the UK, women aged 50 to 70 are generally invited for a mammogram to screen for breast cancer.

In July 2011, The American College of Obstetricians and Gynecologists issued new guidelines calling for mammograms to be done every year from the age of 40. This contradicted the US Preventative Services Task Force in 2009 that shared the current attitude to the UK's policy.

The accuracy of mammograms is debatable, with some researchers suggesting that mammograms miss 25 per cent of cancers in women aged 40 to 49, and 10 per cent in women over the age of 50.[33]

Some authorities suggest that radiation from mammograms may trigger cancer, particularly in those carrying a gene known as oncogene AC; one study suggests that mammograms in women under 35 may cause 75 cases to develop for every 15 cases these tests identify.[34]

Several studies indicate that mammograms in younger women or those with denser breast tissue can lead to up to 90 per cent 'false positives', where mammography leads to invasive procedures such as biopsy or lumpectomy only to find no pathology.

A seminal piece of research published by researchers in Denmark[35] states that tests of more than 200,000 people led to results that were 'unable to find an effect of the Danish Screening Programme on breast cancer mortality'. In other words, mammography may not be all that it has been cracked up to be: it may carry dangers, and it may lead a woman down the path of unnecessary investigations – and yet it remains our gold standard process for investigation into the early stage of disease.

WHO HAS A HIGH RISK OF CANCER?

The following attributes greatly increase your risk of developing cancer:

- Having an immediate family member with cancer
- Having a high number of cancer cases on one or both sides of the family
- Being exposed to ecological risks such as smoking
- Being obese
- Doing too little exercise
- Eating fewer than five portions of organic fruit and vegetables a day
- Working in industry and being exposed to chemical toxins, pesticides, and so on
- Being chronically stressed

Breast ultrasound

There is certainly plenty of evidence that ultrasound may be of benefit in searching for malignant breast masses.[36] Ultrasound potentially runs the risk of providing false positives. However, assessment through ultrasound in the hands of a specialist may be more likely to pinpoint malignant tissue than, perhaps, an expert in mammography who has only one or two views.

One recent paper states that ultrasound appears to be more effective than mammograms when breast tissue is more dense as is the case in women aged 30–39. Ultrasound should be the recommended imaging technique in women ages 30–39 with focal breast symptoms.[37] I would extend that, pending further studies to women under 40 generally and those of all ages who have dense breasts.

One big advantage is that ultrasound does not involve radiation and so carries no risk of triggering cancer. Conclusive evidence comparing ultrasound to mammography has not been put forward. If it had, this cheaper and less uncomfortable technique would be more widely available. This lack of study into whether ultrasound lowers mortality rates for breast cancer baffles me.

Breast thermography

This technology uses a heat-seeking camera in front of which a woman sits comfortably for a few minutes. A technician, after a short while, applies a cold pad to the breasts. The cold sensation causes blood to drain from healthy breast tissue. However, blood continues to circulate through cancerous cells, which means that a tumour shows up as a hot area on the thermograph.

Although the Federal Drugs Administration (FDA) approved breast thermography as an 'adjunct' to mammography, the technique is yet to be accepted as a first-line diagnostic process.

Breast thermography should be considered for all ages, but particularly for those under the age of their country's recommendation for mammography (50 in the UK and USA), especially if there is breast cancer in the family. Women who are known to have dense breast tissue from previous mammography should certainly consider this technique.

Magnetic resonance imaging (MRI)
This expensive process is just too costly for doctors to consider using it for routine screening, although private centres will provide access to those who can afford it. MRI has been shown to be more accurate than mammography and does not deliver a theoretically dangerous radiation dosage.

RECOMMENDED BREAST CANCER SCREENING
1. If you are at low risk or have dense breast tissue, avoid radiation and alternate thermography and ultrasound screening on a yearly basis. This unproven method will need your specialist's approval.
2. If you are at risk (that is, you have a family history, obesity, poor diet, low exercise levels and toxic intake), you should follow the recommendations of your specialist and consider mammography if your healthcare provider offers it, if a specialist recommends it or if a previous thermography or ultrasound suggests an abnormality.
3. If you have very high risk, as well as all the tests above, use the pioneering blood test that isolates cancer cells and measures specific markers as mentioned before.

Advanced investigations and complementary therapies for those diagnosed with cancer

There are thousands of reports of the spontaneous regression of cancer[38] and considerable evidence for the use of complementary treatments for patients with cancer.[39] Many of these treatments are supported with scientific findings, but are not in common or conventional use because we have not yet had evidence from an adequate number of significant trials.[40]

Having reviewed much of the literature on environmental effects and the use of nutritional, complementary and alternative medical (CAM) therapies in cancer cases, I am convinced that natural processes and various protocols are of benefit in supporting the body through orthodox cancer treatment. There is an ever-increasing number of theoretical CAM treatments for supporting those with cancer, and there is even more evidence of effective tests and investigations.

Only individual patient knowledge gives enough information to enable a doctor or other practitioner to set up protocols to support a battle against cancer. Orthodox medicine, however, tends to offer treatment based on statistical analysis.[41]

One researcher reported that the meeting of the American Association of Clinical Oncologists (ASCO) in 2006 gathered some 25,000 doctors to discuss advances in cancer therapy. They were presented with more than 10,000 scientific abstracts. Their conclusion was that new therapies increased survival from 10.8 months to 12.9 months. Progression-free survival (PFS) was changed in another comparison from 7.2 months to 7.6 months. In another comparison, overall survival was changed from 10.2 to 12.5 months, and PFS changed from 4.5 to 6.4 months. In yet another comparison, the overall survival changed from 5.91 to 6.37 months – about two weeks. One week was added to remission-free survival.[42]

By the mid-1980s, treatment had not improved life expectancy in the majority of types of cancer over the previous 30 years.[43] I have yet to see convincing evidence that much has improved in the last 30 years.

Areas to consider

Areas of consideration for investigating and treating cancer include:
1. establishing and removing the cause of cancer;
2. the use of orthodox techniques and medical care;
3. assessment and activation of the immune system;
4. nutritional assessment and dietetic therapy;
5. psychological and healing techniques;
6. reviewing CAM cancer tests;
7. discussing CAM cancer therapy.

1. ESTABLISHING AND REMOVING THE CAUSE OF CANCER

Many cancers have a clear cause: for example, there is the association of lung cancer with smoking, bowel cancer with obesity, harmful UV rays in sunlight with melanoma. We are now seeing that many cancers occur in individuals with a genetic predisposition that leads to immune suppression based on environmental factors such as smoking and nutritional deficiencies, and in this chapter we have already seen the role of nutrigenomics in removing possible causes of cancer.

2. THE USE OF ORTHODOX TECHNIQUES AND MEDICAL CARE

Orthodox medicine has considerable success in the treatment of some cancers and should not be discounted in a holistic treatment plan. The surgeon's knife may be curative, and chemotherapy and radiation treatments improve the outcome in some types of tumour. The 'side effects' of these treatments continue to be a problem – orthodox treatments are often toxic to the system. Full and frank discussion to decide whether the cure is worse than the disease is a prerequisite. Complementary treatments prepare the body for the conventional treatment and can speed healing after surgical and radiation damage.

Complementary support for conventional cancer treatment

When patients undergo conventional treatment for cancer, I provide them with variations based on the following protocols:

Protection alongside chemotherapy

To support the areas that are hit by chemotherapeutic drugs – specifically, liver function, the bowel wall lining, bowel flora, bone marrow and other fast-replicating cells such as hair follicles:

- *Milk thistle (Silybum marianum)*
- *N-acetyl choline*
- *Probiotics*
- *S-adenosyl methionine*
- *L-glutathione*
- *Antioxidants*
- *Shiitake mushroom extract*
- *Vitamin B3*
- *Astragalus*
- *Plant-based immune stimulators*

Preparation for an operation

To promote healing, reduce infection risk and avoid anaesthetic 'hangover':
Homeopathic remedies
- *Nux vomica* – potency 200, take three doses (morning , evening and the morning of the operation), starting one day before the operation.

- *Arnica* – potency 200, take as soon as permissible after the operation, then every 12 hours for three doses.
- *Belladonna* – potency 200, take every 12 hours for 3 doses after fnishing the arnica course.
- Ayurvedic or other herbs that support the liver, such as:
    - *Milk thistle* – 200 mg two or three times daily.
    - *N-acetyl cysteine* – 500–1,000 mgs, two or three times per day for at least two weeks.

Starting one week before the operation and continuing for one month afterward:
- *Vitamin C* – 1–2 g taken three times daily.
- *Zinc with copper* – at a ratio of 15 mg:2 mg taken nightly.
- *Argenine powder* – 15 g taken twice daily (provided you do not suffer from herpes, as this can exacerbate lesions).
- *Calendula- and arnica-based creams* – to apply to the wound or around the edge of bandage two or three times daily.

Protection for radiation therapy

Starting the day before and continuing though the entire course of radiation therapy and for one week afterward:
- *Homeopathic X-ray* – potency 30 (or equivalent remedy), taken two or three times daily.

Starting two days before radiation treatment and continuing through the entire course of treatment and for one month after the last treatment:
- *L-cysteine* – 1,000 mg taken three times daily.
- *Antioxidants* – use natural food state or chelates in combination at maximum dose on the label.
- *Coenzyme Q10* – 30–60 mg taken twice daily.
- *Multivitamin/mineral complex* – use natural food state or chelates in combination at maximum dose on the label.
- *Vitamin K* – 100 mcg taken daily.
- *Blue-green algae* – dosage as on the bottle.
- *Probiotics* – dosage as on the bottle.
- *Isoflavones* – needs to be prescribed.[44]

Most hospitals are unwilling to allow complementary medical care to run alongside orthodox treatment. If such support is not possible, then consider complementary treatment whenever the patient is allowed home and not in hospital receiving treatment.

3. ASSESSMENT AND ACTIVATION OF THE IMMUNE SYSTEM

Cancer may occur when the body's immune system fails and not necessarily because of excessive toxic exposure – most smokers do not get cancer and most people who go out in the sun do not get skin cancers. All of us have cancer cells developing in the body at times, but for the majority of us, the immune system deals with cancer by maintaining a good anti-tumour defence.

The body has specific anti-cancer defenders. Two of the main cellular ones are natural killer (NK) cells and other T-cell white blood cells. Antioxidants are also vital in the battle against cancer. They neutralize free radicals, which are highly reactive compounds formed by environmental pollutants (such as smoke, especially tobacco smoke), by ozone and even by the normal breakdown of ingested fats and proteins in the body. Free radicals attack cell membranes and impair the transportation of oxygen, water and nutrients around the body. They also impact on the efficient removal of waste matter from the cells, subjecting the system to further stress. Obesity, lack of exercise and stress may contribute to free radical production and immune dysfunction.

Antioxidants prevent the formation of these reactive substances before they can damage our tissues. They are also believed to slow down aspects of the ageing process, and research shows that people who consume higher amounts of antioxidants have greater longevity.[45]

Undertake investigations looking at NK-cell and T-cell activation and the nutritional status of the body as a whole – conventional centres will not routinely perform these specialist blood tests, so you will need to seek out laboratories that do them.

4. NUTRITIONAL ASSESSMENT AND DIETETIC THERAPY

Nutritional evaluation can guide doctors or nutritionists toward dietetic changes and supplemental requirements specific to an individual.

There is evidence that diet can inhibit cancer growth and equivocal evidence that diet alone can be a cure.[46] Many doctors and scientists have written books on anti-cancer treatments that are focused purely on diet and supplementation, but the best nutritional programme for each patient is decided through consultation with a nutritionist or specialist in anti-cancer diets. Specific therapies such as Gerson Therapy, macrobiotic diets and fasting options are all worth considering. I particularly draw your attention to Plaskett Therapy, a modified form of the Gerson Therapy. These are natural treatments that stimulate the body's ability to heal using detoxification and high-dose nutritional protocols through diet and supplements (*see* Useful Websites).

There is evidence that cancer is caused by carcinogenic compounds now commonly found in our food chain. The methods by which food is processed and stored may also cause cancer.[47] It therefore makes sense to choose food wisely and to eat natural and organic products as much as possible.[48]

5. PSYCHOLOGICAL AND HEALING TECHNIQUES
There has been considerable scientific research into psychoneuroimmu-nology, the study of the interaction between psychological processes and the nervous system and their control over human immunity.[49] Over the last 40 years or so, positive thinking and sessions of laughter, as well as meditation, prayer and other psychological processes have been proven to benefit survival and the regression of tumours and thereby aid longevity.[50]

The ability of the psyche to influence the nervous system to produce hormones and other compounds influencing the immune system is clear. The use of anti-stress techniques, counselling, hypnotherapy, visualization and meditation techniques all have a place in the treatment of malignant disease, whether that is in dealing with the issues surrounding living with cancer or actually preventing and fighting the disease.[51]

Group therapy has been shown to be beneficial in removing the stress of cancer and to double the life expectancy of patients with terminal cancers. Hands-on therapists and bioresonance computers, magnetic devices and other energy-channelling mechanisms may all be able to offer healing energy treatments. Working on lifestyle, psychology and healing techniques of this sort is essential.[52] Healing has been documented as being effective both as a cure and in relieving pain and discomfort.[53]

6. REVIEWING CAM CANCER TESTS
Studies on the best CAM cancer treatments and supportive therapies are taking place in laboratories all over the world. Researchers are looking at the function of the immune system and capturing cancer cells from biopsies or blood samples. Having grown the individual cancer in the laboratory, they apply chemotherapeutic agents and natural extracts to see which ones kill those individual cells. This specific targeting process is inevitably going to become the normal and preferred choice of treatment (*see* Useful Websites for a broader view).[54]

This technique of isolating cancer cells and growing them in a laboratory is a developing technique known as enrichment and culture. Once a colony of an individual patient's cancer has been cultivated, that specific tumour cell line can be tested against around 40 orthodox drugs and the same number of alternative, natural compounds as well. Such information helps guide oncologists toward the treatments that are most likely to be effective.

There may be many centres researching and providing such tests, but I consider the following to be the forerunners in the field:

- The Research Genetic Cancer Centre, Florina, Greece (www.RGCC-genlab.com), which is providing orthodox and natural treatment options
- Lab 4 More Laboratory (www.lab4more.de), Germany, which does NK cell and T-cell assessment and provides evidence showing which natural extracts and supplements influence the immune system best through a test known as the Full Tumour Immunity Profile

The pioneering developments mentioned above are the best way to support anti-cancer treatment. These tests are currently expensive, but prices will drop as the process becomes more widely utilized and available.

7. CAM CANCER THERAPY

There are many treatments offered throughout the world that may work against some or many types of cancer. Some may not be available in the country in which you live owing to legislation. There is always a risk that travelling far and wide or spending money on treatments offered by specific doctors or clinics that have a vested interest may not necessarily be the best way to formulate a treatment choice.

Testing as indicated above may prevent time and money being wasted.

Revolutionary research work over the last few years suggests that treatments individually tailored to a patient are more frequently beneficial than treatments that are more generally given.[55] For example, some specific tests review the potential benefits of the following natural compounds:

Quercetin	Amygdalin (B17)
Artesunate	Ukrain
Poly MVA	Indole 3 carbinol
Mistletoe	C-statin
Caesium chloride	Samento

Ascorbic acid	Melatonin
Hydrogen peroxide	Selenium
Coenzyme Q10	Carctol
Essiac	Noni juice
Modified citrus pectin	Superoxide dismutase
IP6	IFNa2
N-acetyl cysteine	Niacin
Pancreatic enzymes	L-methionine
Salvestrols	Ellagic acid
Carnivora	Aloe vera extract
L-carnitine	Pawpaw
Vitamin E	Reolysin (reovirus)
Curcumin	Lycopene
Maitake	Green tea extract

Those natural treatments that have most frequently benefited my patients according to the tests I have performed over the last five years are as follows. I hope it is a guide to your senior practitioners if you are unable to access the personalized, individualized test I suggest.

High-dose oral and intravenous vitamin-C therapy
PubMed is a research data service provided online by the United States National Library of Medicine and the National Institute of Health. They cite 45 papers, most of which show efficacy of high-potency vitamin-C therapy in a variety of cancers. Many other papers, journals and websites scrutinized by fully qualified physicians vigorously support such treatment.[56]

Avemar[55]
This is a fermented wheatgerm extract. It has been established in several oncology journals to be effective in many different types of tumours, both alongside chemotherapy and by having direct anti-cancer effects.

Quercetin
This well-researched plant extract brings up more than 900 papers showing its influence on many different types of cancer.[57]

C-statin

This is a plant extract from *Convolvulus arvenis* (field bindweed). It works by blocking the growth of blood vessels – a prerequisite for successful tumour growth.[59]

In conclusion

A professional must always treat cancer. The best approach is to ask your doctor for guidance if you are unsure of your cancer risk or are worried about cancer. He or she must consider the needs of each specific individual in his or her immune-system activity, as well as testing for risk, and – if you are actually dealing with cancer – specific treatments against a particular cancer cell line. Only an oncologist can offer you a prescription, although 'patient choice', as demanded by recent governments in the UK, allows for open discussion of what a patient wants. Any treatment needs to take into account the levels of toxicity and the nutritional requirements of each individual patient. Decide upon the most suitable therapies, general health regimes and psycho-spiritual practices through consultation.

Chapter 10

Other Systems and Organs

THE GASTROINTESTINAL TRACT

Various authors are attributed with the phrase 'Death begins in the colon'. Elie Metchnikoff, awarded the Nobel Prize for Medicine in 1908, is one of the first to be quoted. However, Hippocrates, the so-called father of modern medicine, suggested more than 2,000 years ago that bad digestion is the 'the root of all evil'.

Of course, this does not mean that all reasons for death are to do with gut pathology. However, if we review the basics of what the bowel does, we can see why you could argue that many a fault elsewhere in the body might be considered as being associated with the bowel.

The alimentary canal starts at the mouth and ends at the anus. If you could stretch it out, the long tube would, in effect, look like a complex worm! The bowel is responsible for digestion, turning what we eat and drink into absorbable forms, and our intestine also houses one hundred trillion bacteria that defend us, provide us with nutrients and aid digestion.

The bowel prevents toxins entering the body and is also a repository for the majority of our waste products, via the liver and bile. The surface area of the bowel is greater than any other organ in the body, so faults are more likely to occur here. A failure of the barrier mechanism, a leaky gut, allows molecules and organisms to enter the bloodstream. If the liver does not effectively neutralize these organisms, disease may set in. As we age, our digestive enzymes, stomach acid and bowel wall secretions all diminish, leaving our gut exposed to higher rates of absorption of the toxins we ingest.

It is now perhaps clear to see why physicians in bygone days, who relied upon observation rather than tests and investigations, concluded that the bowel was such an important organ.

Constipation

As we age, our muscles, including the muscles of our bowel, lose their strength and contractibility, which leads to a poor transit of food through the intestine and allows a build-up of faeces. In order not to make matters worse, it is important that we drink good amounts of water and eat plenty of fibre.

Diverticular disease

This disease occurs when weakened muscles of the large intestine allows the colon to herniate in one or several places, leading to 'pouches' in the bowel wall. These can trap faeces.

The presence of diverticula is known as diverticulosis; if the pouch becomes inflamed, a more painful condition known as diverticulitis occurs. This is an increasingly common disorder that may affect up to:

- 10 to 30 per cent of the population over 40;
- 50 per cent of people over the age of 60;
- 66 per cent of those over the age of 80.

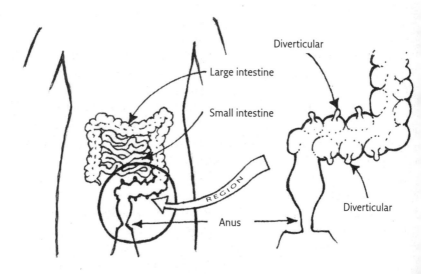

Figure 18: **Diverticular disease in the intestinal tract**

Many of us live with diverticula that never bother us. However, if inflammation does occur, you will need to have a period of fluid-only fasting and to take painkillers to clear the bowel and ease the pain. A slow return to normal eating should include lots of high-fibre foods, and you will probably need to take stool-bulking medication to reduce the chances of recurrence. Surgery is a last resort.

Haemorrhoids

Also known as piles, these protruding veins are present in around 50 per cent of Americans and Britons over the age of 50. Similar to diverticular disease, a haemorrhoid is a projection of engorged blood vessels through the thin rectal wall. Inadequate intake of fibre and roughage, as well as obesity, poor musculature and years of sitting down all contribute to haemorrhoid development.

Haemorrhoids can bleed and if they clot, they are described as 'thrombosed'. Pain is as much an issue as bleeding, although a recurrent bleed can lead to anaemia and runs the risk of infection.

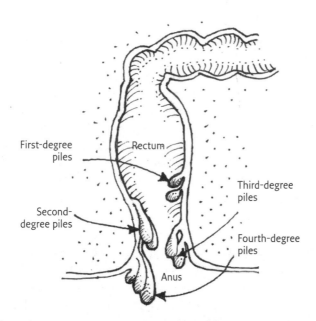

Figure 19: **Haemorrhoids (piles)**

Polyps

An overgrowth of the mucosal lining of the large intestine, polyps are often hard to see, owing to their flat shape. Most project either as lumps or sometimes on a stalk similar to, say, a mushroom. Most polyps are benign, although if found in clusters, they are more likely to be cancerous and are invariably so in a condition known as 'polyposis coli'.

Polyps are theorized as being a reaction to toxic compounds irritating the layers of the colon wall, but they are also known to be associated with deficiencies in calcium and magnesium. They are more common in people over the age of 50 and appear to be associated with bad dietary habits as described in diverticular disease. There is some association with smoking, drinking alcohol, being obese and not exercising enough. Simple changes to diet and lifestyle can overcome the condition relatively easily.

Polyps are usually symptomless. They rarely enlarge to a point of obstruction, and only if they become cancerous are we likely to notice symptoms (such as bleeding, change in stool habit and others described under bowel cancer in Chapter 9).

Reflux, hyperacidity and gastro-oesophageal reflux disease (GORD)

As we age, there appears to be an increase in the prevalence and symptoms of acid reflux.[1]

Most of us recognize which foods or habits cause such reflux and we can change our lifestyle or diet to avoid the problem. It is known that being overweight causes abdominal fat to push acid up the food pipe (oesophagus), especially when we lie down at night. The oesophagus does not have the thick mucus production that protects the stomach lining, so discomfort can easily occur. Hot drinks, especially caffeinated tea and coffee, spicy food, fried foods, anything with a high refined sugar content and alcohol – especially when taken on an empty stomach – all irritate the stomach lining, reduce mucus production and increase stomach acid production.

Orthodox doctors generally prescribe two groups of drugs known as 'antacids' or 'proton pump inhibitors' (most commonly omeprazole and lansoprazole), which cut down acid production. However, such treatment does not get to the underlying cause, although it may reduce symptoms. Stomach acid is there for a reason – predominantly to break down food. I believe that little consideration has been given to the medium- and long-term effects of reducing stomach acid and so hampering these effects.

Proton pump inhibitors are now associated with:
- hip fracture;
- clostridium infection, a serious diarrhoea-inducing organism;
- oesophageal cancer;[2]
- vitamin B12 deficiency, leading to anaemia and arterial disease.

One related, and often underestimated, condition is hypochlorhydria. This is the name for a lack of stomach acid – an inevitability of ageing, when the acid-producing cells in the stomach cease proper function. It is also caused by poor dietary habits, stress and allergy. Its symptoms are often identical to the symptoms of GORD and hyperacidity because the valve at the end of the stomach, the pyloric sphincter, is pH (acid/alkaline) sensitive. Unless we have an acidity of around pH 1 or 2 (very strong acid) in this part of the stomach, the valve does not open, and so the stomach may fail to empty. Poorly digested foods mop up the mucus that protects the stomach lining and then rub against it, leaving areas exposed to normal acid levels.

Overall then, the symptoms of GORD, hyperacidity, indigestion and reflux may, in fact, not benefit from the use of antacids or proton pump inhibitors in the long term – although they may offer relief in the short term.

Instead, and paradoxically, hydrochloric acid capsules taken at meal-times and pancreatic enzymes taken at the end of the meal may, under the guidance and follow-up of an experienced practitioner, tackle the underlying causes of these conditions. These treatments in combination with diet and lifestyle changes may resolve the problem and reduce the need for long-term antacid use.

Investigations

A pioneering test by Acumen Laboratory at Tiverton in the UK has found correlation between stomach-acid production and vascular endothelial growth factor (VEGF), a protein measurable in saliva or blood samples. As research continues, I think it will come to the same conclusions as my practice experience has – namely that many individuals treated with acid-reducing drugs are actually already struggling with low levels of stomach acid.

It is therefore worth considering having the following investigations:
- Stomach-acid VEGF saliva test
- ALCAT food-sensitivity testing
- Food-allergy cellular test or other food-allergy test

How to improve stomach-acid production

NUTRITION
Diets with reduced acid-forming foods, certain natural extracts and supplements can be very beneficial alongside a clear note of the foods you know are your individual causes of reflux.

LIFESTYLE
Simple diet assessment and changes such as chewing more, eating smaller quantities and eating slowly are ways to improve the production of stomach acid.

SUPPLEMENTATION FOR GORD
Try the following:
- L-glutamate
- Liquorice extracts
- Slippery elm (*Ulmus rubra*)
- A fermented soya extract sold as Sano-Gastril®
- Pancreatic enzyme supplements

Maintaining a healthy bowel

When it comes to bowel health, there is a huge amount of information available in books and on the Internet, so rather than repeat all the recommendations in detail, here is an easily digestible summary:

How to help your bowel

NUTRITION
- Eat regularly – three meals with two interim snacks a day.
- Include food from all the major food groups, restricting red meat and fatty or fried foods to two or three times per week.
- Try to eat organic food to avoid the associated toxins found in over-farmed foods or processed foods.
- Ensure that at least one meal a day is high in roughage. Eating porridge for breakfast, having three or four handfuls of vegetable, two or three portions of fruit or juiced fruit or vegetable drinks make this an easier task than many people think.
- Drink plenty of water or herbal teas.

LIFESTYLE

There is a direct association between obesity and a lack of exercise in nearly all bowel conditions. Working on these two areas of health helps prevent the development of colon and rectal cancer in particular.

SUPPLEMENTATION

- Take a combination probiotic nightly and consider changing this every three or four months to prevent overgrowth of any one type of bacteria.
- Use stomach-acid supplementation (HCl betaine or HCl pepsin) – as outlined above, stomach-acid production declines with age, inhibiting the digestive process.
- Pancreatic enzymes also diminish with age, so use a pancreatic digestive supplement either from bovine or porcine sources. For vegetarians, there are plant enzymes formulated to act in a similar way.[3]

First-line investigations

Consider having these tests on a yearly basis, especially after the age of 50.

Stool test

Take a stool test for either of the inflammatory markers: calprotectin or lactoferrin. These markers are possibly more accurate than the conventional search for faecal occult blood. (*See* section on bowel cancer screening on page 261.)

Colonoscopy

Specialists recommend colonoscopy for anyone over the age of 50 but particularly for those with a family history of colon or rectal cancer. This seems like sensible advice! (*See* section on bowel cancer screening on page 261.)

Second-line investigations

Consider the following tests if you have abdominal symptoms such as bloating, infrequent pains or symptoms that have baffled your doctors!

Comprehensive digestive stool analysis with parasitosis

There are many companies offering stool tests that look at beneficial, additional and pathogenic (bad) bowel bacteria. Looking for yeasts, fungi and parasites is also important, as these may cause acute symptoms and also be relevant to longer-term health issues that are often associated with leaky gut syndrome.

Food allergy testing
Without question, the most accurate method of assessing food intolerance or allergy is through food exclusion. Unfortunately, this takes time, with many people finding it extremely hard to maintain. Going onto a Stone Age or palaeolithic diet followed by slow reintroduction of foods and keeping a strict diary of reaction is pretty much infallible.

Many allergy centres use skin-prick or patch testing, which are well-respected and researched diagnostic tools, although it is time consuming.

Many companies offer food-allergy testing through blood analysis. Most conventional doctors and nutritionists test only for immunoglobulin E (IgE; *see* Chapter 2)[4], which is associated with the more marked and aggressive allergic reactions such as anaphylaxis, asthma and hives (urticaria).

Food intolerance
The antigen leukocyte antibody test (ALCAT) is a test measuring the release of compounds from white blood cells activated by foods to which an individual is sensitive. Food allergy cellular testing (FACT) measures the release of a compound called leukotriene from white blood cells in response to the presence of an allergen (a food or molecule that triggers allergy). There is limited research compared with IgE tests and there are some questions over their sensitivity. Nonetheless, some doctors and nutritionists seem to prefer these tests, and they are a popular commercial sale through practitioners.

Food intolerance is not an allergy, and conventional medical practitioners are not as readily open to its diagnosis. Testing for intolerance involves measuring chemicals released by white blood cells (WBC) and by WBC activity. As it goes through more investigation and research, the ALCAT assessment may prove to be a useful methodology for such investigation.[5]

Advanced investigations
Consider the following tests if you have been through the levels of screening described earlier and if your bowel issues have no discernable pathology.

Increased intestinal permeability, or the leaky gut test
This test requires you to drink a small amount of a liquid containing lactulose and mannitol or polyethylene glycol (PEG). The laculose/mannitol or PEG molecules will not pass through an intact and functioning bowel wall. If they do, they pass through the kidneys into the urine. You will then need to collect a urine sample over a set amount of time,

so that it can be tested for the presence of these molecules and in this way diagnose a leaky gut.

Conventional investigation of bowel issues
Discuss any ongoing concerns about bowel symptoms initially with your doctor and, if your symptoms arouse suspicion, ask to be referred to a specialist who can arrange further investigations.

Your doctor will issue you a *colonoscopy* exam (in which a long flexible tube with a camera is inserted into your colon) or *computerized tomography (CT) scanning* (also known as 'virtual colonoscopy'). In the hands of experts the success in spotting a polyp is probably equal in either field. However, virtual colonoscopy is unlikely to spot a flat polyp or cancer and the tube colonoscope may not be able to access all the different folds found in the large bowel. (*See* section on bowel cancer screening on page 261.)

RESPIRATORY SYSTEM

Lungs

The gradual decline in lung function can begin as early as at 30 years of age. The lungs contain bronchial tubes, leading to the alveoli where gaseous exchange takes place. The lungs are an important organ of excretion as well as absorption, removing from our bodies the carbon dioxide we produce at cellular level, as well as other noxious gases that would otherwise harm us.

We develop new alveoli until our early 20s, but thereafter we not only lose lung tissue because of the pollutants we breathe in, particularly cigarette smoke actively or passively, but our body stops rebuilding and replacing it. Ageing damages the elastin (stretchy protein strands) in the lungs and clogs up the small arteries that lead into the lungs.

A loss of muscle tone and bone density in old age causes curvature of the spine that in itself can compress the lungs. As we age, we tend to exercise less, reducing lung capacity. This, along with a weakening of the diaphragm (the main muscle that controls our breathing), means we do not inhale or exhale air at the same rate or quantity.

We go through life picking up coughs and colds, some of which will turn into chest infections – and in a percentage of us, pneumonia – creating further damage. People who smoke not only lose lung tissue, but may also develop the debilitating disease emphysema.

Age-related decrease in immunity (*see* Chapter 9) increases our susceptibility to infection, particularly in the lungs. Inflammation in the bronchial
tubes that lead to the lungs causes bronchitis. If this inflammation lasts a
short time, we have 'acute' bronchitis, but if it persists for three months or
more, it is termed chronic bronchitis or chronic obstructive pulmonary
disease (COPD). This condition is the fourth or fifth highest cause of death
in many polluted or developed countries.

How you can help your lungs

It is not possible to reverse the loss of lung tissue (emphysema), which makes
it all the more important that we take action to protect our lungs as we
age. COPD requires a focus on the immune system and may benefit from
lifestyle changes.

NUTRITION

There is no specific dietetic advice to offer the ageing lung apart from
sensible eating and the following points:

- Avoid food allergens, which may trigger asthma. (I have not included
  asthma in this book, as it is not in itself an age-related condition,
  although asthmatic symptoms are associated with emphysema and
  COPD.)
- Increase your intake of dietary fibre to boost your lung health and
  potentially reduce your risk of developing COPD.[6]

EXERCISES AND BREATHING TECHNIQUES

Maintaining good overall fitness through regular exercise ensures good
musculature in the area of the mid-to-upper spine and increases lung
capacity. The result is improved lung function and reserve (the amount of
air the lungs can hold). Best of all, it is never too late to enjoy these benefits
of exercise – even if you start exercising only later in life.

Most martial arts – including soft ones such as tai chi or chi kung and
hard ones such as karate, judo, and so on – include breathing techniques.
Yoga too has wonderful exercises for improving breathing techniques. And,
like exericse, it is never too late to start. If you have chronic bronchitis or
emphysema, consider specific breathing methods such as Buteko, too.

LIFESTYLE

Do not smoke! Keep your weight to an optimum level and spend as much
of your spare time as possible in areas where there is lower air pollution

(usually outside the city). Keep car windows up if you are driving along busy roads and wear a mask if you are cycling. Visit the countryside as often as you can – even once a week seems to benefit lung function.

SUPPLEMENTATION

Other than the need for vitamins, minerals, essential fatty acids and other nutrients (deficiencies in our soil affect the quality of our food), focusing on specific nutrients does not appear to help our lungs stay healthier for longer.

If you suffer from emphysema or chronic bronchitis or if you are at a high risk of developing either of these conditions (for example, if you smoke), the following nutrients may be of benefit:

- *Vitamins* – A, C and E
- *Minerals* – magnesium, copper with zinc at a ratio of 2:15 mg
- *Essential fatty acids* – lecithin, flaxseed oil
- *Amino acids* – L-carnatene, glutathione (if available by aerosol or inhaler, but otherwise as a lozenge taken under the tongue; swallowing glutathione renders it more or less ineffective)
- *Other nutrients* – N acetyl cysteine

URINARY SYSTEM
Bladder and kidneys

Your bladder is essentially a muscular sack. Its ability to stretch relies upon a tissue protein, elastin. As we age, both our muscles and our elastin levels deteriorate, meaning we more often feel the urge to pee – even when our bladder is not actually full. The weaker muscles also mean that the bladder cannot empty completely, leaving residual urine in which infection can grow.

Men are less likely to suffer bladder infection because their urethra (through which urine travels) lies along the length of the penis and curls around and up, which means that bacteria have quite a distance to travel to reach the bladder. The female urethra is shorter, making the journey for bacteria easier, and as women age, their oestrogen-dependent vaginal secretions, which provide another barrier to infection, reduce.

Because the kidneys filter out the majority of the toxins in the body and the bladder holds the urine that harbours these toxins, kidney failure or an inability to empty the bladder can lead to considerable toxicity.

Although kidney dysfunction does occur as we age (the kidneys lose a percentage of their nephrons – filtering units – and the arteries supplying the kidneys tend to harden and clog up), kidney failure is not something most of us have to worry about – other organs tend to wear out first! However, medications for certain conditions may cause kidney damage. Non-steroidal anti-inflammatory drugs (NSAIDs) used to treat arthritis, ACE inhibitors (for heart problems) and long-term use of any other drug may all impinge on kidney function.

How you can help your bladder and kidneys

Avoiding toxins, maintaining health in the body in general and avoiding drug use are all ways in which you can help protect the health of your bladder and kidneys.

NUTRITION AND EXERCISE

Nutrition and exercise do not play a big part in bladder and kidney issues, although yoga and pelvic floor exercises may help with bladder weakness (urinary incontinence).

SUPPLEMENTATION

- Flowease® – this supplement contains the pollen of the plant *Secale cereal* and can help men maintain bladder health.
- *Berberis and juniper* – these are heralded as kidney-benefiting plant extracts and need to be considered with a herbalist if problems are apparent.

Prostate problems

Composed of muscular and glandular tissue surrounded by a distinct capsule, the prostate wraps around the neck of the male bladder and the beginning of a man's urethra and acts as an involuntary valve; it also makes semen in which sperm live and travel.

I discuss prostate cancer broadly in the cancer section in Chapter 9. The principle symptoms of an enlarged prostate (causing what doctors term 'prostatism') are weak urine stream, bladder urgency (sometimes with incontinence), hesitancy (unable to go when by the toilet) and, most inconveniently, a need to urinate too often, thereby disturbing sleep at night.

Prostatic enlargement (prostatic hypertrophy) is a process of ageing owing to continual use of the muscle fibres that enlarge as the prostate is exercised. Testosterone may have a direct effect on enlarging the prostate's glandular and muscular tissue, and if you are taking testosterone as a supplement, you need to keep an eye on this. [7] Although testosterone is associated with libido and also with an enlarged prostate, having sex frequently does not enlarge the prostate.

To assess the level of problems associated with prostatism so that you can apply an appropriate level of treatment, I recommend a variation on the American Urological Association questionnaire. Answer the following questions on a scale of 0 to 5, where 0 is never and 5 is each time you urinate, for questions one to four, and as described for the remainder.

Over the past month:
1. How often have you had a sensation of not emptying your bladder completely after you have finished urinating?
2. How often have you had to urinate within two hours of going previously?
3. How often do you find that you stop and start when urinating?
4. How many times do you most typically get up to urinate after going to bed?
5. On a scale of 0 (easy) to 5 (difficult), how easy is it to postpone urination?
6. On a scale of 0 (bad) to 5 (good), where do you rate your urinary stream in comparison to the past?
7. Do you have to wait or push to begin urination (0 = no delay, no need to push; 5 = marked delay or have to push)?

Add up the total and score as follows:
- 7 or under – no enlargement
- 8–19 – moderately enlarged prostate
- 20 or more – severe prostatism

How you can help your prostate
NUTRITION
- Increasing your intake of zinc-containing foods such as meat, seafood, wholegrain wheat, pumpkin seeds and eggs may help.
- Choose organic foods because trace metals found in pesticides compete with zinc receptors and may actually reduce zinc absorption; and pesticides may increase levels of testosterone, which may be associated with prostate enlargement.
- Avoid chemicals, particularly bisphenol A (found in many plastics and non-metal tooth fillings), which have been shown to increase

testosterone in studies on men and may also be associated with prostate cancer.

- Oily fish with their omega-3 levels, eaten three times a week, may reduce prostatic hypertrophy.
- Eat broccoli daily. Cauliflower also benefits the prostate. Sulforaphane, which is present in both these vegetables, appears to activate a gene known as PTEN, a tumour suppressor gene that 50 per cent of men carry. Another gene, DSTM 1, may also interact with a compound in broccoli – possibly folic acid – and reduce the incidence of cancer.

SUPPLEMENTATION AND MEDICATION

- *Saw palmetto (Serenoa repens)* – is well known as potentially being able to reduce prostate size.
- *Essential fatty acids* – omega-3 and omega-6 taken at a ratio of 2:1 over three months may help overcome prostate hypertrophy. A 2013 study suggests omega-3 levels are associated with worse prognosis for those with aggressive prostate cancer. This goes against the majority of evidence suggesting benefit, but further research needs to be done to prove an causal link.[8]
- *Zinc with copper* – taken before bedtime, these nutrients may help ease prostatism, but you need to test for metallothionein as a lack of this metal-binding protein may make zinc a problem in prostate cancer. (*See* section on prostate cancer in Chapter 9.)
- *Flowease®* – this is a pollen extract of secale cereal, which has a positive benefit on the function of the bladder and is being researched for its benefits in prostatism.
- *Isoflavones* – these natural plant oestrogen-like compounds have been shown to benefit prostate health and possibly even fight against low-grade prostate cancer.
- *Extract of Pygeum africanum* – provides the plant extract beta-sitosterol which, like saw palmetto, has been shown to offer improvements in prostatism.
- *Drugs* – do not rule out taking conventional medicine. The relief from broken sleep and a disturbed lifestyle can outweigh the potential side effects of taking medication. A doctor will talk you through the benefits and pitfalls of taking drugs known as alpha blockers.

THE MOUTH

Gum disease and tooth decay

Poor dental hygiene shortens your life. It is really as simple as that.

Tooth loss makes it harder for us to chew properly, which, in turn, interferes with the type and amount of food we can eat. Furthermore, the microorganisms that grow in diseased gums and that we swallow and the inflammatory effects of gum disease in the mouth that consequently affect our arteries provide direct links between mouth health and general disease. Dental disease is associated with coronary artery disease, strokes and vascular dementia.[9] Gum disease is also clearly linked to diabetes – diabetes weakens the immune system, which may lead to periodontal (gum) disease. In a vicious circle, inflammation in the gums triggers an increase in tumour necrosis factor-alpha (TNF-alpha), an inflammation control protein, which is associated with an increase in insulin resistance and poor sugar control. The same component, TNF-alpha, is associated with arthritis.[10]

Failure of the parotid and salivary glands leads to a reduction of saliva. The result is dry mouth (xerostomia), which is a problem many people struggle with in their later years. Saliva starts the digestion process and contains many immunoglobulins (defence chemicals). With fewer of these immunoglobulins in the mouth, infection settles into the gums more readily. Infection is liable to speed up the rate of dysfunction of the saliva-producing glands establishing a vicious circle. Furthermore, more than 500 medications that are commonly used to combat age-related illness cause dry mouth – antipsychotics, antidepressants, sleeping pills and blood-pressure tablets among them.

How you can help your mouth

NUTRITION

Avoid sweet foods and snacks such as potato chips (crisps) and biscuits. Refrain from drinking too much fruit juice as the acid in the fruit erodes tooth enamel. Steer clear of hidden sugars that in many foods we think of as savoury, such as tomato ketchup. (West Indian children have splendid teeth as a general rule, and this could be down to the fact that they tend to chew on raw sugar cane as their available sweet food as opposed to the refined sugars available to the developed world. Complex sugar behaves very differently to refined sugar on the tissues in the body.)

Chewing is invaluable in gum health, which means that raw vegetables, *al dente* cooking and fibrous foods are all good for your gums.

LIFESTYLE

Please follow these simple rules:

- Avoid sugars wherever possible and clean your teeth after sweet meals. Chewing sugar-free gum may have some benefit if teeth and gum brushing is not easy to do.
- Ensure you chew your food well, as the repeated pressure on the jaw bones helps to maintain jaw-bone density. Your diet must include chewable foods as much as possible.
- Ideally, clean your teeth morning and evening – after breakfast and just before bed.
- Ask your dentist to show you the ideal technique for tooth cleaning.

DENTAL FILLINGS

Most of the chapters in this book talk about the potential damage caused by heavy metals. The largest exposure to metals such as mercury and cadmium comes from dental fillings and root canal treatments. These metals are known to be highly toxic, and mercury in particular is banned from use in any readily available cosmetic ointment or foodstuff. The authorities will not let mercury touch our skin or be ingested and yet seem to have little concern about putting mercury in our mouths from an early age.

Not all authorities have such a blinkered, commercial view. Norway became the first country to ban amalgam fillings in April 2008 and was shortly followed by Denmark and Sweden. On 11 July 2012, the European Commission contracted an environmental expert group, the BIO Intelligence Service, to prepare a report which has been entitled 'Study on the Potential for Reducing Mercury Pollution from Dental Amalgam and Batteries'. The recommendations are to ban dental mercury by 2018 from all 27 European States.

Mercury has clear connections, as do many other heavy metals, to neurodegenerative and arterial disease, autoimmune disorders, chronic fatigue syndrome and reduced immune function.

One concern is that the alternative fillings, known as resin composites, last about half as long as metal fillings, although that seems to be improving. We need to keep a close eye on whether chemicals (for example, bisphenol A) within these composites may be equally toxic.

The need for dental hygiene cannot be overemphasized in order to avoid the need to have any foreign material put in the mouth.

It is important to get the bristles of your brush into the gaps between the teeth. Electric teeth brushes, which do a good job on the surface of the teeth and at the top of the tooth where they meet the gum, also need to penetrate through the gap between the teeth.

- Floss regularly with wooden dental sticks, 'tipee' brushes or dental cord. Plaque is a bacteria-filled, sticky substance; when hardened, it is called tartar and is difficult to remove from the enamel.
- Do not smoke. This dries the mouth, interferes with immunity and provides high levels of free radicals that directly damage the gums.

SUPPLEMENTATION

A wealth of research has shown that glutathione and other antioxidants treat and protect against periodontal disease. Obtain a glutathione spray or open a capsule and place the contents under your tongue. Force the saliva formed in response to this through the teeth like a mouthwash.

Mouthwashes themselves may do more harm than good as they kill off a lot of protective bacteria. Glutathione and soluble antioxidants such as selenium (dissolved in water and used as a mouthwash two or three times a day) will have a beneficial effect as they neutralize free radicals and encourage white blood cell response.

EYES AND VISION

The eye is one of the more amazing designs of nature. Given the complexity of its delicate features, it is surprising that not more things go wrong with it. Unfortunately, the more we age, the more you will have exposed your eyes to environmental toxins, so the greater the risk that something will go wrong. The result is that the eye is subject to a few age-related conditions.

Cataract

As we age, the lens of the eye, which has no blood supply of its own and so takes oxygen directly from the atmosphere, begins to cloud over, creating cataracts. Approximately 50 per cent of people over the age of 65 struggle with some level of symptoms of cataract: foggy vision, scattering of sunlight or car headlights, perhaps blurred vision and, if the cataracts are not treated, obstructed blindness.

Diabetes and malnutrition can lead to earlier development of cataracts, as can infection. Once the problem has reached a critical point, your doctor will offer you surgery. That attitude may change and operations may be offered at an earlier stage, as we become more confident about lens replacement, which is now being performed to help people avoid the use of spectacles.

How you can help deal with cataracts

NUTRITION

There is some evidence that milk sugars such as lactose and galactose encourage cataract formation. There is certainly evidence that galactose causes an acceleration of cell ageing (senescence). Diabetics have an increased risk of 'sugar cataracts' and should avoid dairy produce, as should anyone with a suspected or known intolerance showing elsewhere such as bloating, nausea or diarrhoea.

Antioxidants have been shown to help slow down the onset of cataracts, so eat plenty of fruit and vegetables, particularly if you have cataracts in the family as you may be genetically predisposed to getting them.

SUPPLEMENTATION

There are few conventional studies into natural treatments for cataracts. However, the use of the amino acid N-acetylcarnosine as eye drops, with a combination of some of the supplements below, may be of benefit.[11] Many of these will appear in combination supplements aimed at eye health. I do not give specific dosages as these may vary in such combinations. Follow instructions on the label and take the maximum dose recommended.

Vitamins
- Vitamin B2 – riboflavin
- Vitamin C
- Vitamin E

Minerals
- Zinc
- Selenium

Amino acids
- N-acetyl cysteine (NAC)
- Taurine – protects against sugar cataracts

Other nutrients
- Quercetin

Dry eyes, conjunctivitis and blepharitis

As we age, the lacrimal glands that make tears lose function. The result is 'dry eye', which tends to precede the inflammatory conditions blephari-tis (the inflammation of the blephora – the eyelid) and conjunctivitis (the inflammation of the conjunctiva, the mucus membrane that lines the inner eyelid and attaches to the periphery of the eyeball).

Blepharitis can be divided into two different types. Anterior blephari-tis is the inflammation of the area where the eyelashes are attached to the eyelid; whereas posterior blepharitis describes inflammation deeper within the eyelid in the meibomiam glands. These secrete an oily film that coats our tears, stopping them from evaporating and from easily spilling over the eyelids. For the sake of being thorough, I should mention goblet cells, also found in the eyelids, which produce mucin, a mucous layer that lies directly over the cornea (lens) and which encourages the tears to spread across the whole eyeball.

Infection or toxic inflammation of the conjunctiva worsens as we age, as the lacrimal glands secrete fewer tears. The delicate membranes of the con-junctiva are then exposed to toxins, pollutants and bacteria, which causes conjunctivitis.

Conventional treatment

An optician or an eye doctor will recommend that you use commercially developed compounds to help remove frequently found waxy deposits that block the gland ducts in the eyelids. They may also recommend topical antibiotics, and sometimes steroids. Conventional treatments are not par-ticularly harmful although long-term use of antibiotic or steroid drops can lead to bowel flora disturbance as your tears will drain via your nose into your throat where you swallow them. Although the amounts of steroid that reach your stomach are very small, they can cause a problem.

How you can help avoid dry eye and infections

NATUROPATHY

- *Euphrasia eyedrops* – use at the dose recommended on the bottle.
- *Vitamins C and A, and colloidal silver* – if the eyedrops above do not work, make up a solution using the following ingredients in approximately 20 ml of once-boiled, cooled water:
  - *Vitamin C*: 1 ml of concentration 150 mg/ml
  - *Vitamin A*: 1 ml of 5,000iu/ml
  - *Colloidal silver*: 4 parts per million, 2 drops

Apply this solution as drops or by blinking into an eye bath three to four times daily, until you notice an improvement. After that, reduce frequency until the problem has cleared completely for three to four days.

SUPPLEMENTATION
• *Alpha lipoic acid* – this is very well researched in diabetes where eye issues are common.

Glaucoma

Glaucoma is an increase in pressure within the eye. There are two types: acute (closed angle) glaucoma and chronic (open angle) glaucoma. Acute glaucoma generally presents with a severe pulsating pain in the eye, blurred vision and often nausea or vomiting. The pupil dilates and fixes and does not respond to light. *This is an emergency and you need to get into hospital rapidly to save your sight.*

Chronic glaucoma may show no symptoms for many years and often is noticed as a gradual loss of peripheral vision. There is a genetic link, so if anyone in your family has been affected, have regular eye checks after the age of 40.

Standard treatment utilizes drops do not cure glaucoma, but reduce the pressure in the eye. Daily use of these drops therefore is a long-term requirement and generally prevents the risk of blindness.

How you can help reduce glaucoma
NUTRITION
There are many studies that relate free-radical activity or oxidative stress to glaucoma.[12]

NATUROPATHIC TREATMENTS
The use of various antioxidants has been shown to reduce glaucoma, and high fruit and vegetable intake is likely to be protective, if not therapeutic.

Some studies suggest that food sensitivity or intolerance, allergies or sensitivity to chemicals such as monosodium glutamate (MSG) may cause chronic glaucoma, in which case you may need to avoid other chemicals, too.

EXERCISE
Brisk walking (100 steps per minute for 40 minutes) or more intensive aerobic exercise may prevent worsening of glaucoma.[13]

SUPPLEMENTATION
The following supplements have been found to be useful. Many of these will appear in combination supplements aimed at eye health. I do not give specific dosages as these may vary in such combinations. Follow instructions on the label and take the maximum dose recommended.

Vitamins
• Vitamin C

Minerals
• Magnesium

Essential fatty acids
• Omega-3

Amino acids
• Taurine

Other natural supplements
• Gingko biloba
• Coleus – an Ayurvedic medicine
• Alpha lipoic acid

Macular degeneration (MD)

The macula, at the centre of the retina at the back of the eye, is a conglomeration of rods and cones – the nervous system's receptors for light – and is responsible for fine vision. Age-related macular degeneration (AMD) is mostly a condition where the macula area is damaged, usually by decreased blood supply through the ageing of arteries, arteriosclerosis, diabetes or high blood pressure. There are two types of AMD: dry AMD and wet AMD.

Dry AMD, the most common form, occurs in about 90 per cent of those with the condition. Yellow material called 'drusen products' form in the retina, although we do not yet really know why. The most likely explanation is reduced blood flow, which reduces the oxygen levels to the back of the eye and encourages free-radical (oxidative) damage to occur. Dry AMD may have very few symptoms in the early stages, but as the disease progresses, you will experience blurred vision and things may not appear as bright as they used to be. You will need more light for reading or visual control of delicate finger manoeuvres. As the condition gets worse, people come to rely more on peripheral vision, turning their heads to look at things from a side angle.

In wet AMD, abnormal blood vessels develop behind the retina and under the macula. Ten per cent of people with the dry form will go on to develop the wet form. These new blood vessels probably form in an attempt to increase failing blood flow, but tend to be fragile and leak blood. This causes the macula to swell and puts pressure on the nerves, causing irreparable damage.

Treatment options

Injections
In wet AMD, abnormally high levels of a compound known as vascular endothelial growth factor (VEGF) is found in the eyes. This substance promotes the growth of new abnormal blood vessels. Anti-VEGF injection therapy blocks this. You may need frequent and repeated injections, possibly monthly.

Laser therapy with or without photodynamic therapy
A drug called verteporfin is injected into a vein in the arm. The drug travels to new, abnormal blood vessels and highlights those in the eye. A laser beam is then shone into the eye to activate this drug and destroy the new blood vessels in the hope of slowing the rate of vision loss. The procedure takes about 20 minutes.

It is extremely important to have any visual deterioration examined by a specialist as soon as you notice it. *Do not delay* – an earlier diagnosis leads to earlier treatment and improved prognosis.

How you can help against AMD
NUTRITION
Aim for a low-fat, low-sugar diet full of vegetables to provide antioxidant benefit and encourage improved blood vasculature. Cherries and blueberries (bilberries) contain anthocyanidins, antioxidants that are increasingly thought to help in the prevention of AMD.[14]

SUPPLEMENTS
Vitamins
- Vitamin A and beta carotene
- Vitamin C
- Vitamin E

Minerals
- Selenium – 200 mcg taken daily.
- Zinc – 10 mg taken three times a day.

Amino acids
- Taurine

Other natural supplements
Specially trained, medically qualified practitioners can offer intravenous (IV) infusions of some of the supplements below, possibly at frequent dosages. There are no longer-term or large studies to attest to the efficacy of IV administration, but I believe in prescribing IV treatment sooner rather than later for this condition, as do many other centres.
- Lutein
- Zeaxanthin
- Anthocyanadins
- Ginkgo biloba

A special mention should be made of Melatonin. Either form of AMD seem to benefit from Melatonin, the naturally produced sleep hormone, and it appears more affective than current injection treatments which are the gold standard.[15] Specially trained, medically qualified practitioners can offer intravenous infusions of some of the above nutrients possibly at frequent dosages. No long-term or large studies have been published, but many, many centres offer this and it is one of those conditions that I prescribe IV treatment for sooner than later.

THE SKIN

The skin is a multifunctional organ:
- It encases, waterproofs and insulates the tissues and organs of the body.
- It acts as an organ of elimination (sweat has a similar composition to urine).
- It provides sensory information through nerves.
- It protects against infection.
- It helps control body temperature.
- It protects us from the damaging rays of the sun and environmental toxins.

The skin is constantly exposed to the environment, and its good health depends upon good nutrition and hygiene. A failure in the function of the skin leads to disease or dysfunction of the body. The skin may be the first organ to show signs of underlying internal problems.

The structure of the skin

The outermost layer of the skin is the epidermis. The epidermis becomes thicker toward the surface as a protein called keratin is laid in and between the cells. This keratinized layer offers the greatest protection from the elements, including making the skin waterproof. Below the keratinized layer lies the dermis. This is made up of many different tissues, but predominantly protein chains known as collagen and elastin. These work as a

---

LOOKING AFTER YOUR SKIN

You can slow down and possibly reverse skin changes by:
- exposing yourself to adequate and safe levels of sunshine;
- avoiding refined sugars;
- avoiding obesity;
- not smoking;
- avoiding toxins through regular showering or bathing;
- sweating often through exercise and ensuring that you bathe or shower off the sweat before the toxins have a chance to be reabsorbed;
- using saunas as often as possible.

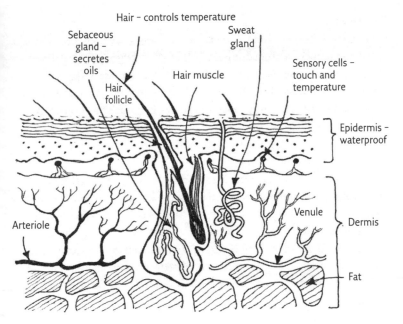

Figure 20: **The skin**

mesh, promoting elasticity to keep the skin as firm and springy as possible.

The skin contains two types of gland: the sweat glands that help keep us cool through the evaporation of sweat, and the sebaceous glands that produce sebum-containing moisturizing oils and immune-defence compounds called immunoglobulins.

Certain cells in the skin known as melanocytes contain a chemical called melanin, which darkens when absorbing what would otherwise be harmful rays of the sun, in particular ultraviolet light. The more melanocytes there are, the darker the skin and the better the protection.

What causes the skin to age?

As our skin ages, it becomes thinner and less elastic, causing wrinkles. We might notice changes in patches of skin colour, including conglomeration of melanocytes leading to 'age spots' (also known misleadingly as liver spots), and we may experience a loss of function, including reduced sensation or dryness, because we are not producing enough sebum, our skin's natural moisturizer. Inflammation, arterial dysfunction, nutritional deficiencies and toxins all contribute to this ageing process.

Inflammation

Environmental toxins and toxic organisms constantly bombard the skin, as do damaging rays from sunlight. All of these trigger an inflammatory response, which is a sign that the skin is trying to heal itself. However, if the inflammation persists, the cell wall becomes damaged and there is a breakdown of proteins and other structural molecules, so eventually the signs of ageing appear.

Capillary dysfunction

Chapter 6 describes why our arteries clog and close up. When this happens, the necessary oxygen and nutrients do not reach the skin, which has very small capillaries as its main supply route. These small vessels are particularly exposed to radiation damage from the sun and therefore tend to diminish in patency and function more quickly than the capillaries deeper inside the body. A loss of nutrients, particularly essential fatty acids and proteins, leads to skin wrinkling and to thinning at a faster rate.

Nutritional deficiencies

A loss of nutrition through arterial blockage and deteriorating absorption from the gut is highly visible in the skin. I list later a variety of essential vitamins, minerals and nutrients that will be of benefit.

Toxins

We are back to free radicals. These positively charged molecules caused by a variety of toxins, natural waste products, stress and poor diet damage all parts of the body. When settled into the skin, they interfere particularly with the formation and maintenance of collagen and elastin, leading to the changes associated with ageing.

How you can help your skin

LIFESTYLE

Do not smoke. Smokers take in more toxins, not just through the lungs but through smoke contact with the skin that permeates throughout the body. The face is most exposed to cigarette chemicals, and most of us can recognize the more marked lines and wrinkles on the faces of long-term smokers.

Stay out of the sun at its most fierce times of day, between 11 am and 3 pm. However, remember that we need some sun exposure in order for our bodies to manufacture vitamin D. So, instead of constantly covering

THE SUN AND VITAMIN D

More than 50 per cent of the adult population have insufficient levels of vitamin D and 16 per cent have severe deficiency during winter and spring.[16]

up, hiding in the shade and using suncreams, stay in the sun for just less time than it takes for your skin to start reacting to the UV light. In some skin types, this may be as little as ten minutes in strong sunlight, whereas darker skin may be able to expose itself all day. We need to establish our own individual tolerance and then expose the skin to direct sunlight for our personal safety timeframe. After that, the use of suncream, protective clothing or staying in the shade is, of course, important to avoid the risk of developing skin cancers.

You can read about our different skin shades on scales as broad as 1–16,[17] but while this may be useful to dermatologists or cosmetic skin specialists, it is perhaps a little too detailed for easy use. Basic trial and error can indicate how long you should be exposed to the sun and be safe.

Alternatively, invest in a UV exposure wristband suitable for your skin type. This will change colour to warn you before you have too much sun exposure.

NUTRITION

Adjust your diet and exercise more to lose some weight if necessary. Those with more subcutaneous fat will have toxins closer to the surface of the skin where fat-soluble toxins lie. Sun rays potentially activate chemical changes in these toxins and trigger inflammatory responses. Higher fat levels under the skin also lead to an increase in surface temperature encouraging sugar 'caramelization', which influences arterial and lymph flow to and from tissue, in those of us who eat more sugars.

Stay hydrated. The keratonized outer epithelial layer of the skin holds water in as much as it keeps it out. Regardless of the lotions and potions you may consider using, you have to ensure good hydration from within, so aim to drink 1.5 litres (3 pints) of water per day.

Ensure you have a good protein intake and an adequate supply of essential fatty acids. These are as important as the fruit and vegetables that provide the high levels of antioxidants needed to protect against free radicals.

Avoid refined sugars and fats as much as possible if you wish to keep your skin healthy.

Dr Sharma's Programmes

Preferably, supplementation to promote healthy skin should start before signs of skin ageing occur, but you will see benefits at any stage. You should be able to find the following range of supplements in combination rather than having to take a plethora of different ones.

Dr Sharma's Maintenance Programme

In order to maintain the health of your skin, which should be a vital part of your anti-ageing regime, take the following.

MINERALS

- *Zinc* – this has an anti-inflammatory effect, and zinc deficiency is associated with faulty collagen production and failure to maintain smooth skin.[18]
- *Silicon* – this is found in wholegrains, vegetables and fruit. Supplementation with silicon improves elasticity of the skin and reduces rough texture.
- *Iron* – this plays an important role in hair follicle health.

VITAMINS

- *Vitamin C* – this has an antioxidant effect and is reported to decrease the appearance of wrinkles.[19]
- *Vitamin E* – protects against sunburn and UV light damage, especially in combination with carotenoids.[20]
- *Carotenoids* – particularly lutein, zeaxanthin and astaxanthin.

ESSENTIAL FATTY ACIDS

- *Omega-3 and -6* – Take a supplement with a ratio of 1:4 omega-3 to omega-6.

AMINO ACIDS

- *Hyaluronic acid (HA)* – strictly speaking, this is not a pure amino acid, as it is combined with natural sugars. It attaches to collagens and elastin to form cartilage, but also holds water in the skin, helps wounds to heal more quickly and may help smooth out wrinkles. It is involved in the health of hair follicles, gives structure and plumpness to the lips and is found surrounding most cells, acting as a matrix in which many of the body's structural proteins sit.

OTHER NUTRIENTS
- *Resveratrol* – this is found in red grape skin, red wine, chocolate and many berries

Dr Sharma's Advanced Programme
If you have damaged skin, take the following supplements:

- *N-acetyl glucosamine* – this is one of the building blocks for hyaluronic acid. Taken orally, it may enhance HA production at a faster rate.
- *Collagen* – this protein complex makes up 95 per cent of the more superficial layers of the skin. A lack of collagen leads to the wrinkling, thinning and skin dysfunction associated with ageing. Many cosmetics contain collagen, but as these are large molecules, skin penetration is neither easy nor likely. Taking collagen orally seems to work, although it is essential that it is taken in a hydrolized form as this is more likely to bypass the digestive processes.
- *Grape seed extract* – this supports collagen production, has a powerful antioxidant effect and may have a direct antibacterial action.

The use of cosmetics
To achieve healthy and younger-looking skin, avoid skin damage (such as as a result of sunburn, smoking and exposure to chemicals) and maintain the underlying structure of your skin through good nutrition and appropriate supplementation.

Cosmetics are effective only in the short term. No cosmetic on the market appears to be designed to offer a long-term benefit. I have no major objections to the use of cosmetics, and indeed the phrase 'look good, feel good' reflects the importance of a person's psychological state on their health as a whole. However, I do have some concerns.

Antiperspirants block the pores located directly beneath the sweat glands in the armpits. This is one of the body's most important methods of detoxifying and elimination. Moreover, antioxidants have been linked with causing some forms of cancer.[21]

Ointments and creams may block pores, reducing detoxification capability and also interfering with the natural function of the sebum, which the skin depends upon for moisture and protection.

Rehydrating or anti-wrinkle creams hold water in the superficial layers of the skin and may 'teach' the body that further moisturizing is not necessary.

When you stop using the cosmetic, the body may take a while to rehydrate the area naturally as local reflexes will have been suppressed, closing off blood vessels and possibly sebum production. The same principle applies to lip balms. These easily become addictive, and it may take several weeks (and a period of sore lips) to wean yourself off them.

Rather than using chemically enhanced creams, switch to those that are made using natural ingredients. While these will still have the potential to damage your skin reflexes and hydration, their lack of chemical ingredients minimizes that risk. Your body has already evolved to manufacture enzymes that break down natural products, whereas it struggles with chemicals. There is plenty of evidence to suggest that aloe vera and calendula can repair damaged skin, and that it is, arguably, more effective than any pharmaceutical-grade ointments, which tend to be based on antibiotics or steroids.

Cancer of the skin

There are three main forms of skin cancer:
- Basal cell carcinoma (BCC), also known as a rodent ulcer
- Squamous cell carcinoma (SCC)
- Melanoma

Basal cell (BCC) and squamous cell carcinoma (SCC) are named after the cell from which the cancer initially developed. BCC and SCC are less dangerous than melanoma because BCC spreads only locally and SCC is slower growing and only rarely spreads through the body. Both also respond well to chemotherapy and radiotherapy. Melanoma is the most aggressive form of skin cancer, but also the most rare. It can spread to other parts of the body and is treatable only if it is caught early – which is why it is imperative that you see your doctor if you have any cause to suspect you may have skin cancer of any kind. Go to your doctor if you have:
- any lesion such as a mole or freckle that grows;
- any lesion that changes colour or has different colours within it;
- a persistently itchy or painful lesion that lasts more than 2–3 weeks;
- a lesion that bleeds;
- any lesion that recurs;
- any lesion that has an associated swollen lymph gland.

Basal cell carcinoma (BCC)
Also known as rodent ulcer, BCC develops from the innermost layer of the skin, tends to be slow growing and does not spread. A rodent ulcer looks like a rough or scaly bump, or a small ulcer. These ulcers generally occur on parts of the skin exposed to the sun and are the most common lesions found where skin meets membrane (such at at the corners of the eye or mouth). The ulcers are flesh-coloured, painless lesions that rarely grow beyond 1 cm (½ in) in diameter before you notice and deal with them.

Squamous cell carcinoma (SCC)
SCC usually arises as a result of skin damage from heat, ultraviolet light, chronic infection or compromised blood flow such as in association with arteriosclerosis or venous ulceration. This tumour invades local tissues, ulcerates easily and appears as a friable lesion that bleeds easily. SCC can metastasize (spread) and may settle in the lymph glands and other parts of the body.

Melanoma
Malignant melanoma, more commonly known simply as melanoma, is a cancer that is initiated in the melanin-containing cells in the lower layer of the skin. It is characterized by a brown or black mole-like lesion. However, lesions are not always the same to look at and can, very rarely, be pale and quite unnoticeable.

Individuals who have many moles have no greater risk of any mole becoming a melanoma – they just have more to keep an eye on.

A malignant melanoma may remain localized for a few months, but if left unattended, it will generally spread and grow rapidly in other parts of the body. Melanomas are occasionally spotted in routine eye examinations as they can form in the retina, but, like most internal cancers, they may not show symptoms until late in the day when they have already spread.

Investigations

You will need your doctor to investigate any lesions that look suspicious. He or she will organize a biopsy and then, if necessary, for you to have the lesion removed. At the time of writing, we do not yet have a means to identify dangerous melanoma other than under a microscope, so there is presently no way to avoid having suspicious lesions removed.

Blood tests are not in mainstream use, but please review the section on cancer in Chapter 9 and particularly the predictive potential of the gene expression tests. I think we are not too far away from having the ability to screen and test for melanoma and other cancers through blood tests, well before we spot them by looking at our bodies, or with scanners.[22]

Meanwhile, use the Internet to find a melanoma screening clinic in your area. Find one that will provide expert examination of suspicious moles and take photographs of your skin that you can compare at future appointments – high-definition cameras are essential.

Treatment options for skin cancers

For non-melanoma skin cancer you will first receive topical anti-cancer drugs. However, if these are not effective, your doctor will probably recommend that you have surgery to remove the lesion.

There have been recent exciting studies on the potential of solasodine glycoside extract from a plant called Devil's apple (*Solanum linnaeanum*), a nightshade plant related to the aubergine (eggplant).[23] Available as topical Curaderm cream, I suggest that you try this first in treatment of non-melanoma skin cancers.

With regard to melanoma, keep an eye out for good news about ongoing research to produce a vaccine that triggers an effective body response to attack this dangerous disease.[24]

There are also emerging immunotherapeutic regimes that may offer treatment even in late stages of the disease, but only to selected and specific individuals. Much more work is ongoing in this area.[25]

References

Introduction

1 Source: Permission gratefully received from Dr Damien Downing, President of the British Society of Ecological Medicine, 2012

2 Viña, J, Borrás, C, Miquel, J, *International Union of Biochemistry and Molecular Biology*, Apr–May, 59 (4–5): 249–54, 2007

3 Terman, A, Redox Rep, vol 6 (1): 15–26, 2001

4 Aubrey D N J, de Grey, R G Landes Company, Austin, Texas, USA, Copyright © 1999

5 Lippman, Dr Richard, *Stay 40: Without Diet or Exercise*, Outskirts Press Inc, Denver, Colorado, 2008

Chapter 1

1 Jakubowicz, D, *et al*, *Steroids*, vol 77, issues 8–9, pp887-889, July 2012

2 Chan, June M, *et al*, *Cancer Causes Control*, August, 20(6): 835–846, 2009; and *Cancer Epidemiology, Biomarkers and Prevention*, a journal of the American Association for Cancer Research, 2012

3 Stolarz-Skrzypek, *et al*, *JAMA*, 305 (17): 1777–17852, 2012

4 Gaziano, J Michael, MD, MPH, *et al*, *Multivitamins in the Prevention of Cancer in Men: The Physicians' Health Study II Randomized Controlled Trial*, *JAMA*, 308 (18): 1871–1880. doi:10.1001/jama.2012.14641, 2012

5 Bjelakovic, G, *et al*, *JAMA*, 297(8): 842–57, 28 February 2007

Chapter 2

1 http://www.hsph.harvard.edu/nutritionsource/what-should-you-eat/pyramid-full-story/index.html#intro)

2 www.who.int/nutrition/databases/en/

3 www.stewartnutrition.co.uk

4 Pearce, S H S, Cheetham, T D, *Diagnosis and management of vitamin D deficiency*, British Journal of Nutrition, 340: b5664, 2010

5 Chris Irvine, *The Daily Telegraph*, UK, 7 November 2009

6 Jackson, *et al*, *British Journal of Nutrition*, vol 133, no 5: 1557S-1559S, 1 May 2003

7 Community Nutrition Mapping Project, 29 July 2009

8 Werbach, M R, MD, *Alternative Medicine Review*, 5(2): 93–108, 2000

9 Niloofar, PhD, and Bauchwa, MD, *American Journal of Psychiatry*, 160 (2): 221–36, 2003; National Health Service, 2009

10 www.cdc.gov/cfs/general/index.html

11 Allard, *et al*, Public Library of Science, PLoS One 3(9): e3211. doi:10.1371/journal.pone.0003211

12 Vallardy and Hellerstein, *American Journal of Clinical Nutrition*, 86 (1): 7–13), July 2007

13 Vallardy and Hellerstein, *American Journal of Clinical Nutrition*, 86 (1): 7–13), July 2007

14 Bishop and Guarente, *Nature* journal, 447, 545–549, May 2007

15 Poehlman, E T, *et al*, Gerontology A Biol Sci Med Sci, 56: 45–54, 2001

16 Asnawi, Abdullah, *et al*, *International Journal of Epidemiology*, August 2011

17 Calle, E, *et al*, *NEJM*, 348; 625–38, 2003

18 Gill, T, Cancer Detect Prev, 27: 415–21, 2003

19 Van den Brandt, Piet A, *American Journal of Clinical Nutrition*, vol 94, no 3, September 2011

20 Arch Intern Med, 172 (7): 555–563, 2012 doi:10.1001/archinternmed.2011.2287 http://archinte.ama-assn.org/cgi/content/abstract/archinternmed.2011.2287

21 *Homeopathy* journal, 96 (3): 175–82, July 2007

22 Grandjean A C, *Journal of the American College of Nutrition*, vol 19, no 5: 591–600, October 2000

23 Wang J, Chemosphere, 75 (8): 1119–27; May 2009; Epub 8 February 2009

24 http://edugreen.teri.res.in/explore/water/health.htm

25 Janna, H, Environ Sci Technol, 45 (9): 3858–3864, 2011

26 William L. Wolcott and Trish Fahey, *The Metabolic Typing Diet*, Doubleday, January 2000

27 D'Adamo, Dr Peter, *Eat Right 4 Your Type*, G P Putnam's Sons, New York, 1996

28 Trichopoulou and Vasopoulou, *British Journal of Nutrition*, 84, suppl 2, S205±S20), 2008

29 Bohn, H L, McNeal, B L, and O'Connor, G A, *Soil Chemistry*, pp5–13; 68–80, 87–90, 116–120, Wiley-Interscience, New York, 1985

30 Taiz, Lincoln, and Zeiger, Eduardo, *Plant Physiology* (edition 5), http://5e.plantphys.net/index.php, 2010

31 Cohen, Suzy, RPh, *Drug Muggers*, Roedale Inc, New York, 2011

32 Gaby, Alan R, MD, *Alternative Medicine Review*, vol 7, no 5, 2002

33 Sharma, Dr R, *The Element Family Encyclopedia of Heath*, Thorsons/Element, UK, 1998

34 Li, J, *et al*, Breast cancer res, 13: 49, 2011

35 Kasperzyk, J, Journal Nat Canc Int, 103: 876–84, 2011

36 Santos, C, *et al*, J Alzh Dis, 2010

37 Lawrence, B, Riggs, Heinz W, Inc, *Dietary Calcium Intake and Rates of Bone Loss in Women*, 0021-9738/87/10/0979/04, vol 80: 979-982, October 1987 http://www.ncbi.nlm.nih.gov/pmc/articles/PMC442335/pdf/jcinvest00094-0065.pdf

38 Eaton, Russell, *The Milk Imperative*, DeliveredOnline.com, 2006

39 Butler, Dr Justine, *White Lies*, http://www.vegetarian.org.uk/campaigns/whitelies/wlreport01.shtml

40 Lampe, J W, *Journal of the American College of Nutrition*, 30 (5 suppl 1): 464S–70S, October 2011; Plant, Professor Jane, *Your Life in Your Hands*, Virgin Books Ltd, London, 2006

41 Smith, Justin, *$29 Billion Reasons to Lie About Cholesterol* (www.29billion.com), Matador, UK, 2009

42 Han, L, Am J Alz, 25: 367–71, 2010

43 http://www.exploreenumbers.co.uk/How-Safe-are-E-Numbers.html

44 Stebbing, J, *Postgraduate Medical Journal*, 73:863 606 doi:10.1136/pgmj.73.863.606-b), September 1997

Chapter 3

1 Lynn, *et al*, Arch Int Med, 168{2} 154–58, 2008

2 Calvert J W, *et al*. Int J Vasc Med, 2012: 396369, 2012

3 Barres, R, *et al*, *Cell Metabolism*, vol 15, issue 3, 405-411, 7 March 2012

4 Ben-Ari, Elia, The National Cancer Institute, 2011

5 Tymchuk, Christopher N, *et al*, *Journal of Urology*, vol 166, issue 3, September 2001

6 Singh, M A F, *Journal of Gerontology: Medical Sciences*, vol 57A, no 5: M262–M282), 2002

7 I-Min, Lee, and Jr, Ralph S, *Am J Epidemiol*, 151: 293–9, 2000

8 Bussle, J B, *et al*. Am J Prev Med, 2009

10 Jakicic, J M, *JAMA*, 290(10): 1323–1330. doi:10.1001/jama.290.10.1323, 2003

11 Buchfuhrer, M J, *Journal of Applied Physiology*, vol 55 no 5 1558–1564, November 1983

12 Pupka, A, *Medicina Sportiva*, vol 12, no 4, December 2008

13 Wen, C P, *The Lancet*, 378:1244–1253, 2011

Chapter 4

1 Cutolo, M, Sulli, A, Straub, R H, Auto Immune Rev, 11 (6–7), May 2012

2 Pimentel, David, Jagric Environ Ethos, 8 (17–29), 1995

3 Jacobs, Marjorie (revised), http://healthliteracy.worlded.org/docs/tobacco/Unit4/1whats_in.html, 1997

4 Beever R, *Canadian Family Physician*, vol 55 (7): 691–6, July 2009

Chapter 5

1 Cohen, Suzy, RPh, *Drug Muggers,* Roedale Inc, New York, 2011

2 Trombetti, A, *et al*, Osteoporos Int, 2002 Sep; 13(9): 731–7, September 2002

3 Russo, Allison, MPH, Holmquist, Laurel, MA, and Elixhauser, Anne, PhD, US Hospitalizations Involving Osteoporosis and Injury, 2006 and 2009

4 Patrick Haentjens, MD, PhD, *et al, Annals of Internal Medicine*, vol 152, no 6: 380-390, 16 March 2010

5 Kanis, *et al*, Osteoporos Int, 18 {8}: 1033–46, August 2007

6 Melton, *et al*, Osteoporos Int, 9 {1}: 29–37, 1999

7 Sornay-Rendu, E J, *Journal of Bone and Mineral Research*, 20(10): 1813–9, October 2005/Epub 20 June 2005; and Ross, Dr Philip D, and Knowlton, William, *Journal of Bone and Mineral Research*, vol 13, issue 2, pp297–302, February 1998

8 Taal, Maarten W, Nephrol Dial Transplant, 14 (8): 1917–1921, 1999

9 Nelson, *et al*, 2001

10 Larkin, Ann, http://www.dimond3.org/Dublin%202006/2%20DEXA%20QA%20Training%20for%20Physicists/7%20Accuracy%20of%20DEXA%20&%20other%20methods.pdf

11 Lehrer, S, Montazem, A, Ramanathan, L, *et al, Journal of Oral and Maxillofacial Surgery*, vol 67, issue 1, pp159–161, January 2009

12 Cramer, J A, Gold, D T, Silverman, S L, Lewiecki, E M, Osteoporos Int, 18 (8): 1023–31, August 2007

13 Park-Wyllie, Laura Y, *et al, JAMA*, 23 February 2011; Green, Jane, *et al, Oesophageal Cancer, British Medical Journal*, 341: c4444, 2010.

14 Bolland, *et al, British Medical Journal*, 341: c3691, 2010

15 McCullagh, *African Journal of Ecology*, vol 7, issue 1, pp85–90, August 1969

16 Lee, John R, MD, and Hopkins, V, *What Your Doctor May Not Tell You About Menopause*, Warner Books, New York, 1996

17 Grant, Dr Ellen, http://www.npis.info/wddtycancer.htm

18 Wagner, Dr Josh, http://lifehousechiropractic.com/got-milk-the-real-facts-on-milk-consumption-and-osteoporosis/, 2012

18 Prevent disease.com, http://preventdisease.com/news/10/111810_dangers_pasteurization_homogenization.shtml 18 November 2010

19 Weiwen, Jiang, *et al*, *Journal of Leukocyte Biology*, January 2008

Chapter 6

1 Frieden, T R, NEJM.org, 13 September 2011

2 Kendrick, Dr Malcolm, *The Great Cholesterol Con*, John Blake Publishing Ltd, London, 2007

3 Di Renzo, Eur Rev Med Pharmacol Sci, 11(3): 185–92, May–June 2007

4 Ross, Julie A, *Annual Review of Nutrition*, vol 22: 19–34, July 2002

5 Rautiainen, S, *Stroke*, doi 10.1161, 2011

6 Ahluwalia, A, *Hypertension*, 2010

7 Tanaka, K, *Journal of Nutritional Medicine*, 139: 1333–8, 2009

8 Boekholdt, *British Journal of Nutrition*, 96(3): 516–22. 96 516, September 2006

9 Nicolosi, *American Journal of Clinical Nutrition*, vol 70, no 2: 208–212, August 1999

10 Goyal, R, *American Journal of Clinical Nutrition*, 34: 824–9, 1981

11 Micha, R, *Circulation*, June 2010

12 Wu, J, *et al*, *Food Chemistry*, 129: 155–61, 2011

13 Talya Lavi, *Journal of the American College of Cardiology*, 55: 2283–7, 2009

14 Liya, Li, Navindra, P Seeram, *Emerging Trends in Dietary Components for Preventing and Combating Disease*, Chapter 18, pp.323–333, 2012

15 Basaraba, S, *European Heart Journal*, 31: 1616–23, 2010; *Hypertension*, 46:398-405, 2005

16 Wieslander, G, Fabjan, N, *et al*, *Tohoku J Exp Med*, 225(2): 123–30, 2011

17 Naito, Y J, *Cardiovasc Pharmacol*, 54(5): 385–90, November 2009

18 Wofford, M R, Rebholz, C M, *et al*, *European Journal of Clinical Nutrition*, 28 September 2011

19 Guo, Z, Chen, W, *et al*, *Nutr Metab Cardiovasc Dis*, 17 September 2011

20 The Mayo Clinic Staff: http://www.mayoclinic.com/health/alcohol/SC00024

21 Sacco, R L, *et al*, *JAMA*, 281: 5360, 1999

22 Szmitko, Paul E, BSc, and Verma, Subodh, MD, PhD, *Circulation*, 111: e10–e11, 2005

23 Larson, S C, *et al*, *Stroke*, 42: 908–12, 2011

24 Sugiyama, K, *et al*, Arterio Throm Vasc Bio, 2010

25 Brown, C A, *et al*, *Journal of Epidemiology and Community Health*, 47: 171–175, New England, 1993

26 Hospitality Institute of Technology and Management www.hi-tm.com/facts@tips/decaff.html

27 Hodis, H N, Mack, W J, LaBree, L, *et al*, *JAMA*, 273: 1849–1854, 1995; Stephens, N G, *et al*, *The Lancet*, March 23, 1996; 347: 781-786, 23 March 1996; Hemila, H, Kaprio, J, *Age Ageing*, 40(2): 215–220, 2011

28 Wang, L, *Arch Intrn Med*, 168: 459–65, 2008

29 Wang, J, *American Heart Association*, 16 November 2009

30 Zacharski, L R, *JAMA*, 297(6): 603–610, 2007

31 Ahluwalia, N, J NUT 140:812-816, 2010; and J VAS Surg, 51(6): 1498, June 2010

32 Pool, G F, *Atherosclerosis*, 161(2): 395–402, April 2002

33 Kiechl, S, *British Medical Journal*, 314: 793–794, 1997

34 http://www.drcranton.com/chelation/study6.htm

35 Keon, W J, *Canadian Medical Association Journal*, vol 131, 15 September 1984

36 Whitaker, Julian, *The Pros and Cons of Bypass Surgery*, Hay House, London, 2000; Ozner, Dr Michael, *The Great American Heart Hoax*, Benbella Books, Inc, Dallas, Texas, 2008

37 Coupland, Carol, *British Medical Journal*, 343: 4551, 2011

38 Schmidt, M, *et al*, *British Medical Journal*, 343, 2011

39 Gorelick, Philip B, MD, MPH, FACP, Weisman, Steven M, PhD, *Stroke*, 36: 1801–1807, 2005

40 Bhaskaran, K, *British Medical Journal*, 343: d5531, 2011

41 Astrand, 1960

42 Suprko, H R, Am J Cardiol, 88: 260–64, 2001

43 www.arteriograph.hu\english\index\php

44 Coronary Artery Surgery study, 1975–79; Pálinkás, A, *et al*, *European Heart Journal*, 23(20): 1587–95, October 2002

45 Hak, A E, 2002, and Micheli, A, 2007

46 Wilders-Truschnig, M, *Exp Clin Endocrinol Diabetes*, 116(4): 241–5, April 2008; Epub 10 December 2007

Chapter 7

1 Babizhayev, M A, *et al*, Drugs R D, 3(2): 87–103, 2002

2 Millen, *et al*, *Arch Ophthalmol*, 129(4): 481–489, 2011

3 Chiu, C J, *American Journal of Clinical Nutrition*, 86: 180–8, 2007

4 McGwin, 2010; G Jr Arch Otolaryngol Head Neck Surg, 136(5): 488–92, May 2010

5 Alzheimer's Society 2011, published 1 March 2011, http://alzheimers.org.uk/site/scripts/news_article.php?newsID=918

6 Erkinjuntti, Timo, *New England Journal of Medicine*, 337: 1667–74, 1996

7 Croisile, B, Auriacombe S, Etcharry-Bouyx, F, Vercelletto, M, Rev Neurol, Paris, 12 May 2012

8 Alzheimer Association, USA, http://www.alz.org/downloads/facts_figures_2011.pdf, 2011

9 Yasui M, Kihira T, Ota, K, *Neurotoxicology*, 13(3): 593–600, 1992

10 Wirdefeldt, K, *European Journal of Epidemiology*, suppl 1: S1–58, 26 June 2011

11 Willis, Allison W, *American Journal of Epidemiology*, October 2010

12 Wang, A, *et al*, *European Journal of Epidemiology*, 26(7): 547–55, July 2011

13 Dhillon, A S, *Journal of Agromedicine*, 13 1 37–48, 2008

14 Kedar, N, Prasad, PhD, *et al*, *Journal of the American College of Nutrition*, vol 18, no 5: 413–423, 1999

15 Evatt, Marian L, MD. *Archives of Neurology*, vol 68, March 2011

16 do Nascimento, José Luiz M, Indian J Med Res, 128: 373–382, October 2008; Ghoshal, N, *American Journal of Pathology*, 155: 1163–72, 1999

17 Mercola, Dr, http://emf.mercola.com/sites/emf/emf-dangers.aspx

18 Moulder, John, Medical College of Wisconsin, http://large.stanford.edu/publications/crime/references/moulder/moulder.pdf, 2005

19 The International Society for Neurofeedback and Research, www.isnr.org

20 Seshadri, Sudha, MD, New England Journal of Medicine, 346: 476-483, 2002; hyperlink: http://www.neurology.org/search?author1=K.H.+Masaki&sortspec=date&submit=Submit; Masaki, K H, *Neurology*, vol 54, no 6: 1265–1272, 28 March 2000

21 Fogarty, J, Nolan, G, Department of Community Care, Western Health Board, Gahvay, *Irish Medical Journal*, vol 85, March 1992

22 Riggs, K M, *American Journal of Clinical Nutrition*, vol 63, no 3: 306–314, March 1996

23 Belkacemi, A, Expert Rev Mol Med, 13: e34, 4 November 2011

24 Fiocco, Dr Alexandra, *Neurobiology of Ageing*, 22 August 2011

25 Gelber, R P, J Alzheimer's Dis, 23(4): 607–15, 2011

26 Vieth, Reinhold, *American Journal of Clinical Nutrition*, vol 69, no 5: 842–856, May 1999

27 Sánchez-Barceló, E J, *et al*, Curr Med Chem, 17 19: 2070–95, 2010

28 Galasko, Douglas R, MD, *et al*, *Arch Neurol*, (): 1–6, 2012

29 US National Library of Medicine National Institutes of Health, http://www.ncbi.nlm.nih.gov/pubmed?term=antioxidants%20dementia

30 Goebels, Norbert, MD, Soyka, Michael, MD. *The Journal of Neuropsychiatry and Clinical Neurosciences*, 12: 389–394, 2000

31 www.ecomed.org.uk or, in the USA, visit http://theneuronetwork.com/ Those in Eastern or Central Europe can review Dr Bieber and Miltz's comments on www.dr-bieber.de/englisch/index/html.

32 Geng, J, Dong, J, Ni, H, *et al*, *Ginseng for cognition. Cochrane Database Syst Rev*, 12, CD007769, 2010

33 Hansen, I L, *et al*, *Research Communications in Chemical Pathology and Pharmacology*, 14(4): 729–38, 1976

34 Shults, C W, Arch Neurol, 59(10): 1541–50, October 2002

35 Baskys, Andrius, and Hou, Anthony C, Clin Interv Ageing, 2(3): 327–335, September 2007

36 Ha, Wong and Zhang, 2011

37 Kasture, S, *et al*, Neurotox Res, 15(2):111-22, February 2009; Epub 20 February 2009

38 Katzenschlager, R, *et al*, Parkinson's Disease study group, 2004; J Alt Comp Med, 1: 249–55, 1995; Katzenschlager, R, *et al*, *J Neurol Neurosurg Psychiatry*, 75: 1672–1677, 2004

39 Suravarapu, S, *et al*, Alzheimer Dis Assoc Disord, 20(3): 138–40, July–September 2006

40 Giardino, I, *et al*, *Diabetes*, 47(7): 1114–20, July 1998

41 Fox, Chris, MD, *Journal of the American Geriatrics Society*, vol 59, issue 8, pp1477–1483, August 2011

42 Public citizen, www.worstpills.org

43 Ellul, J, *et al*, *J Neurol Neurosurgery Psychiatry*, 78: 233–9, 2007

44 Treloar, A, *British Journal of Psychiatry*, 197(2): 88–90, August 2010

45 Wadsworth, Emma J K, *Human Psychopharmacology: Clinical and Experimental*, vol 20, issue 8, pp561–572, December 2005

46 Kobayashi, Katsunori, *et al*, http://www.mindandmuscle.net, 4 February 2012

47 Coupland, C, *British Medical* Journal, 343, 2011

48 Steffens, D C, *et al*, *Stroke*, 39: 857–62, 2008

49 Wagstaff, L R, *et al*, *Pharmacotherapy*, 23: 871–80, 2003

50 Bethold, *et al*, Curr Pharm Des, 17(9): 877–93, 2011

51 Adverse events, www.adverseevents.com, 12 March 2012

52 Graff-Radford, N R, Alzheimer's Res Ther, 3(1): 6, 28 February 2011

53 Crizzle, Alexander Michael, MPH*; Newhouse, Ian J, PhD, *Clinical Journal of Sport Medicine*, vol 16, issue 5, pp422–425, September 2006

54 Van Praag, Henriette, *Neurosciences*, vol 32, issue 5, pp283–290, May 2009

55 Ahlskog, J E, et al, Mayo Clin Proc, 86(9): 876-84, September 2011

56 Delp MD, et al. June 15, 2001 *The Journal of Physiology*, 533, 849–859

57 Pattillo, Robin, PhD, RN, *Education*, 35(2): 78, March 2010

58 Christos, G A, *Medical Hypotheses*, 41(5): 435–9, November 1993

59 Pagnoni, G, Cekic, M, *Neurobiological Ageing*, 28(10): 1623–7, October 2007; Epub 25 July 2007

60 Hu, X, *et al*, *Medical Hypotheses*, 77(2): 266–9, August 2011

61 Hyperlink http://apt.rcpsych.org/search?author1=Ola+Junaid&sortspec=date&submit=Submit Ola Junaid
Hyperlink http://apt.rcpsych.org/search?author1=Soumya+Hegde&sortspec=date&submit=Submit Soumya Hegde
Advances in Psychiatric Treatment, 13: 17–23, 2007

62 Craik, F I, Bialystok, E, Freedman, M, *Neurology*, 75(19): 1726–9, 9 November 2010

63 Kamer, Angela R, *Alzheimer's and Dementia*, vol 4, issue 4, pp242–250, July 2008,

64 Hyperlink http://oem.highwire.org/search?author1=E+Cardis&sortspec=date&submit=Submit Cardis, E, *Occupational environmental medicine*, 68(9): 631–640, 2011

65 Epel, Elissa, *Annals of the New York Academy of Sciences*, vol 1172, pp34–53, August 2009

66 Hitt, Emma, PhD, *Medscape Education Clinical Briefs*, 5 October 2011

67 Riemersma-van der Lek, R F, *et al*, *JAMA*, 299: 2642-55, 2008

68 Hanser, S B, Thompson, L W, *Journal of Gerontology*, 49: 265, 1994

69 Guetin, S, *et al*, Encphale, 35: 57–65, 2009

70 Chartier-Harlin, Marie-Christine, *American Journal of Human Genetics*, vol 89, issue 3, pp398–406, 9 September 2011

71 Hughes, John R, MD, PhD, John, E Roy, PhD, *The Journal of Neuropsychiatry and Clinical Neurosciences*, 11: 190–208, 1999

72 de Weerd, A W, Perquin, W V M, Jonkman, E J, Dement Geriate Cogn Disord, 1: 115–118, 1990

Chapter 8

1 Engelmann, Mario, Landgraf, Rainer, Wotjak, Carsten T, *Frontiers in Neuroendocrinology*, vol 25, issues 3–4, pp132–149, September–December 2004

2 Park J K, *Journal of the American Geriatric Society*, 59(5): 944–7, May 2011

3 The Mayo Clinic Staff: http://www.mayoclinic.com/health/growth-hormone/HA00030

4 Hertoghe, Thierry, MD, *The Hormone Handbook*, International Medical Books Publications, USA, 2006

5 Sklar C. Horm Res 2004; 62 suppl 3: 30–4

6 Ditzen, Beate, Schaer, Marcel, Gabriel, Barbara, Bodenmann, Guy, Ehlert, Ulrike, and Heinrichs, Markus, http://www.psychologie.uni-freiburg.de/abteilungen/psychobio/team/publikationen/BiolPsychiatry-CoupleConflict09.pdf, 2008

7 Changxian, Yi, *Annals of the New York Academy of Sciences*, vol 1057, 384–392, December 2005

8 Mills, *et al*, J. Pineal Res 39 {4}: 360–6

9 Sánchez-Barceló, E J, *et al*, Curr Med Chem, 17(19): 2070–95, 2010

10 Pierpaoli, Dr Walter, www.melatoninznse.com

11 Pierpaoli, Dr Walter, *The Melatonin Miracle*, Simon and Schuster, New York, 2010

12 Pearson, *et al*, *Cell Metabolism*, 8 {2}:157–68

13 Hontela, Alice, *Environmental Toxicology and Chemistry*, vol 14, issue 4, pp725–731, April 1995

14 www.iodine4health

15 Androbalance: http://www.androbalance.co.uk/testing-saliva.htm

16 Innes, K E, Selfe, T K, Vishnu, A, *in Maturitas*, 66(2): 135–49, June 2010; Epub 18 February 2010

17 Nedrow, A, Miller, J, Walker, M, Nygren, P, Huffman, L H, Nelson, H D, Arch Intern Med, 166(14): 1453–65, 24 July 2006

18 Zitnanova, I, Rakovan, M, *et al*, *Menopause*, 15 September 2011

19 Labrie, F, *et al*, *J Steroid Biochem Mol Biol*, 99(4–5): 182–8, June 2006; Epub 18 April 2006

20 Morley, *et al*, *Metabolism*, 49, pp1239–1242, 2000; *The Ageing Male*, 2012

21 Wilson, Dr J L, *Adrenal Fatigue: The 21st Century Stress Syndrome*, Smart Publications, Petaluma, California, 2000

22 Medline Plus, www.mlm.nih.gov, 7 July 2011

23 Yanase T, *et al*, *Endocrine Journal*, 43(1): 119–23, 1996

24 Levin, Pamela, RN, http://www.mlo-online.com/
   articles/1207/1207clinical_issues.pdf

Chapter 9

1 Jefferson, et al, Cochrane Acute Respiratory Infections Group,
   17 February 2010

2 Kwok, Roberta, Nature, 473, 436–438, 2011

3 Simpson, R J, Ageing Res Rev, 11(3): 404–20, July 2012

4 Fan, Y, Tang, Y Y, Ma, Y, Posner M I, J Altern Comp Med, 16(2): 151–5,
   February 2010

5 Dhondup, L, Husted, C, Ann N Y Acad Sci, 1172: 115–22, August 2009

6 Hofmann, S G, Grossman, P, Hinton, D E, Clin Psychol Rev, 31(7):
   1126–32, November 2011; Epub 26 July 2011

7 Davidson, Richard J, Psychosomatic Medicine, 65: 564–570, 2003

8 Calder, Phillip C, Journal of Nutrition, vol 136, January 2006

9 Graaf, Matthijs R, Jounal of Clinical Oncology, vol 22, no 12: 2388-2394,
   15 June 2005

10 The International Network of Cholesterol Skeptics, http://www.thincs.
   org/unpublic.UR3.htm

11 Ferlay, J, Annual Oncology, 18(3): 581–592, 2007

12 Mistry, M, Parkin, D M, Ahmad, A, Sasieni, P, Cancer Incidence in the UK:
   Projections to the Year 2030, British Journal of Cancer, vol 105, pp1795–1803,
   2011

13 National Cancer Institute: http://www.cancer.gov, March 2012

14 Orsini, N, Mantzoros, C S, and Wolk, A, British Journal of Cancer,
   98: 1864–1869, 2008

15 Sankpal, U T, Tumour Biology, 22 May 2012

16 Lillberg, K, American Journal of Epidemiology, 157(5): 415–423, 2003

17 Ames, Bruce N, and Wakimoto, Patricia, Nature Reviews Cancer,
   2, 694–704, September 2002

18 American Cancer Society: www.cancer.org/cancer/prostatecancer,
   27 February 2012

19 Clark, L C, et al, British Journal of Urology, vol 81, issue 5, pp730–734,
   May 1998

20 Cancer Active: www.canceractive.com

21 Varsavsky, M, Reyes-García, R, et al, Endocrinological Nutrition,
   18 October 2011

22 Worldwide breast cancer, http://www.worldwidebreastcancer.com/learn/
   breast-cancer-statistics-worldwide/

23 Wise, J, et al, British Medical Journal, 342: d808, 2011

24 Pala, V, International Journal of Cancer, 129(11): 2712–9,
    1 December 2011

25 Chan, Andrew T, and Lippman, Scott M, The Lancet, vol 378, issue 9809,
    pp2051–2052, 17 December 2011

26 Sasieni, PD, British Journal of Cancer, 105(3): 460–5, 2011

27 www.lab4more.de

28 Mohammed, S I, Springfield, S, Das, R, Methods of Molecular Biology,
    863:395–410, 2012

29 Lerner, Michael, Choices in Healing, MIT Press, Cambridge, MA, USA,
    May 1996

30 American Cancer Society. Colorectal Cancer Facts & Figures 2011-2013.
    Atlanta, American Cancer Society, 2011

31 National Cancer Institute, USA 25 Juy 2013 http://www.cancer.
    gov/cancertopics/pdq/screening/colorectal/HealthProfessional/
    Page3#Reference3.5

32 Accuracy of CT colonography for detection of large adenomas and
    cancers. N Engl J Med 359 (12): 1207-17, 2008

33 Epstein, Dr Samuel S, The Politics of Cancer, October 1998

34 The National Cancer Institute, www.draxe.com/mammograms-cause-
    cancer/, 2009

35 Jørgensen, Karsten Juhl, Zahl, Per-Henrik, Gøtzsche, Peter C, British
    Medical Journal, 340: c1241, 2010

36 Gordon, Paula B, MD, Goldenberg, Larry S, MD, Cancer, 76: 626–30, 1995

37 Lehman CD, Lee CI, Loving VA, Portillo MS, Peacock S, Demartini
    WB. 2012. Accuracy and value of breast ultrasound for primary imaging
    evaluation of symptomatic women 30-39 years of age, Am. J. Roentgenol.
    5:1169-77

38 Everson, Tilden C, Be Careful What You Wish For, 1966; Dossey, Larry,
    Spontaneous Regression of Cancer, 1998

39 The National Cancer Institute: http://www.cancer.gov/cam/about_us.html

40 Lynes, Barry, The Healing of Cancer (ISBN 0-919951-44-9); Walker,
    Martin J, Dirty Medicine, Slingshot Publications, London

41 CA: A Cancer Journal for Clinicians, vol 60, issue
    5, pp277–300, September/October 2010

42 Wysong, Dr Randy, http://dr-randy-wysong.wrytestuff.com/swa57770.
    htm

43 Feldman, Allen R, MD, et al, New England Journal of Medicine,
    314: 1226–1232, 8 May 1986

44 Prasad, K N, PhD, Cole, W C, PhD, and Haase, G M, MD, The British

Journal of Radiology, February 2004

45 Cutler, R G, *American Journal of Clinical Nutrition*, vol 53, 373S–379S

46 Greenwald, C, Clifford, K, Milner, J A, *European Journal of Cancer*, vol 37, issue 8, pp948-965, May 2001

47 Bates, 1979; Farlow, 2004

48 Farlow, Christine H, DC: http://www.healthyeatingadvisor.com/9cancer-causingchemicals.html, 2004; Bates, R R, IARC Sci Publ, (25): 93–9, 1979

49 Irwin, Michael, Vedhara, Kavita, *Human Psychoneuroimmunology*, Oxford University Press, Oxford, 2005

50 Kiecolt-Glaser, J K, and Glaser, R, *European Journal of Cancer*, vol 35, issue 11, pp1603–1607, October 1999; Antoni, M H, *Brain Behav Immun*, 17 Suppl 1: S84–91, February 2003

51 Musial, F, *et al*, *Forsch Komplementmed*, 18(4): 192–202. doi: 10.1159/000330714, 2011; Epub 8 August 2011; Hirshberg, Carlyle, and Barasch, Marc Ian, *Remarkable Recovery: What Extraordinary Healings Can Teach Us About Getting Well and Staying Well*, Riverhead Books, Penguin Group, USA, 1995

52 Health Creation: www.healthcreation.co.uk

53 Astin, John A, PhD, *et al*, *Annual of Internal Medicine*, vol 132, no 11: 903–910, 6 June 2000

54 Lab 4 More: www.lab4more.de; Research Genetic Cancer Centre: www.rgcc-genlab.com

55 Is My Cancer Different?: http://www.ismycancerdifferent.com/about/, June 2012

56 Gordon Research Institute: www.gordonresearch.com, 2012; MedPage Today: www.medpagetoday.com, 2012

57 Avemar.Com: http://www.avemar.com/avemar.php

58 http://www.ncbi.nlm.nih.gov/pubmed?term=quercetin percent20cancer)

59 Meng, X L, *et al*, P R Health Sci J, 21(4): 323–8, December 2002

Chapter 10

1 Becher, A, Dent, J, *Ailment Pharmacol Ther*, 33(4): 442–54, February 2011

2 Poulsen, A H, *British Journal of Cancer*, 100(9): 1503, 5 May 2009

3 Saltzman, John R, Russell, Robert M, *The Ageing Gut: Gastroenterology Clinics of North America*, vol 27, issue 2, pp309–324, 1998

4 Mullin, G E, *Nutr Clin Pract*, 25(2): 192–8, April 2010

5 ALCAT Worldwide: www.alcat.com

6 Kan, H, *et al*, *American Journal of Epidemiology*, 1, 167(5): 570–578, 1 March 2008; published online: doi: 10.1093/aje/kwm343, 5 December 2007

7 Yavuz, B B, *Ageing Clin. Exp* res, 20(3): 201–6, June 2008

8 Brasky et al, 2013 http://mynorthwest.com/11/2312013/
   Seattle-researchers-confirm-link-between-fish-oil-and-prostate-cancer

9 de Oliveira, C, *British Medical Journal*, 340: c245, 2010

10 Bastos, M F, Lima, J A, Vieira, P M, Mestnik, M J, Faveri, M, Duarte, P M,
   Oral Diseases, vol 15, issue 1, pp82–87, January 2009

11 nacetylcarnosine.com 2012; http://www.nacetylcarnosine.com/
   published_information_about_can-c.htm
   International Anti Ageing Systems: http://www.antiageingsystems.com/
   search.php?orderby=position&orderway=desc&search_query=Can-c

12 Izzotti, A, Bagnis, A, Sacca, S C, *Mutation Research*, vol 612, issue 2,
   March 2006

13 Johns Hopkins Health Alerts: 23 February 2007 (reviewed June 2011)

14 Winston J. Craig, *Journal of the American Diatetic Association*, vol 9,
   issue 10; 199–204, October 1997

15 *Annals of the New York Academy of Sciences*, Volume 1057; 384-392,
   December 2005

16 Baumann, L, *The Skin Type Solution*, Bantam Dell, New York, 2006

17 Aggett, P J, *Clin Endo metab*, 14(3), August 1985

18 Hyperlink: http://www.ajcn.org/search?author1=Maeve+C+Cosgrove&s
   ortspec=date&submit=Submit Cosgrove, Maeve C, *American Journal of
   Clinical Nutrition,* October 2007

19 Hyperlink: http://www.ajcn.org/search?author1=Wilhelm+Stahl&sortsp
   ec=date&submit=Submit Stahl, Wilhelm, *American Journal of Clinical
   Nutrition*, vol 71, no 3: 795–798, March 2000

20 Darbre, Philippa D, Breast Cancer Res, 11, suppl 3: S5, 2009

21 www.rgcc-genlab.com

22 Cham, B E, Daunter, B, Evans, R A, *Cancer Letters*, 59(3): 183–92 BEC5,
   September 1991

23 Sznol, M, *Semin Oncology*, 39(2): 192–203, April 2012

24 Atallah, E, Flaherty, L, *Current Treatment Options for Oncology*,
   6(3): 185–93, May 2005

Useful Websites

Contact details for Dr Rajendra Sharma
www.drsharmadiagnostics.com

References in support of statements made by Dr Sharma.

Research library:
Vitasearch: www.vitasearch.com

Adverse events:
www.adverseevents.com March 12th 2012

Allergy and immune testing:
UK Regenerus Labs: www.RegenerusLabs.com www.regeneruslabs.com

USA Cyrex Laboratories: www.cyrexLabs.co www.cyrexlabs.co

Alzheimer's and dementia:
The Alzheimer Association (US): http://www.alz.org/downloads/facts_
figures_2011.pdf

Cancer:
American Cancer Soc.: www.cancer.org/cancer/prostatecancer, 02/27/2012.

UK Cancer Care and Support Health Creation: www.healthcreation.co.uk

Cancer Therapy, The Plaskett Therapy: www.thetherapyofcancer.co.uk

MelanomaMobile: http://melanomamobil.co.uk/about-us-2/
statement-of-purpose/

National Cancer Institute, March 2012: http://www.cancer.gov

National Cancer Institute http://www.cancer.gov/cam/about_us.html

Is My Cancer Different: http://www.ismycancerdifferent.com/about/

Riordan, Dr Neil. San Juan, Costa Rica: www.medisteminc.com

Ann Larkin, St James's Hospital, Dublin Cancer Research UK, Nov, 2011

The National Cancer Institute, 2009: www.draxe.com/
mammograms-cause-cancer/

The Times, London, 29 February 2008

Worldwide Breast Cancer: http://www.worldwidebreastcancer.com/learn/
breast-cancer-statistics-worldwide/

The Pfeifer Protocol. Cancer Active: www.canceractive.com

Chelation:
http://www.drcranton.com/chelation/study6.htm

Information re research on chelation therapy: http://www.drcranton.com/
chelation/study6.htm

Cholesterol:
www.29billion.com and Statin Nation

The International Network of Cholesterol

Drug adverse events:
www.adverseevents.com March 12th 2012

Electromagnetic dangers:
Dr Mercola: http://emf.mercola.com/sites/emf/emf-dangers.aspx

Hormonal:
Androbalance: http://www.androbalance.co.uk/testing-saliva.htm

The Iodine Group: www.iodine4health

The Mayo Clinic Staff: http://www.mayoclinic.com/health/growth-hormone/
HA00030

Dr Ellen Grant: http://www.npis.info/wddtycancer.htm

Milk:
http://www.vegetarian.org.uk/campaigns/whitelies/wlreport01.shtml

Dr. Josh Wagner 2012: http://lifehousechiropractic.com/
got-milk-the-real-facts-on-milk-consumption-and-osteoporosis/

Nutritional:
Healthy Eating Advisor: http://www.healthyeatingadvisor.com/9cancer-
causingchemicals.html)

http://ec.europa.eu/food/food/labellingnutrition/vitamins/
comm_reg_en.pdf

http://www.exploreenumbers.co.uk/How-Safe-are-E-Numbers.html

www.hi-tm.com/facts@tips/decaff.html

www.stewartnutrition.co.uk

www.who.int/nutrition/databases/en/

Decaffination Hospitality Institute of Technology and Management:
www.hi-tm.com/facts@tips/decaff.html)

Toxic environment:
http://edugreen.teri.res.in/explore/water/health.htm

http://healthliteracy.worlded.org/docs/tobacco/Unit4/1whats_in.html

Mayo Clinic Staff: http://www.mayoclinic.com/health/alcohol/SC00024

Medline Plus www.mlm.nih.gov 07/07/2011

Public Citizen: www.worstpills.org

The Anarem Report by the US Department of Agriculture

Melatonin:
US National Library of Medicine National Institutes of Health: http://www.ncbi.nlm.nih.gov/pubmed?term=melatonin%20antioxidants

Walter Pierpaoli, M.D.: www.melatoninznse.com

Neurological:
inc QEEg and Neurofeedback: www.londonscientificneurotherapy.com

www.121neurofeedback.com

The International Society for Neurofeedback and Research: www.ISNR.org www.isnr.org

US National Library of Medicine National Institutes of Health:

http://www.ncbi.nlm.nih.gov/pubmed?term=antioxidants%20dementia

Laboratory Websites, Contact Details and Suppliers

Cancer tests:
Cancer risk testing and treatment: The Research Genetic Cancer Centre, Florina, Greece. Worldwide: www.RGCC-genlab.com UK: www.RGCC-uk.com

Full Tumour Immunity Profile

(Lab 4 More www.lab4more.de)

Candida antibodies:
www.RegenerusLabs.com

www.biolab.co.uk

Comprehensive stool analysis:
www.RegenerusLabs.com

ww.gdx.net

DNA adducts; acumenlab@hotmail.co.uk

Far InfraRed Therapy : www.get-fitt.com

Food allergy testing:
ALCAT Worldwide www.alcat.com. UK : www.RegenerusLabs.com

FoodAllergyCellularTest: USA www.GDX.net | www.metametrix.com

Genomics testing:
Worldwide: www.RegenerusLabs.com

Lab Reunis : www.labo.lu

www.glx.net

Hormone testing inc. sex and neurohormones, stress testing:
www.RegenerusLabs.com

www.glx.net

Immune system testing:
Lab 4 More Laboratory, Germany, www.lab4more.de

Leaky Gut Testing

www.Biolab.co.uk

www.RegenerusLabs.com

Nutritional studies mentioned or alluded to in text:
UK, USA and worldwide nutritional studies: www.RegenerusLabs.com

Wide-ranging and specifically the health risk profile: www.Biolab.co.uk

Wide-ranging and specifically NutrEval and NutrEval Plus USA: www.GDX.
net | www.metametrix.com

Mitochondrial and ATP/ADP studies:
acumenlab@hotmail.co.uk

Phospholipid exchange:
UK The British Society of Ecological Medicine: www.ecomed.org.uk and
www.genesiswellness.com

USA: http://theneuronetwork.com/ and those in Eastern or Central Europe:
www.dr-bieber.de/englisch/index/html

Toxicity testing inc. metals:
www.RegenerusLabs.com

www.Biolab.co.uk

White blood cell metal sensitivity:
Acumenlab@hotmail.co.uk

www.mellisa.com

Nutritional Supplement Suppliers

The Dispensary. Worldwide distribution (for all Dr Sharma recommended
products): dispensary@accountingbureau.co.uk

Also: Citrate Supplement Suppliers UK: www.nutrigold.co.uk

Specific Anti-ageing Supplements / International Anti-ageing Systems http://
www.antiagingsystems.com/search.php?orderby=position&orderway=de
sc&search_query=Can-c

Index